To AL

The Laparoscopic Surgery Revolution

Thanks for a special Cape Cod fishing experience— and for an opportunity to rekindle our friendship —

All the best,

Dave
8.31.2022

The Laparoscopic Surgery Revolution

Finding a Capable Surgeon in a Rapidly Advancing Field

David W. Page, MD, MFA, FACS

Foreword by Carol E. H. Scott-Conner, MD, PhD, MBA

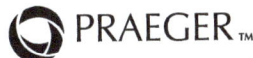

PRAEGER™

An Imprint of ABC-CLIO, LLC

Santa Barbara, California • Denver, Colorado

Library of Congress Cataloging-in-Publication Data

Names: Page, David W., 1943– author.
Title: The laparoscopic surgery revolution : finding a capable surgeon in a rapidly
    advancing field / David W. Page, MD, MFA, FACS ; Foreword by
    Carol E. H. Scott-Conner, MD, PhD, MBA.
Description: Santa Barbara, California : Praeger, an Imprint of ABC-CLIO, LLC, [2017] |
    Includes bibliographical references and index.
Identifiers: LCCN 2016044322 (print) | LCCN 2016045293 (ebook) |
    ISBN 9781440844775 (hardcopy : alk. paper) | ISBN 9781440844782 (ebook)
Subjects: LCSH: Laparoscopic surgery. | Surgeons.
Classification: LCC RG104.7 .P34 2017 (print) | LCC RG104.7 (ebook) |
    DDC 617.5/50597—dc23
LC record available at https://lccn.loc.gov/2016044322

ISBN: 978-1-4408-4477-5
EISBN: 978-1-4408-4478-2

21 20 19 18 17   1 2 3 4 5

This book is also available as an eBook.

Praeger
An Imprint of ABC-CLIO, LLC

ABC-CLIO, LLC
130 Cremona Drive, P.O. Box 1911
Santa Barbara, California 93116-1911
www.abc-clio.com

This book is printed on acid-free paper ∞

Manufactured in the United States of America

To Gloria

And to the surgical residents past and present at Baystate Medical Center

And to the leadership and guidance provided by the following organizations in their efforts to assure excellence in surgical education and patient safety:

The American College of Surgeons
The Association for Surgical Education
The Association of Program Directors in Surgery
The Society of American Gastrointestinal and Endoscopic Surgeons
The American Board of Surgery

The rapid adoption of laparoscopy has led to the development of a new sub-specialty area in surgery . . . minimally invasive surgery. This has fostered much basic and clinical research and innumerable papers published on all conceivable aspects of minimally invasive surgery. While this expansion of knowledge has been desirable, the sheer bulk of it has made it difficult for the individual surgeon to keep abreast of the most recent advances.

Layton F. Rikkers, MD, FACS
Professor Emeritus
Department of Surgery
University of Wisconsin
School of Medicine and Public Health

Contents

Foreword

"Belly-button" or "laser" gallbladder surgery took American surgeons by surprise in 1988, when the first laparoscopic cholecystectomy—as we surgeons call it—was performed in the United States. The old operation, open cholecystectomy, which I had learned (and taught), required a long incision and weeks of painful recovery. There were no randomized prospective clinical trials to demonstrate the superiority of the new technique. There were no organized training programs, no simulators, not even any textbooks. But by 1990, as Dr. Page eloquently explains in this clear and lucid history, the "tipping point" had been reached, and thereafter laparoscopic cholecystectomy became the operation of choice. Dissemination of the technique was so rapid that instrument makers could not keep up with demand; hospitals often had to wait six months or more to get the new equipment. And buried in this revolution was the uneasy knowledge that some patients suffered tragic, even fatal, complications.

Surgeons were operating with their hands outside the belly and watching a video monitor instead of looking directly into the incision. The view was seductively clear, magnified so that every capillary seemed to glisten. But the view was different and so were the perils. Now, several decades later, Dr. Page meticulously dissects and analyzes the factors that led to success (and problems) with the rapid, uncritical adoption of this new surgical technique.

This is important reading, because the lessons in this book remain relevant to today's constantly changing world. Newer, less invasive techniques for spine surgery, varicose veins, even heart valve replacement are now available. If you are facing surgery for yourself or a loved one, how should you evaluate the effectiveness of these new techniques? How can you be sure that your surgeon is trained in a new procedure? Is your surgeon fairly presenting all alternatives? If you are a practicing surgeon or a teacher of young surgeons, how do you adapt to this constantly shifting environment? How do you learn a new technique and apply it safely? And a related problem: When everyone is a specialist, who will provide general surgery—the surgical equivalent of primary care?

Read on!

Carol E. H. Scott-Conner, MD, PhD, MBA
Professor Emeritus
Department of Surgery
University of Iowa Carver College of Medicine
Iowa City, Iowa

Preface

Even within a specialty such as general surgery different physicians seldom provide equivalent services. Although most general surgeons receive comparable training leading to Board-certification, the services they provide in practice may be highly variable.

> Karen B. Stitzenberg, MD, MPH, and George F. Sheldon, MD, FACS, *Journal of the American College of Surgeons*, 2005

Nowadays, becoming the consummate general surgeon is difficult—some would say impossible—with the expanding range of surgical diseases, disciplines, and the development of new therapies and techniques.

> Said C. Azoury, MD, *Bulletin of the American College of Surgeons*, 2014

Writing about patient safety, like performing intricate surgery, has moral consequences. Readers and patients must be able to trust the practitioner to do the right thing. The practice of surgery has always carried with it the freighted obligation to do only that with which the surgeon has extensive experience. True informed consent requires that the individual surgeon's actual expertise—as contrasted with the profession's overall claim of mastery—be shared with the patient. In today's cluttered practice of general surgery, the obligation to be transparent about personal training and experience stands out as the biggest challenge for practicing surgeons. Thus, the topics I have chosen to discuss regarding surgeon capability, such as surgical innovation and learning curves, hinge on the deeper meaning of our moral obligation as surgeons to communicate honestly with our patients.

My primary goal in writing this book is to reveal what has not been adequately discussed with the public: that there are new risks patients may be exposed to when seeking a surgical operation. I will describe how this occurred and why surgical expertise continues to be available but frequently in a different distribution than in the past. Therefore, the dilemma for you, a potential surgical patient, is how to determine whether the surgeon to whom you have been referred is well trained to do the particular operation you need.

From the outset of the laparoscopic revolution (a laparoscope is a lighted telescope pushed through a "sleeve" into the belly cavity; the surgical field is displayed on an overhead TV screen), surgical educators have known that the addition of large numbers of minimally invasive (laparoscopic) operations to the plethora of traditional open procedures already in use would pose almost insurmountable challenges for our profession. I will shed light on the opaque corners of modern general surgical practice and will chronicle the impact of the laparoscopic innovations of the last three decades. Foremost, my concern is that the relatively swift shift to less invasive laparoscopic "keyhole" operations from scalpel-based procedures has thrown the daily practice of surgery, our education methods, and patient safety into a state of uncertainty.

It was said some years ago regarding pressing issues of 21st-century surgical practice that individual capability "is the issue of mounting pressure for physicians to demonstrate their competence and ability to deliver high-quality patient care."[1] Referring to the value of documenting that surgeons have good outcomes (low rates of wound infections, pneumonia, deep vein clotting, etc.), the author added, "The question is, are there other methods which we can use to evaluate the competence of the surgeon?"[2] There are, and I will examine why this is important and describe methods you may use to check a surgeon's track record.

But first let's look at the big picture.

In most locations in America, you have available to you the most sophisticated surgical care in the world—if you know where to look for it. That's the key issue. Surgical talent abounds in the United States. But not every surgeon possesses the same capabilities. Before the laparoscopic revolution arrived in 1990, general surgeons were more alike in skills and knowledge than today. Now, you must discuss what operations your surgeon does frequently. So remember that almost nothing is the same in the world of 21st-century surgery as compared with 20 or 30 years ago.

In the last two-plus decades, ragged pockets of incomplete training have found their way into the otherwise tightly knit fabric of the U.S. surgical community. A quick statistic speaks volumes to the challenges facing 21st-century surgical educators. There are 121 operations considered essential to the field of general surgery. Our current graduates will *not* have performed or observed (scrubbed in the operating room) on even one case of 50 percent of those basic operations. In other words, *newly minted general surgeons will have been exposed to only half of their specialty*. And they will have done very few of many of the other essential operations on the list.[3] Keep these statistics in mind when I challenge the notion that our general surgery graduates are capable of starting out in practice as competent practitioners in all aspects of general surgery.

Prior to 1990, general surgeons provided care for a large variety of diseases. The scope of a general surgeon's practice formerly included all aspects of the care of traumatic injuries, cancer care, and the management of infectious and inflammatory diseases. Major diseases involved the skin, thyroid gland, breast (endocrine surgery), lungs and bronchi (thoracic surgery), all types of blood vessels (vascular surgery), and all diseases of organs in the abdomen (liver, spleen, gastrointestinal tract). In the 1970s and 1980s, specific specialty areas broke away from the main body of general surgery. Vascular surgery is a prominent example of a collection of operations—most commonly on abdominal aortic aneurysms ("ballooning" and weakening of the body's biggest artery), blocked carotid arteries in the neck (clogged with fatty deposits), and procedures to bypass narrowing (blockages) in the lower extremity—that require specific technical skills.

Then, with unusual reluctance at the outset of the decade of the 1990s, general surgeons joined their gynecologic and urological colleagues and began to learn how to perform less invasive but nonetheless complex laparoscopic operations. A decade and a half later, a prescription for failure crept into the daily workings of surgical education in the form of work-hour restrictions for trainees. These two cataclysmic changes—the imperative to learn a large number of complex new laparoscopic operations during less training time—arrived with the laparoscopic revolution. These changes were not only disruptive to our practices, but the two diametrically opposed forces also completely revolutionized how we train and educate young surgeons.

These forces explain why we are not as easily able to train general surgeons to do the wide scope of operations that you, the public, expect of them. Although some surgeons will disagree with my thesis, the data is compelling. It all began in the 1990s when our professional obligations multiplied as the technical challenges imposed by laparoscopy confronted general surgeons with a harsh reality: our specialty abruptly underwent a mitosis-like doubling; traditional open operations became retooled in order to be performed with tiny incisions and a laparoscope. The less invasive operations forced us to accept the indisputable fact that general surgery had divided in two, just as one cell splits into two cells in the process of mitosis. A long list of laparoscopic operations quite suddenly was added to the bread and butter caseload of daily general-surgery practice. Specialty surgery—if not already utilizing less traumatic procedures (arthroscopy, pelviscopy, cystoscopy, etc.)—soon followed suit.

For example, in 1988, 0 percent of gallbladder removals were done laparoscopically. By 1992 over 80 percent of cholecystectomies were performed with the innovative less invasive operation. Now, that is the consequence of a revolution. *Laparoscopic cholecystectomy* (minimally invasive removal of the gallbladder) didn't creep up on surgeons; it exploded onto the general surgery scene. Other organs were assaulted with the laparoscope as the 1990s plunged us into a world of chaos.

How we got to this juncture in the ever-evolving history of modern surgery is the subject of this book. And as you will discover, the chaotic early history of laparoscopic general surgery is as fascinating as it is frightening. Most of the innovations we'll discuss, including those in use currently, are *transitional* forms of technology. We don't know what will confront us next. It may involve robots or no-incision surgery; operations will no doubt continue to be miniaturized. Thus, the story of minimally invasive surgery is far from complete.

Through my pursuit of the history of laparoscopic general surgery, as well as the almost-forgotten story of earlier innovations by gynecologists and urologists, I am seeking to tease out the historical threads of surgical competence. These threads have led to the formation of the current strong cable of overall general-surgery capability in the United States and around the world specifically using less invasive operative techniques. Yet at the outset of the laparoscopic revolution, in a 1995 book on complications of laparoscopic operations, the internationally recognized surgeon Dr. Hiram C. Polk Jr. stated, "The initial excitement among surgeons regarding the proliferation of various forms of less invasive access is giving way to a more reasoned and organized analysis of the potential pitfalls and perils of such approaches."[4] Without a doubt, not all was smooth sailing at first.

Thus, my aim is to imagine what sorts of insights into the constantly shifting approaches to surgical disease modern patients might need to assure their personal safety. In order to do so I have reviewed countless scientific studies on the evolution of minimally invasive general surgery. The studies of how laparoscopy evolved, what problems were encountered, and how they were solved involves more detail than can be addressed in this book. However, I will attempt to document as many points of contention as possible in support of my own convictions about the implications of the laparoscopic revolution.

It would be impossible to give credit to all the historic innovators that figure prominently in the expansive story of laparoscopic surgery. To be certain, this is a story with complex characters, a twisted plotline, complications, resolutions, and a denouement you must appreciate to be an informed patient. I have ferreted out those scenes and sequences, fragments of tales, and entire stories that have interested me in doing this project. In particular, I have paid special attention to the messages the historical record offers that seem to be most important in understanding where you may find your surgeon's capability along the continuum of surgical expertise today. That is, it is my contention that you must inquire about the practical experience of any given surgeon you may encounter.

Mitosis.

One cell divides into two cells. Open surgery is now joined by laparoscopic (minimally invasive) operations—surgical skills and knowledge mitosis.

The consequence of this immense tangle of surgical innovation and the information explosion that ensued is that no single general surgeon can perform all these operations in a capable manner now designated as part of our specialty. The political, cultural, psychological, and sociological issues will be addressed as the backdrop to my primary discussion of the issue of surgeon capability (studies quoted often use the term *competence*, which I deem equivalent to *capability*).

I will develop five themes which when seen in combination create the challenging environment in which modern surgical care is practiced. The *central theme* as articulated above is that the multiplication of new operations—most notably those performed using minimally invasive techniques—and ever-changing and increasing complexity of surgical technology, when added to the existing traditional body of open general-surgery procedures, precludes practitioner capability in all domains. No one can do it all.

A *second theme* involves the reality that the new surgical education paradigm requires creating a "pretrained novice" (a surgical resident who learns basic skills before going to the operating room) through skills lab learning on models. Nonetheless, some surgical educators remain committed to the notion that competence is strongly anchored to memorizing minutiae. Newly discovered genetic, molecular-biological, and other facts rarely have immediate clinical application and can and should be retrieved on a digital device in seconds—behavior we witness daily with our residents and medical students. While memorizing esoteric scientific information to some degree translates into becoming a competent surgeon, being *capable of retrieving information* and applying it to clinical cases must become the new learning paradigm. We must also remember the disturbing fact that the *human factors* scientific principle of relying on memory—an enduring, unshakable part of all medical education—is a major reason for the creation of medical errors.

A *third theme* involves the unfortunate but politically motivated idea that fatigue is the new enemy and a prime cause of surgical errors—despite the absence of studies to support this notion. There is no doubt about the adverse effect of fatigue on all sorts of human performance, including technical skills. Data abounds on the subject. Detailed scientific literature on the impact of fatigue and sleep deprivation on performance remains unassailable. Fatigue can lead to mistakes. But what the public has not been made aware of is the need for multiple handoffs, or patient information transfers, that appear to be more dangerous than sleep deprivation itself. A handoff involves an informed doctor passing on information to a rested physician coming on duty; just as with the old telephone game where the message gets distorted, patient information transfers have proven to be dangerous as vital facts are lost or changed. The real issue (supported by a new study of surgical resident work hours) regarding patient safety remains buried beneath reams of laboratory data on sleep deprivation.

The profession of surgery, while greatly improved in terms of how surgeons interact with the public, has not developed a zero tolerance for the disruptive features of the surgical personality. Thus, my *fourth theme* is that narcissistic surgeons who continue to coerce patients, intimidate nurses from acting independently, and discourage medical students from entering our profession by virtue of their behavior should be severely sanctioned. This includes the all-too-often tolerated sexual harassment of female surgical residents by their male faculty who feel untouchable. As a consequence of these players, too many surgical residencies are marred by an inexcusable and smoldering toxicity.

Finally, my *fifth theme* concerns the urgent need to transform the informed consent process to reflect the new reality of uneven surgeon capability now in evidence. The urgent demand for true transparency (informed decision making) in surgeon-patient communication, including surgeons' *revealing their personal training and operative experience with a particular operation*, reflects the public's growing awareness of the real magnitude of surgical errors. That individual general surgeons possess significantly different surgical skills sets is the new challenge facing patients today. We, as practitioners, must accept that our patients need to know what our true experience is with the operation that a particular patient needs. As a patient, you must recognize that *this idea is transformational* and will be resisted by some surgeons in practice. Not that we haven't always performed a variable collection of common operations using individualized methods—a different kind of suture here, a drain tweaked daily there. In fact, surgeons routinely perform specific operative procedures in their own way following basic steps and guidelines.

The laparoscopic revolution has muddied the dialogue regarding the benefits and risks for our patients. Scars have shortened to postage-stamp length. In this regard, you will also learn how the idea of "natural orifices" surgery—operating through the mouth, anus, vagina, and so forth without a scar—crept into the surgical imagination. Paradoxically, this state of affairs stands in absurd contrast to the decade of the 1980s, a perilous period in modern surgical history for general surgeons. Ignoring the unstoppable trend toward less invasive operations driven by gynecologists and urologists, general surgeons risked becoming extinct. As surgeons plunged into heroic cancer and other major incision-based operations, leaving a swath of pain and disfigurement in their wake, creative radiologists and gastroenterologists quietly stole our bread and butter. Notably in this regard, the gallbladder and its truckload of stones very nearly escaped our hands. With little fanfare, gallstones fell into the waiting arms of nonsurgeons plying them with medical treatments such as shock waves to smash and pass stone pieces, as well as the use of bile salt pills to dissolve them. In the mid-1980s nonsurgical interventions exploded in number, and our aggressive incisions and bloody operations seemed increasingly outdated. And the addition of less invasive operations threw surgical education into a mess.

Here's a concrete example of the training challenges surgical educators currently face: although today laparoscopic gallbladder removal is one of the most common general surgery operations performed in practice, according to some national leaders in surgical education, 30 percent of graduating surgical trainees are not capable of performing this basic operations safely.[5] In the same survey of recent surgical graduates who were evaluated by the program directors of advanced surgical fellowship training programs, it was noted that 66 percent of recent graduates were deemed unable to operate for 30 minutes on their own, unsupervised, while performing a major case. Over 50 percent couldn't do basic laparoscopic suturing, and 25 percent of recently trained surgeons in that study were unable to identify the signs and symptoms of certain postoperative complications. These surgical residents were the products of certified five- to seven-year surgical training programs in the United States. Their program directors had signed them off as prepared for practice.

Grim statistics?

Not if you know the rest of the story. Placed into perspective, these statistics reflect the new reality for general-surgery residents training under work-hour restrictions with an ever-increasing number of operations to learn. It is the sobering reality faced by millions of patients undergoing surgery every year in the United States. The unresolved question for potential surgical patients is how to deal with what are, in effect, partially trained surgeons.

Above all, this book is not a screed against surgeons. Rather it is an attempt to redefine the meaning of surgical competence for patients as well as for surgeons. In a very real sense, surgical patients must be more cautious and better informed than ever when choosing a surgeon. I will use the example of how laparoscopic gallbladder surgery was introduced into practice as a cautionary tale for all of us. Five years after the first laparoscopic gallbladder removal in the United States, Dr. Polk, quoted above, added: "The progress of surgery has been marked by a sequence of forward charges, followed by plateau periods during which surgeons have assimilated and reassessed the real value of the surgical advance. . . . Such intellectual and technical plateaus—whose physical and temporal bounds are set only by the limits of our imagination as scientists and clinicians— provide the staging areas from which the future forward advances will be launched."[6]

Now, 20 years later we are indeed in need of a "plateau" period to reassess the current forward advances involving less invasive procedures such as robotic surgery and no-incision operations. Just as important in this pause for professional self-reflection is the imperative to acknowledge and identify the redistribution of surgical talent in the United States, as well as define the variability of individual surgeon capability. Competent surgeons abound. But the one you meet may or may not have the credentials necessary to perform your particular operation safely.

Our core of American general surgeons represents to my mind the hardest-working members of the medical profession. They are skilled and competent. However, some are frustrated and burned out. Remarkably, stress in surgeons was identified as a real issue at the *beginning* of the laparoscopic revolution in 1990![7] And it's more prevalent today.[8] Therefore, I'll provide you with information you'll need on this and other concerns in order to understand the current status of general surgery.

To repeat: the new reality is that many of our freshly minted general surgeons are not ready for independent practice. And surveys show that the residents themselves are acutely aware of their deficiencies.[9] This is why 80 percent of graduating surgical residents pursue their training further in a variety of fellowships typically lasting one or two years.

The chaotic introduction of laparoscopic surgery into general surgical practice in the 1990s is, in and of itself, a fascinating tale. Referring to this phenomenon, one educator stated, "The latter was introduced in an inappropriate manner, which has led to the evolution of teaching of technical skills away from the apprenticeship-based activity toward more formal skill-based training programmes."[10] Additionally, describing the miscues and successes of the laparoscopic revolution is the best way to explain why, despite the triumph of less traumatic operations, the public remains at risk in the hands of some practicing surgeons today. I'll spell out in detail what to expect if you must deal with surgeons without scalpels.

It isn't a matter of bad surgeons having poor skills. Rather, the issue revolves around some really good surgeons having inadequate training and too little experience with many of the complex new operations making up the technical and knowledge overload challenging today's general surgeons. As I mentioned a moment ago, it is why graduates often do surgical fellowships for one, two, or three additional years. When they enter surgical practice after fellowship training, they do so with remarkable technical talent. Additional training in the form of "transition to practice," as established in the form of guidelines by the American College of Surgeons, as well as by some independent residency programs, also assures the public of finding a capable general surgeon. Thus, a uniform and broadly accepted definition of surgical practitioner competence is no longer available.

In their 2009 book, *The Coming Shortage of Surgeons*, doctors Williams, Satiani, and Ellison remarked on the experimental method of a less invasive type of surgery known as NOTES (natural orifice transluminal endoscopic surgery). It refers to operating through the mouth, vagina, anus, or another natural body opening and thus leaves no scars. The authors ask, "Will there be enough general surgeons to perform these procedures and lead the way to further innovation directed towards making procedures less invasive, painless, and safe?"[11] How far the issue has progressed in the few years since that book was published. As I indicated, our graduating trainees feel inadequate about their *basic* surgical skills and in no way in the immediate future can they expect to master robotic operative skills, let alone the exquisite operative challenges of NOTES.

How did this happen? Is less invasive laparoscopic surgery always the best way to go? And how can you find a surgeon with the skills your particular operation requires?

The remarkable thing about the laparoscopic revolution is that it contains all the practitioner errors, miscues, prejudices, invective, ridicule, self-importance, and bitter bile that have characterized every major advance in medicine. For years general surgeons ridiculed gynecologists for their "Mickey Mouse" keyhole operations, performed deep in the half-hidden recesses of the pelvis. Then, in the decade of the 1990s, surgeons acknowledged, red-faced and embarrassed, the need to learn that very challenging minimally invasive technological innovation themselves. Our patients wanted less pain and a faster recovery. But, sadly for the public, the initial results of laparoscopic gallbladder removal were frightening.

At first, little was said publicly about surgeon error at the beginning of the laparoscopic revolution. The good news is that today surgeons overall have remarkable skill with the less traumatic operations, and they are readily available in most parts of the United States. Nonetheless, Americans still know little or nothing about the current strengths and deficiencies of our surgical workforce. The public also is poorly informed about the negative forces degrading the surgical practice environment. These and other factors conspire to complicate the availability of safe surgery in the United States.

My vantage is that of a surgical educator with a unique background and experience with coaching and skills teaching. Throughout the book I will return to core ideas critical to patient safety and weave them together, because they are interdependent. These include innovation, learning curves, innate talent, aspects of gaining and losing technical competence, individual surgeon training and testing, and the educational theory related to our current concepts of surgical education.[12,13]

The laparoscopy gallbladder course I took in 1990 was one of several offered across the United States. It marked the beginning of a modern surgical revolution. It launched a redirection of my personal journey as an active participant in the changing world of surgical education. Through the telling of the story of the rise of laparoscopic general surgery, I will explore the history of surgical competence and the variability of individual surgeon capability at the beginning of the 21st century. It's not entirely what you might imagine.

Acknowledgments

A book that spans the history of a revolution owes immeasurable debt to many creative minds, all of whom saw different parts of the transformation of general surgery by minimally invasive operations. Throughout this book I have attempted to document the work of other researchers in each area of inquiry that I found myself drawn to from the bigger picture of the laparoscopic revolution. To these individuals I owe a debt of gratitude for their published work, and any errors are entirely mine.

In this regard, I am especially indebted to Grzegorz Litynski for his 1996 classic, *Highlights in the History of Laparoscopy*. Through journals (many in German), interviews, telephone conversations, and other communications, Dr. Litynski documented the rise of general surgical laparoscopy within the larger story of the history of laparoscopy. Without his work—which I have quoted from liberally and with gratitude—this book would have been incomplete.

My thanks to the following national leaders in surgical education who read and critiqued the manuscript and made invaluable comments and corrections: Dr. Richard H. Bell, MD, FACS, past chair, Surgical Council on Resident Education, and adjunct professor of surgery and senior surgical educator, Temple University (Dr. Bell was instrumental in the activities of the Surgical Council on Resident Education [SCORE], which—as a nonprofit initiative to provide high-quality educational materials for surgical residents and a structured program for self-learning—has been arguably the most significant contribution to modern surgical trainee competence); Dr. James C. Hebert, MD, FACS, Mackay-Page Professor of Surgery, University of Vermont College of Medicine, former president of the Association for Surgical Education, for his important suggestions, especially the need for added federal funding for surgical education; Dr. Carol Scott-Conner, MD, PhD, MBA, emeritus chair, Department of Surgery, University of Iowa

Carver College of Medicine, former president of the American Association of Clinical Anatomists, for her critique of the manuscript and valuable suggestions and for the foreword to this book.

I wish to thank the two Baystate Medical Center chairmen of the Department of Surgery who ushered me through a career that would have been considerably less successful without their mentorship and guidance. In the early years, Dr. Paul Friedmann, MD, FACS, encouraged my nascent educational interests. In the later years, Dr. Richard B. Wait, MD, PhD, FACS, provided me with the support and endless opportunities I needed to explore and evolve as a surgical educator. Both of these superb, nationally known surgical leaders were also accomplished clinical surgeons, and they have contributed in countless ways to this book.

I am indebted to my colleagues and the surgical residents at Baystate Medical Center (BMC) for their contributions and support for this project. My gratitude especially goes out to my colleague and friend, Dr. John Romanelli, director of Bariatric and Robotic Surgery and director of our MIS Fellowship Program at BMC. John not only led me to Litynski's book early in my research, but he also improved the work with careful editing. John also offered valuable operative photo opportunities and innumerable suggestions regarding the book's content and tone.

Over my many years of teaching at Baystate, my medical students and our residents have educated me about how to engage them with enthusiasm and to listen to them with care. I am especially thankful for the contributions to the book by the following residents: to Saiqa Khan for her editing and contributions to the work-hour discussion; to Erica Kane for her help with the photos and diagrams; and to Ruchi Thanawala for introducing me to the work of Ray Kurzweil and its profound implications for the future of surgical education.

Thanks to my editor at Praeger, Debbie Carvalko, who gently led me through the rock-strewn waters of editing and publication with understanding, encouragement, and insight. I offer my enthusiastic gratitude. And thanks to Rashmi Malhotra, project manager with Westchester Publishing Services for her expertise and grace in directing my edits.

My family has been a source of support, encouragement, and love over the many years during which I wrote this and other books, as well as practiced general surgery—night and day. They have tolerated my physical and cognitive absences with kindness and forgiveness. Thanks, guys!

Above all who have supported me in this endeavor, my wife, Gloria, has served as my life-support system in good times and during life's inevitable challenges. Supporting a husband who added a writing career to the challenges of practicing and teaching surgery requires the courage Gloria possesses in large measures. Mostly, when a good idea needs redirection and sometimes even abandonment, Gloria has been gentle and supportive of my excess self-criticism. I truly could never have survived the process of delivering this book without her ever-present help.

Abbreviations

ABS
American Board of Surgery: founded in 1937, the ABS offers board certification in general surgery and vascular surgery, as well as secondary certificates; an independent nonprofit organization designed to establish qualification of surgeons; board certification demonstrates the surgeon's commitment to professionalism, lifelong learning, and quality patient care.

ABSITE
American Board of Surgery In-Training Examination: given to all general surgery residents in training; used to assess depth of knowledge and clinical reasoning and as a guide to promotion.

ACGME
Accreditation Council for Graduate Medical Education: a private professional organization responsible for assuring quality in 9,600 resident and fellowship programs that include over 120,000 trainees; relies on experts to make accreditation decisions; consists of Residency Review Committees for each specialty; institutes site visits to assess programs including clinical learning environment reviews and milestones or competency-based developmental outcomes.

ACS
American College of Surgeons: founded in 1913, the ACS is a scientific and educational organization whose primary goal is to improve the quality of surgical patient care by setting high standards for surgical education, training, and advocacy; it is the foremost organization for providing a variety of educational opportunities for trainees and practicing surgeons, including courses in leadership for surgeons as teachers and residents as teachers.

APDS
Association of Program Directors in Surgery: founded in 1977, the APDS provides a forum for the exchange of ideas about postgraduate surgical education,

maintains high standards in surgical residency training, provides advice and support to program directors, and supports research in surgical education.

ASE
Association for Surgical Education: formed in 1980, the ASE promotes, recognizes, and rewards excellence, innovation, and scholarship in surgical education; the ASE Foundation secures grants to fund research into better ways to teach the complex field of surgery.

ASGE
American Society of Gastrointestinal Endoscopy: promotes safe patient care related to endoscopy as well as all aspects of digestive health; promotes research in endoscopy and its applications.

ERCP
Endoscopic retrograde cholangiopancreatography; endoscopic and X-ray (fluoroscopic) evaluation of the bile ducts (tubes), pancreatic duct, common bile duct; also used to remove stones, remove small tumors, treat bile duct strictures, diagnose postoperative problems, and so forth.

FES
Fundamentals of Endoscopic Surgery; teaches and evaluates knowledge and skills related to the use of an endoscope for diagnosis and treatment of digestive diseases; similar to FLS regarding content and test completion before graduation from surgical residency.

FLS
Fundamentals of Laparoscopic Surgery skills course; knowledge and skills must be mastered and a test passed before graduation from residency.

FUSE
Fundamental Use of Surgical Energy: an interactive Web-based, multimedia-enhanced educational program designed to teach the use of a variety of energy-based devices such as electrocautery in the OR, endoscopy suite, and elsewhere.

LC
Laparoscopic cholecystectomy; laparoscopic removal of the gallbladder.

MIS
Minimally invasive surgery; the term is used interchangeably with laparoscopic surgery.

NOSCAR
Natural Orifice Surgery Consortium for Assessment and Research: oversees research on NOTES surgery and associated new technology.

NOTES
Natural orifice transluminal endoscopic surgery: endoscopic surgery through the mouth, vagina, anus, or any other natural body opening (orifice); requires putting a hole in an internal organ, such as the stomach or colon, in order to reach,

for example, the appendix or gallbladder and remove it through the stomach wall and then through the mouth without an incision.

RRC-S

Residency Review Committee for Surgery; a member of the ACGME; oversees residency programs in surgery and sets standards and requirements for graduation and training.

SAGES

Society of American Gastrointestinal and Endoscopic Surgeons: the mission of SAGES is to improve the quality of patient care in the realms of endoscopic surgery, including the use of endoscopic imaging and energy sources; to provide education and leadership; and to encourage research in gastrointestinal and endoscopic surgery.

SCORE

Surgical Council on Resident Education: a high-quality nonprofit initiative to provide training surgeons with educational materials and a structured program for self-learning; includes textbook material, videos, journal articles, and so forth.

SILS

Single incision laparoscopic surgery; many names apply to this technique, which uses a single belly-button incision with special trocar/cannulas with three to four openings for laparoscopic instruments; requires a special set of technical skills.

PART 1

The Third Great Revolution in Surgery: A Trail of Chaos from Heroic Scalpels to a World of Scopes

CHAPTER ONE

"Dry Lab on Saturday, Pig Lab on Sunday, Grandma on Monday"

There is nothing more difficult to plan, more doubtful of success, nor more dangerous to manage than the creation of a new order of things.
Niccolò Machiavelli, *The Prince*

The specialty of general surgery has recently undergone a revolution. The application of video-guided surgery to cholecystectomy led to the greatest post-graduate training effort in the history of general surgery.
Edward H. Philips and Raul J. Rosenthal, *Operative Strategies in Laparoscopic Surgery*, 1995

Chopsticks—1990

In a dimly lighted operating room in a conference center in Marietta, Georgia, I huddle in blue scrubs with two of my colleagues and a couple dozen strangers. The room smells like a pig farm. The dank porcine stench clings to my scrubs and pokes into my nose like soiled fingers. Before us a huge boar lies stretched out on its back on the special operating room table. Out of its mouth protrudes a breathing tube taped to its fleshy snout. Corrugated plastic tubing loops from the breathing tube to a nearby sighing anesthesia machine. A veterinary technician preps the swine's belly with brushstrokes of brown antiseptic solution. The pig's legs are tied down and the animal is draped, leaving a square of belly skin exposed as if this were a regular human operation.

We're all board-certified general surgeons standing quietly in the shadowy room. And something's in the air. Something akin to excitement punctuated by raw dread. We're starting a training course we didn't expect to take, didn't ask for, didn't really want. But we're here in this classroom with the pig and a table strewn with strange-looking instruments.

Moments earlier, we had witnessed a video showing a country-singing general surgeon named Eddie Joe Reddick sneak a pig's gallbladder out of its body without a large incision. In our blissful ignorance we watched this huge man with a drooping mustache and wearing Farmer John overalls grasp long instruments and perform a laparoscopic operation. He made it look easy—like plucking a guitar.[1] After a few hours of lectures about the new equipment and specific technical maneuvers, I try it myself in the darkened operating room. And when I do, the reality of how difficult laparoscopic gallbladder surgery is strikes me like a blow to the ribs.

As a consequence of that minicourse I took to learn how to remove a porcine gallbladder in 1990, my professional life changed overnight, as did the lives of surgeons all over the United States.

Gallbladder removal is one of the most common general surgery operations done in the United States; about 700,000 are done a year. Surgical patients around the country quickly discovered that a less traumatic gallbladder operation had become available. They wanted it—*now*. The truth hidden from these eager patients was that virtually no one in the field of general surgery knew how to perform the minimally invasive operation. Not at first. And not until too many patients had been injured as a consequence of our poor laparoscopic skills.

On that day in 1990, I realized with disbelief that my surgical practice and my career were about to undergo disorienting changes. The less invasive operation I was attempting to learn on the pig would be tried by thousands of general surgeons in the United States and around the world. Some surgeons never did the pig training. They just watched videos, listened to lectures, and instructed their hospitals to order the new equipment. Some surgeons weren't particularly skilled in using the awkward laparoscopic "chopsticks" while staring at a TV screen (Figure 1.1). And what would not become evident for years during the subsequent transformation of general surgery was the disturbing incidence of surgical errors that would arrive with the new, less invasive surgical territory.

Gradually, in that first year of attempts to master the new laparoscopic gallbladder operation, surgeons would become obsessed with what the public only much later came to know about as *learning curves*. General surgeons henceforth would no longer look at their scalpels with the same sense of familiarity. An unfettered urgency to hoist the laparoscope grew. There was now another way to enter the abdominal cathedral. The door was minuscule, the view unfamiliar. And soon other less invasive doors to the chest, the brain, and other body cavities would squeak open as well.

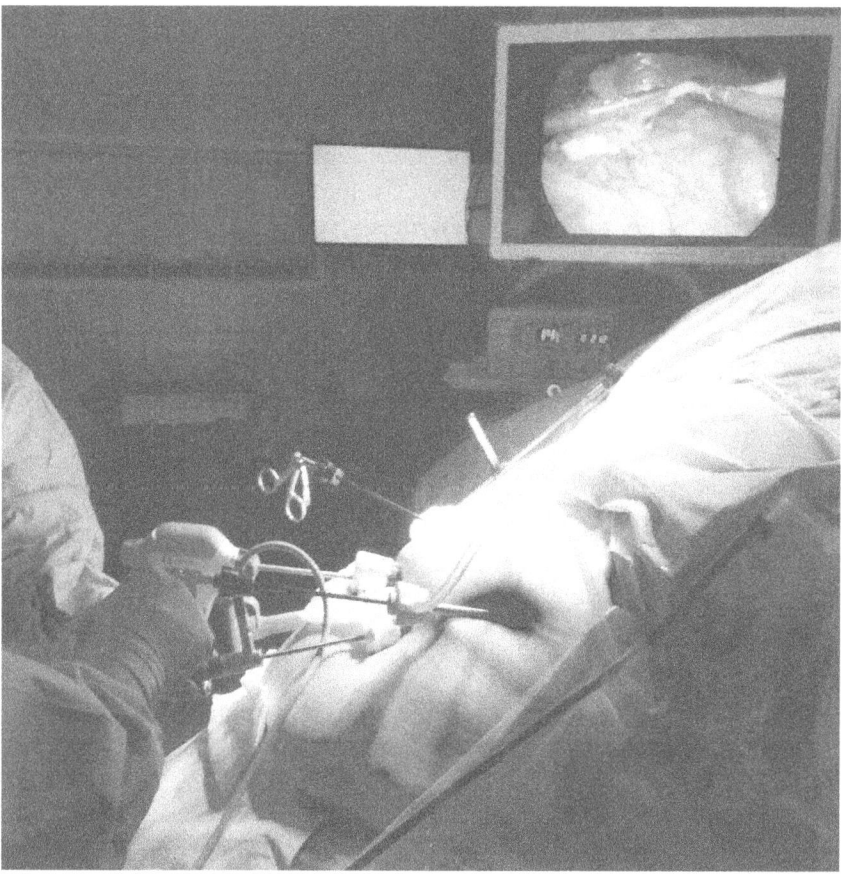

Figure 1.1 Darkened Environment of Laparoscopic Operating Room (photo by David Page, MD)

As news of the laparoscopic gallbladder operation spread, our patients begged for the less invasive procedure. Under time constraints to introduce laparoscopy into surgical practice around the country (the financial benefits of being the first on the block with a shiny new laparoscope were thought to be considerable), surgeons sprinted to the few available courses to learn the chopsticks operation. Few of us completed enough training. Some of the early gallbladder patients suffered serious complications and unnecessary death.

In 1991, a report identified the key issues with the introduction of laparoscopic gallbladder removal. The authors stated, "Initial reports on the laparoscopic procedure were followed by an unprecedented (at least for biliary tract surgeons) rush by surgeons to learn the new technique, advertisements and/or promotions by both manufacturers of the required equipment and health care providers, and consumer demand for the new procedure. . . . This fundamental change in technique for the most commonly performed general surgery procedure in the United States has occurred despite very little published data to substantiate that the laparoscopic approach is superior to the traditional procedure."[2] The authors suggested that establishing guidelines would be difficult because of the explosive arrival of the new laparoscopic operation.

To our shame, laparoscopic incompetence went unacknowledged in our professional surgical circles, but not in the media. By 1992, Lawrence Altman wrote in the *New York Times*, "The learning curve is a complex policy issue. It involves the tangled web of medical politics—turf battles between specialties, and town-gown conflicts between professors in teaching hospitals and practicing surgeons in community hospitals."[3] He had identified the unusual circumstance that laparoscopic cholecystectomy's birthplace was the community hospital, not the academic medical center. In the *Washington Post* in the same year, Judy Licht opined, "Nicknamed 'Nintendo surgery', laparoscopy is performed by specially trained surgeons who avoid opening a patient and cutting through muscles and tissue to reach inside the body. Using a miniature video camera, doctors operate through tiny holes."[4]

Indeed, we were not very "specially trained surgeons"!

In some cases, we were not really trained at all (but as you will often hear, surgeons may be wrong but not often in doubt). The powerful drive to succeed as well as a sense of impenetrable confidence led us into the laparoscopic fray with few skills and little practical experience. To the credit of general surgeons everywhere, their laparoscopic skills became refined (in most hands) remarkably quickly.

Thus, in the dawning hours of the laparoscopic revolution, the flame had been lit. And no one was going to blow it out. In those early days of minimally invasive laparoscopic gallbladder removal, professional excitement pulsed like electricity from Marietta, Georgia, and Nashville, Tennessee, from Los Angeles, California, and on around the country in expanding waves of practitioner curiosity. It seemed at the time as though equal doses of disbelief and dismissive condescension were spreading in surgical circles as news about the mysterious new operation reached U.S. surgeons. Of course, most of us were tradition-bound, and our collective thinking was summarized in specific reports documented in a variety of surgical journals.

The goal of the hardbound *Yearbook of Surgery* is to reproduce leading articles that were published in other journals that year and gather them in disease-related chapters to summarize advances critical to general surgery.

For example, in the *Yearbook* for 1988, studies on lithotripsy (shock-wave destruction of gallstones) as well as on the use of endoscopy through the stomach and into the duodenum to retrieve common bile duct stones were popular topics. These topics appeared again in 1990 along with a report on the problem of damaging the common bile duct during open cholecystectomy.[5] Interestingly, in the 1991 *Yearbook*, Philippe Mouret in France reported on the laparoscopic treatment of perforated (burst) peptic ulcer disease, a novel application of the less invasive laparoscopic techniques.[6] Yet there was no mention of his research on laparoscopic cholecystectomy despite the fact that he was one of the very first innovators. Mouret was also one of several distinguished authors writing of the European experience with laparoscopic cholecystectomy that year.[7] The *Yearbook* chose not to review that landmark report. However, the reviewer of the 1991 article on perforated ulcer treatment, Dr. J. C. Thompson, stated, "Just because something can be done, there is no reason to conclude that it should be done. As a result of the explosive popularity of laparoscopic cholecystectomy, I am sure we will see attempts to perform nearly every intra-abdominal procedure by laparoscopy (or as our circulating nurse calls them, operations by remote control)."[8] He concluded that the various aggressive patterns of peptic ulcer disease led him to support an open operation because a definitive ulcer operation could then be performed for complicated disease. Those open operations and virtually all ulcer procedures have all but disappeared today because of pharmaceutical advances.

What was less than subtle was the reviewer's disdain for laparoscopic surgery. This was often expressed at the time by leaders in many academic medical centers. The 1991 *Yearbook* covered such gallbladder issues as the difficulty taking out an acutely inflamed gallbladder, minilaparotomy (small incision) cholecystectomy, and dissolving gallstones with chemicals—all arguments waiting in the wings to be battled over as the laparoscope danced its way into the hearts of general surgeons on the big stage. Only in the 1992 *Yearbook of Surgery* did laparoscopic cholecystectomy receive its due recognition as an established procedure.[9,10,11,12] Indeed, this recognition was a necessary acknowledgment of the overwhelming success of "operations by remote control."

American Genesis

A German general surgeon performed the first laparoscopic cholecystectomy in the world in 1985. This entry into the realm of gynecologists was followed in 1987 by three Frenchmen who have subsequently and erroneously been given credit for the first laparoscopic cholecystectomy.

To be fair, with fewer available communication capabilities and before the advent of the Internet, it is understandable that the flurry of laparoscopic activity in the mid- to late 1980s would not be sorted out until years later. Also, the technological approaches these general surgeons used to create a less invasive gallbladder operation were innovative and variable.

In early 1988, a general surgeon, Barry McKernan (who had an unusual background in urology, including cystoscopy), and a gynecologist and superb laparoscopist, William Saye, together performed the first laparoscopic gallbladder removal in the United States. Neither was known as a hepatobiliary specialist (an expert in surgery of the gallbladder, bile ducts, and liver). But they possessed special skills well beyond the technological training of most general surgeons. McKernan also possessed the needed skills with open gallbladder removal should the less invasive operation have failed.

There wasn't anything normal about the surgical procedure I performed on the anesthetized pig on that career-changing day in Marietta. I had never done the strange operation before. Nearby, in other rooms set up as operating suites, dozens of equally naive surgeons struggled to insert and manipulate skinny instruments through hollow sheaths or sleeves poked through the pig's belly wall. No one in the room had ever seen, let alone performed, the awkward operation before Dr. Reddick's demonstration that day. In the hushed darkness we stared up at a television screen on which colorful 2-D images of the pig's interior anatomy darted by—pink loops of intestines, yellow streaks of fat, the brown, chunky liver with its green gallbladder hanging on for dear life. Within weeks we would be performing the operation on our first patients.

We all experienced a sense of foreboding. We couldn't quite grasp the idea of removing a sick, stone-caked gallbladder with glorified sticks. We couldn't touch it. We couldn't *grasp* the gallbladder with our hands.

I had traveled with two colleagues to Georgia from my institution, Baystate Medical Center, the Western Campus of Tufts School of Medicine, in Springfield, Massachusetts, to learn the new surgical procedure. Through tiny stab wounds we pushed hollow, cigar case-like sleeves called trocars to reach the pig's abdominal cavity (Figure 1.2). Then we slipped the soda-straw graspers and tiny scissors through the trocars and looked up at the TV screen. The tip of the instruments darted in and out of our field of vision. The person holding the camera often lost control of the telescope, and the surgical field jiggled, creating chaos. The laparoscopic operation defied every surgical instinct I had acquired through years of training and practice. Suddenly I couldn't hold the tissue in my hand, couldn't

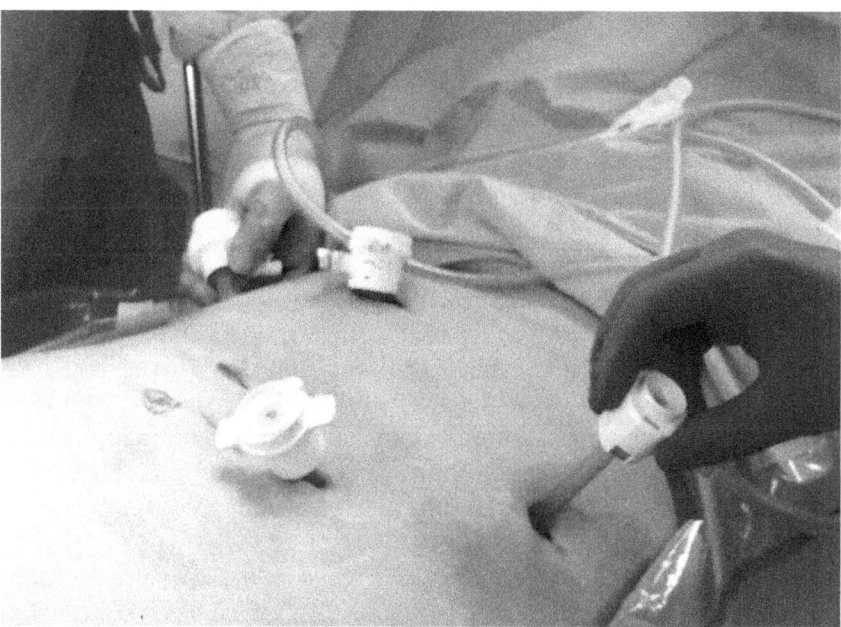

Figure 1.2   Trocar/Sleeves (Sheaths) through Abdominal Wall (photo by David Page, MD)

manipulate, squeeze, rotate, pull, or push it. I could only stab at it with the blunt end of those damned little sticks.

What no one at the Marietta course appreciated at the time was that the new "Band-Aid" surgery would quickly become an overwhelming hit with the public. It would spread like proverbial wildfire. This occurred long before the operation could be researched or tested or could acquire a credible track record. In fact, to this day no prospective scientific study has ever been performed to prove that laparoscopic gallbladder removal is superior to the traditional open operation. But then again, no one has done a prospective study randomizing parachute versus no parachute to prove the device's value.[13]

We approached laparoscopic gallbladder removal all wrong at first. In fact, it was noted in 1991, "We can hope that with the future expansion and application of laparoscopy, critical analyses of *prospective* trials on the outcome of such procedures will be accomplished before reliable techniques or procedures of the immediate past are abandoned."[14] No prospective study was ever done.

While the operation lacked scientific proof of its effectiveness and safety, that little lapse didn't stop us from applying the difficult operation in our practices. No sooner had we arrived home from our brief weekend training excursion than we offered the operation to the next gallstone sufferer. The public quickly caught on to the benefits of less surgical trauma. But it would take years before patients learned about the downside of general surgeons attempting to learn the new gallbladder operation.

For example, disadvantages noted by Soper in 1991 included that (a) most general surgeons at the time were unfamiliar with laparoscopy and the "lever" effect and how to manipulate the sticks inside the abdomen; (b) 3-D depth perception was degraded to 2-D, and the surgeon wasn't familiar with such cues as shadowing to work back to a 3-D view of the pathology; (c) patients had to be good candidates for general anesthesia; (d) poor operative candidates included obese patients, those with excessive inflammation around the gallbladder, and those who had had previous surgery with adhesions (organs stuck together); and (e) the challenge of how to handle common bile duct stones (many surgeons lacked the skill to remove them laparoscopically).[15]

This lack of skill changed within two or three years. Soper also described a rising problem with credentialing, writing, "Anecdotal reports of bile duct injuries and deaths have surfaced, and rumors have circulated that gynecologists, urologists, and gastroenterologists are performing laparoscopic cholecystectomy with general surgeons on 'standby' call to take care of possible complications."[16] Commenting on the potential for inadequate training, which alarmed members of the Society of American Gastrointestinal and Endoscopic Surgeons (SAGES), Soper concluded, "The Society considers the procedure to be investigational and that only those surgeons who are able to perform open biliary surgery should be allowed to perform laparoscopic cholecystectomy."[17]

The Third Surgical Revolution—Risks and Benefits

Four tiny scars.

These nearly invisible skin incisions would signal the advent of minimal postoperative pain for patients undergoing the less invasive gallbladder operation. In no time patients were being sent home after only a few days in the hospital. Soon, they would be discharged on the same day as their laparoscopic operation. This, instead of a week in the hospital with a huge slash across the upper abdomen, a nasogastric tube dribbling bile for days, an inability to get out of bed and walk independently, constipation from huge doses of narcotics, and more often than not, a urinary bladder catheter that too often resulted in a urinary tract infection.

To be sure, the new gallbladder operation was not just an improvement. It was revolutionary. And unsuspecting people die in the chaos of revolutionary fervor.

Today, more and more often in the nation's operating rooms, the scalpel is nowhere in sight. For the most part that's a good thing. *For the most part.* If you know why you are being offered a particular operation. And by whom. And especially if you know the surgeon's experience with the operation. Less invasive surgery is the gold standard in most cases. But to be safe in the hospital, you have to have an appreciation of the radical changes in surgical technology that have occurred. Also, it's crucial that you realize that more changes are coming toward you just down the pike.

The phrase *minimally invasive surgery* (MIS) joined such other well-known revolutionary words as *anesthesia* and *antisepsis*, two ideas that over a century ago transformed the art and science of surgery. It was also known as *minimal access surgery.* Whatever it would ultimately be called, the innovative operation I learned in Marietta promised to end the tradition of huge surgical incisions and the exquisitely choreographed, gloved handiwork that had marked decades of heroic cures—and, yes, immeasurable patient suffering. Yet those huge operations represented general surgery at its very best. And they still play an essential role in surgical care today. Back in the day we felt secure with our mastery of the scalpel.

In the pig lab in 1990 for the first time we clutched the porcine bile bag with long, skinny instruments instead of with our hands. The pistol-grip handles of the long instruments felt strange. The tiny grasping tool at the end of the chopstick jerked erratically inside the belly cavity. The performance played out on an overhead TV screen. Our every uncertain move glared out at us from the unforgiving screen on which every passerby could peer through the OR window at the "lap chole" show.

In the pig lab we often misdirected the long laparoscopic sticks through the inner space of the bovine belly cavity. At first our hands trembled. We awkwardly tore tissue. We swore and grasped the gallbladder more desperately and teased out bloody structures attached to the pig's liver. And at long last we tugged our first ragged green gallbladder—appearing much like a child's tattered and deflated balloon—out of the pig's belly through one of the trocar tubes.

Apparently, this crazy gallbladder operation was just the beginning of profound technological change. As R. David Rosin stated in the preface of his 1993 book, *Minimal Access: Medicine and Surgery, Principles and Techniques,* "Laparoscopic cholecystectomy exploded onto the general surgical scene like no other procedure before it. Embraced by the public, and promoted by technologic advances, it rejuvenated general surgery. Although there were a few skeptics, the rush to learn minimal access surgical techniques was phenomenal and took surgical trainers by storm."[18]

My message for you is that, as a potential surgical patient (Americans tend to undergo three to four major operations in a lifetime), you must be keenly aware of today's patient-safety issues, as well as changes in surgical technology and surgeon training, experience, and attitudes. The story of how laparoscopic surgery revolutionized our profession includes successes and failures as we struggled through the last decade of the twentieth century. But we haven't seen the endgame of this pioneering shift to all things surgical becoming smaller. Many risks for patients remain. So, my prime theme is that general surgery and surgical subspecialties are in a state of flux; *uncertainty about who should be doing what operation to which patients is of unprecedented importance because we are still learning about the challenges of less invasive operations.*

Consider the issues surrounding the training of capable surgeons suggested by two quotations made over two decades apart. The sobering first quotation, from a laparoscopic gallbladder surgery atlas written during the introductory phase of laparoscopy in general surgery in 1990, is by doctors Alfred Cuschieri and George Berci: "There are few surgeons in the US who graduate residency as accomplished endoscopists or even have more than a passing familiarity with diagnostic laparoscopy. It is difficult therefore, to comprehend how such practicing physicians in this country feel comfortable incorporating laparoscopic cholecystectomy (gallbladder removal) into their therapeutic armamentarium with this unsatisfactory background."[19] Clearly, in 1990 these authors felt the need to caution surgeons that their lack of formal training in laparoscopy could well produce unintended complications.

Compare this statement about the training of general surgeons at the *beginning* of the laparoscopic revolution with the following statement made by Dr. Layton F. Rikkers two decades later in the preface of a 2012 laparoscopic surgery atlas: "The rapid adoption of laparoscopy has led to the development of a new subspecialty area in surgery . . . minimally invasive surgery. This has fostered much basic and clinical research and innumerable papers published on all conceivable aspects of minimally invasive surgery. While this expansion of knowledge has been desirable, the sheer bulk of it has made it difficult for the individual surgeon to keep abreast of the most recent advances."[20] In 1990, the warning was clear: most general surgeons were not formally trained in laparoscopy. The idea of introducing laparoscopic cholecystectomy into their practices was seriously challenged by Cuschieri and Berci. In 2012, the warning continued: general surgeons were struggling to keep up with a laparoscopic surgical field that had exploded with new and complex operations, as well as an uncontrollable amount of required knowledge. Thus, two major sources of technical advice and special knowledge regarding the practice of minimally invasive procedures were hedging their bets about the wisdom of widespread adoption of laparoscopy. In the 2012 atlas mentioned above, Dr. Jeffrey L. Ponsky added his concern: "The field of minimally invasive surgery has grown geometrically in the last two decades. Beginning with the birth of laparoscopic cholecystectomy, it has since expanded dramatically in many directions. . . . *The literature is also hard to keep up with* [my italics] and the value of particular approaches is in some ways unproven and untested."[21]

So, just a few years ago, in addition to reservations about how a general surgeon might master less invasive operations, we were additionally warned that not all the new laparoscopic operations had been tested for safety. Like the trend to push the proverbial envelope to continue to innovate and refine less invasive operations, the risk to unwary patients grows. No prospective clinical trials had been done for the new applications of laparoscopy in general surgery. These cautionary statements by academic surgeons two decades apart make it clear that, if an operation looms in your future, you must make certain you understand how to assure your own safety. These authors were visionary. And so in subsequent chapters, I will explain how pockets of surgical incompetence sneaked unannounced into our midst.[22,23,24]

Our health care system remains cloaked in a satin shroud of silence. So far, transparency hails more as a concept than as a commitment. Surgeons know that technical mistakes happen early in a practitioner's experience with a new operation. Less experienced surgeons have more complications than experts until they've logged a significant number of cases. And large numbers of operations available in the hands of general surgeons means fewer actual cases performed by any surgeon in each category.

The training landscape today's young surgeons face seems incomprehensible to practicing surgeons who trained as I did in the 1970s or earlier. It's worth repeating what I mentioned earlier: in the first few years of our experience with laparoscopic technology, surgeons around the United States and elsewhere began a dangerous trend of operating on one or two pigs over a weekend course—some courses had no actual skills training, just lectures—and returned home to offer the operation to their patients the next week. It was the beginning of the laparoscopic revolution, and the onset of a staggering maldistribution of surgical talent in the United States.

One surgical educator, Dr. Leigh Neumayer (I owe her the title of this chapter), described the early approach to laparoscopic gallbladder removal as "Dry Laboratory on Saturday, pig on Sunday, and Grandma on Monday," which "probably was not the best training method, especially when proctoring was not available."[25] Unfortunately, this phrase correctly describes how laparoscopic cholecystectomy found its way onto the general surgery menu. Thus, the real dilemma facing surgical patients today involves finding experts who perform specific modern minimally invasive or traditional open operation that they need.

The issue isn't that there is a lack of surgical expertise per se in the United States. The problem centers on identifying the *location and distribution of surgical capability*. And as I have suggested, two solutions to the problem of surgical capability include additional fellowship training or proctoring by experienced surgeons in actual practice. This story will educate you about some of these defects in the magnificent fabric of American surgery.

My Scalpel Has No Voice

I must rely on my pen to awaken you to the fabulous, yet uneven world of surgical expertise in the United States right now at the beginning of the twenty-first century. Periodically, a member of a group must speak up about the shadowy elephant in the room.[26] And so I feel compelled to identify the uncertainty birthed by a revolution that has otherwise brought major improvements to how surgery is performed. This book honors the trust patients have placed in surgeons everywhere and provides information about the new minimally invasive world of surgery. I'm convinced that these sensational operations have created a dilemma for surgical patients: increased case complexity combined with less surgical experience in some hands has placed true informed consent on trial. I wonder if explaining a complicated operation, as well as stating a surgeon's experience, is possible in the claustrophobically squeezed minutes of an office visit. Patients must know what questions to ask a surgeon and how to pose them in order to receive safe and effective care in this era of evolving surgical technology.

The telescope we used for the first time in Georgia, referred to as a *laparoscope*, was originally used by skilled European internists and gynecologists (Figure 1.3). Then, two decades ago, a few general surgeons like me began to survey the inside of the abdomen for diagnostic purposes. I had

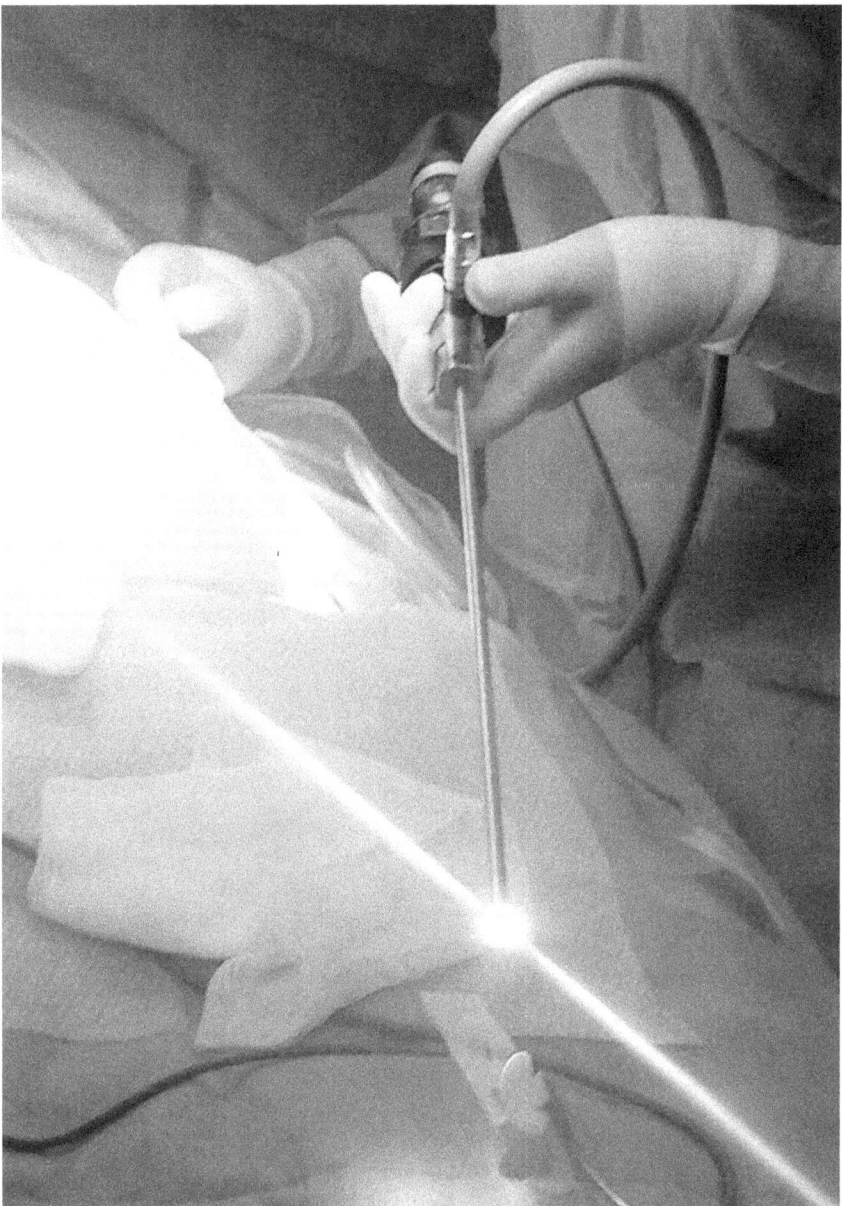

Figure 1.3   The Laparoscope (Telescope) and Camera (photo by David Page, MD)

been doing diagnostic laparoscopy for a few years before I attended the Marietta, Georgia, laparoscopic gallbladder course in 1990. But I did it without the digital camera, microchip, and TV technology. The transition we embarked on in Georgia—actually *operating* through tiny trocar sleeves with Lilliputian instruments—was an intrepid leap of faith for incision-bound surgeons. The timing of the arrival of the laparoscopic revolution was as remarkable as it was unexpected.

The future of general surgery looked grim indeed in the 1980s. However, the demise of our beloved surgical specialty had been predicted before. Maybe we could escape with our practices intact this time after all. So we whittled and wept and bemoaned our shrinking professional futures as the pilfering of our cherished cases accelerated.

Then, an odd thing happened to the scalpel.

The knife lost its iconic allure. Steadily, the laparoscope nudged its way into the general surgeon's toolbox. No longer could we sneer in derision at our gynecologic colleagues. Suddenly, we needed *their* skills.

There is no shortage of irony in our early and vehement rejection of the laparoscopic technology that would save our specialty of general surgery. And today as cultural and political battles rage in academic departments and in private-practice circles, the scalpel lies quietly on the scrub tech's back table, its future uncertain.

CHAPTER TWO

The First Sounds of a Revolution

The most conscientious historian must deal with legends, and legends grow rapidly. Even the passage of a day begins to turn facts into fanciful and entertaining stories. Interestingly told, these tales combine truth and ridiculousness in such delightful and charming proportions that they are bound to last for a long time.

Loyal David, *Fellowship of Surgeons*, 1960

At the turn of the twentieth century, a Dresden surgeon used a cystoscope to observe the abdominal organs of dogs. Ninety years later, surgeons across the United States have started distributing videotapes of laparoscopic surgery; some patients even invite friends in to watch their surgery on a screen while munching potato chips.

Grzegorz S. Litynski, *Highlights in the History of Laparoscopy*, 1996

Death in the Afternoon

Early in 2010, Egyptian president Hosni Mubarak traveled to Germany to have his gallbladder (and a small intestine tumor) removed at the Heidelberg Hospital. His surgery was performed through a traditional open incision. He did well. But he left the hospital with pain and a large gash on his belly. A year earlier in 2009, Ed Koch had had his gallbladder laparoscopically snatched out of his belly with fanfare but without incident at New York Presbyterian Columbia Hospital. Mr. Koch's discomfort was fleeting.

Congressman John Murtha's gallbladder story was sadly very different. Murtha died on February 8, 2010, at age 77, a few days after readmission following a routine laparoscopic gallbladder operation at the National Naval Medical Center. Reportedly, the surgeon hit his intestine, leading to uncontrolled infection. The surgeon's technical mistake was presumably that he or she poked a hole in Murtha's large intestine with a sharp trocar (designed like a knife to cut through the belly wall), made a hole with the cautery, or crushed it with a retractor. Presumably, feces spilled into Murtha's sterile abdominal cavity.[1] What a sad irony for a veteran who earned a Bronze Star and two Purple Hearts.

Presumably. Because despite repeated reminders that this is an era of transparency in health care, no one has explained publicly how this tragedy happened. Murtha's death highlights an unpleasant reality: despite the availability of excellent surgeons in the United States, Americans may be subjected to less than capable surgical care in certain areas of practice. My concern about the level of technical competence of graduating surgeons isn't new. But the importance of the issue has accelerated in recent years.

Ironically, laparoscopic gallbladder surgery is one of the operations with which general surgeons have a great deal of experience. That reality makes Murtha's death all the more regrettable. This sad event occurred to a national leader 20 years after general surgeons trained for the first time at weekend courses to learn laparoscopic gallbladder removal. And today, after operating on a pig or two, some surgeons like their 1990 brethren return to their practices and attempt the unfamiliar robotic operation on human patients.

The Cult of the Scalpel

We held the knife gently as if it were a feather, the handle against the palm, the razor-like blade protruding beyond the index finger. The grasp of a scalpel mimics no other tool-holding hand position, save perhaps the delicacy of a composer's embrace of his baton. The scalpel is, anthropologically speaking, tool use in the extreme. Anthropologists describe chimpanzees, the animal we share greater than 98 percent of our DNA with, fishing for termites with sticks. Now, imagine a surgeon dissecting the thyroid gland in the neck or performing robotic telesurgery across the Atlantic Ocean with the surgeon in New York City and the patient in France.

A chilling sense of wonder washes over me whenever I pick up a scalpel and carve deeply into another's flesh. It melds privilege with urgency, obligation with uncertainty. There are no easy cases. And the touch of the knife against tissue necessitates knowledge of that tissue, of that anatomy, of that particular pathology. The surgeon's work merges from novice to master skill only after years of training and practice.

And that reality must infuse and inform any conversation regarding the credentialing of capable surgeons and the educational challenges involved in teaching and learning technical skills.

Since the discovery of anesthesia and asepsis, surgeons have excised diseased tissue with the knife, cured intestine perforations, and stanched massive stomach hemorrhage. It was how we declawed deadly cancers and triumphed against overwhelming flesh-eating infections. This modern paradigm of aggressive cutting was ushered in by such innovations as Halsted's radical mastectomy in the late 19th century, an operation that was to endure and disfigure despite its lack of superior effectiveness over less aggressive procedures. Throughout most of the 20th century, radical mastectomy flourished in the hands of heroic surgeons. A modified form of the operation (called modified radical mastectomy or some variant) survives in more rural practice pockets where multidisciplinary breast-cancer care is less available. And while some types of aggressive open abdominal, chest, and pelvic operations continue to represent a necessary part of our daily life-saving activities, overall general surgery has transformed itself into a less invasive endeavor.

Before the Laparoscope

The hands of surgeons are legendary. Sensing and pressing. Applying a precise knife swipe, a delicate scissors squeeze. Directed. Skilled. Iconic. And nothing if not heroic in the therapeutic scope of the effort. In the day, surgeons thrust their hands deep into their work, controlling massive diseased-based as well as self-inflicted bleeding—the master surgeon lunging with a clamp, grabbing a bleeding artery or vein in the instrument's crude teeth. Slithering like an anaconda into the depths of a belly, the talented gloved hand advanced with its own radar, touching the liver, the spleen, coils of intestines. The hand ballet pirouetted through artistic maneuvers, teasing tissue planes, delicately inserting sutures and sealants with therapeutic precision—through a gaping incision.

That is, actually touching human tissue was possible until recently.

At the beginning of the 19th century, fear of inflicting pain and provoking infection and uncontrolled hemorrhage restrained surgeons from entering the body's mysterious cavities where growths and traumatic damage lay concealed. Survival was only occasional when surgeons tampered with the abdomen. Entering the chest or head was taboo. Suffering was extreme with or without surgical intervention.

In 1809, Ephraim McDowell performed the first ever planned abdominal operation (laparotomy) in Danville, Kentucky, for what turned out to be a 20-pound ovarian cyst. He conducted the operation before the availability of general anesthesia and before the medical profession understood bacteriology. McDowell completed his remarkable technical feat on his kitchen table while ignoring a raucous lynching crowd swirling in anger outside his kitchen window, brandishing a hanging rope in case he had failed.

The operation was completely successful. No major bleeding. No subsequent infection in the belly or in the wound. Thus, McDowell's courage signaled the advent of abdominal surgery.[2]

By the end of the 19th century, solutions to effective anesthesia, sepsis (infection), and bleeding were well in hand. Such pioneers as Kock, Pasteur, and Lister unraveled the mysteries of bacterial infection. Observing fermentation, setting up creative experiments, and using new microscopes to identify "animalcules," each of these great men contributed to the new discipline of bacteriology and snuffed out the theory of spontaneous generation.[3] Spraying carbolic acid about the operating room, Lister began a revolution that concluded with the control of surgical infections and overwhelming sepsis. His was a transformational idea that crashed into the stubborn stone walls of medical dogma, preconception, and prejudice before becoming self-evident.[4]

At the same time, such names as Horace Wells, Crawford Long, William Clark, Charles Jackson, William Thomas Green Morton, and Dr. John Collins Warren became 19th-century magnates. These various practitioners swarmed over the country in a stew of ego, claims of primacy of discovery, and lunatic behavior—all of which characterized the early history of inhalation (general) anesthesia. This dubious yet innovative cast of dentists, chemists, and surgeons brought forth the use of ether, nitrous oxide, and chloroform in what Oliver Wendell Holmes Sr. named anesthesia.[5]

The practice of surgery had somehow stumbled to the margins of science.

Reflecting on the state of 20th-century surgery, in 1955 Isidor S. Ravdin, professor of surgery at the University of Pennsylvania, wrote, "Daily the entire stomach is being removed, the entire pancreas, half a liver, and large sections of the most important blood vessels, and a host of other operations of great magnitude are being performed that only a few years ago were operative curiosities or were not being done at all."[6] *Operative curiosities.* Ironically, most of these operations now have a less invasive laparoscopic twin. And, for example, although gastric surgery for ulcer disease is almost extinct today because of the discovery of a bacterium (*Helicobacter pylori*) treatable with antibiotics, we still remove the stomach for cancer and weight control. I marvel with equal admiration as did Dr. Ravdin when I reflect on how a few of today's surgeons engage in modern operative curiosities, for example, removing the pancreas with a laparoscope.

However, the third revolution in modern surgery—the invention of less invasive laparoscopic and robotic operations, and the focus of this book— had to await major discoveries in several scientific domains. Interestingly, today laparoscopic surgery is considered a translational operative technique. In other words, what we are doing at the outset of the 21st century will transform itself into the next, yet undefined method of performing surgery. It's a continuation of the journey from Bozzini's 19th-century cystoscope using candlelight and mirrors to the current visual-spatial and range-of-motion improvements of the robotic wrist and lens system (Figure 2.1).

But before we discuss the introduction of less invasive operations into surgical practice, travel with me on an imaginary voyage. I'm going to describe how it felt to do a major open operation back in the day. Because as we progress through the book we'll be measuring everything we do in the operating room today that is *less* invasive against this traditional open surgical experience.

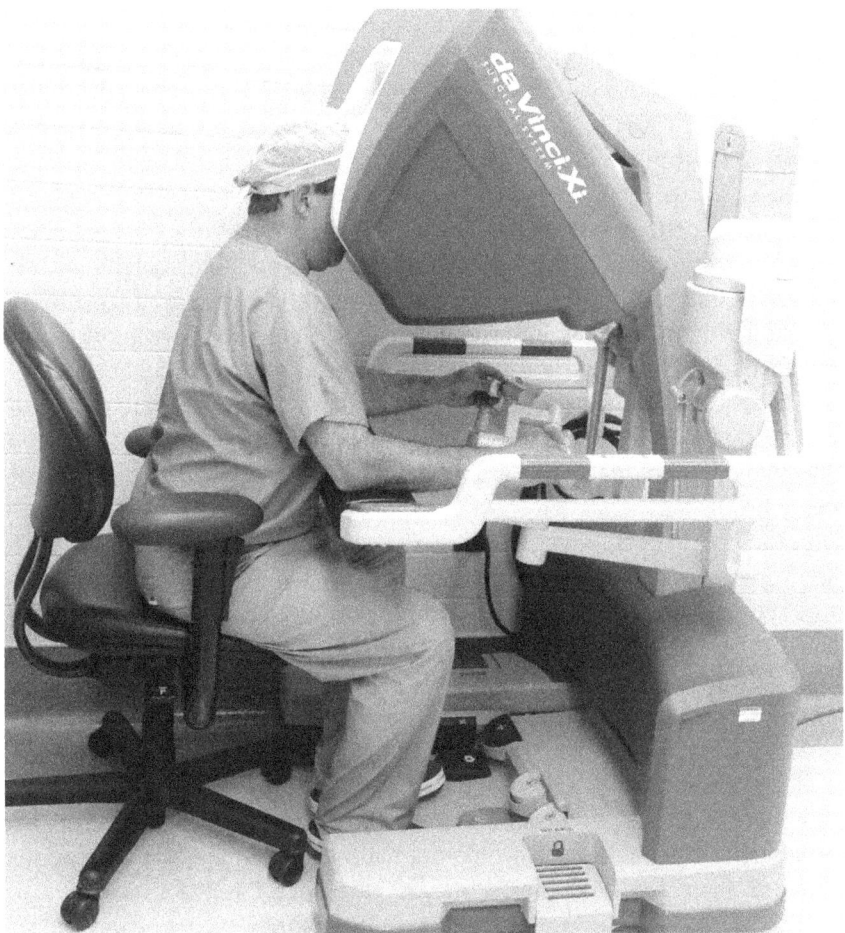

Figure 2.1   Da Vinci Robot Console (photo by David Page, MD)

So follow me now into that hallowed room, the operating theater of three decades ago with its brilliant overhead lights and hushed atmosphere.

Scrubbing On a Traditional Open Abdominal Operation

The operating room of three decades ago was not democratic.

As anthropologists have shown, surgeons then (as many still do today) viewed themselves as heroic curers of uncontrolled disease.[7,8,9] In the operating room, we tolerated few challenges to our authority as captain of the ship. As a stepping-stone into the new world of darkened operating rooms, flickering TV screens, and indirect minimally invasive surgery, imagine you are standing with me in an operating room of the 1980s. You are my assistant. I am the conductor and you, the scrub tech, the circulating nurse, and the anesthesiologist and his team are the orchestra. But there is no team concept in play here.

We'll perform a colon removal for cancer. We're gloved and gowned, beginning the case together. I nod to the scrub tech. The exposed patch of belly skin is brown with antiseptic paint, cordoned off with sterile blue drapes and illuminated by brilliant scooped-out overhead lights.

The scrub tech hands me the scalpel.

I don't ask the anesthesiologist if he's ready. We have not talked about the case. We have not communicated about the possible anesthetic techniques he might use or about the patient's risk factors. I nod to you, my assistant, with nothing more informative than a grunt. We are 30 years and hundreds of publications away from checklists, time-outs, and debriefings. The term *medical error* lies dormant in the minds of only a few prescient physicians. Surgeons back then would scoff at the touchy-feely notion of effective interpersonal communication. In the 1970s and 1980s era, a philosophical chasm separated most surgeons from a habit of self-reflection.[10] And the notion of thinking about quality improvement resided in a future seemingly measured in geologic time.

On this day I take charge of the case. I am the captain of the ship. You stand there and don't move for worry of contaminating yourself. Standing across from me, you might not sense my fleeting unease, an erasable moment of uncertainty. In any case, I would disavow it if asked.

I'll tell you how it feels to be a surgeon. Watch me wield the blade. I will make the unkind cut into another's flesh knowingly inflicting pain, praying for success, for cure. I will not hesitate in the act of cutting. The remarkable thing is that you would not pause either. Medical students crave that first cut. They do not fear it as you have been told.

The moment of cutting into another's flesh surges into a powerful feeling of godlike control. A brief moment of doubt is banished to the outer ionosphere of my consciousness. That I might lose it if things unravel quickly is a flicker of dread quickly buried in a swell of excitement.

My hand moves in a flash.

The knife slits open the belly layers as blood wells up and is controlled by cautery and snug suture ties. The stench of burning flesh drifts up from the belly cavity and lurches you toward nauseated disgust. Deep in the wound, I push aside loops of pink small intestine and reveal the deadly cancer biting down like a crab on the colon.

I dissect around the cancer. Suddenly, the surgical field floods with blood. Something is wrong. I swallow a trickle of bile rising in the back of my throat.

Quietly, I ask for a hemostat. An artery you didn't see spurts up and sprays my glasses. The maroon veil drips away my visibility. Across from me you stare at the delicate blade in my hand . . .

My knife has a conscience. It sits in my gloved palm. It awaits the slightest movement of my fingers. One swift flick of the wrist and the scalpel's keen edge cuts deep into another's flesh. Repairing torn flesh, excising cancerous growths for cure, dramatically preserving life—just like that.

Healing with intent.

That is how it went in the day. Big incisions. Angry cancers. And acceptable cures. We went on night and day. Case after case. No restrictions on work hours. We ignored the pain we inflicted on our patients in order to avoid our own.

Surgeons struggle to perfect their craft. During decades of progress in the art of surgery, we have experienced self-satisfaction and have pranced proudly in our hallowed masks and gowns, unruffled in our self-control, princes in sterile armor, gowned statues in well-lighted operating rooms. Back then we withstood many challenges alone under hot lights, invading the body temple, opening the abdomen and chest and skull.

Look at our instruments. Dozens of them lined up with handles. Hand tools. Clamps, scissors, grabbing instruments all to be applied directly to the flesh. Crude metal tools wielded through a huge slash in the abdominal wall, poking and prodding and dripping with blood, soaking sponges and lap pads red. For a while, open abdominal operations defined general surgery. Then, slowly, less painful replacements appeared on the clinical scene. At first we didn't pay much attention. But when our wallets began to empty, general surgeons began to wake up.

Today, radiologists drain abscesses almost anywhere in the body with thin catheters, replacing the surgeon's scalpel. Appendicitis is thought in certain circumstances to be amenable to antibiotics alone. Removing lymph glands under the arm in the treatment of breast cancer has been mostly replaced by observation alone or with axillary radiation. And those painful, pulsating aortic aneurysms, whether in the chest or abdomen, are now treated in a special operating room where the ballooning blood vessel is controlled by an endovascular (placed from inside the artery) graft repair of the aneurysm (EVAR). No incision on the belly is required.

But none of these changes occurred quickly. Or quietly.

Throughout the transition from aggressive operations performed in the 1970s and 1980s and into the 1990s, to the less intrusive, less invasive procedures that characterize modern general surgery, surgeons retooled themselves without ever undergoing formal testing of their new skills. As remarkable as this may sound, it was the way of the land and still is to a large extent. To their credit, most surgeons obtained the experience and skills necessary to make the transition from incision to laparoscope without creating too much damage to their patients.

It was in the incendiary year of 1990 that we plunged into unfamiliar territory. In the flash of a television screen, the laparoscopic revolution was born. Our aggressive surgical approaches started to unravel in 1985 when a German general surgeon started thinking small.

A Glitch in Medical Education—The Decline in Physical Examination Skills and the Rise of Invasive Imaging

As a consequence of this technological invasion of medicine, medical educators found themselves facing a new reality. The rapid advance in diagnostic instruments was accompanied by a decline in young doctors' diagnostic clinical skills. This loss of the ability to competently examine an abdomen, for example, creates a disturbing sidebar to the laparoscopic revolution. There can be no doubt that young physicians possess significant deficiencies in their examination skills. The iconic stethoscope so prominently draped about the medical student or resident's neck promises something perhaps anchored more in history than in today's clinical reality.

In the case of surgery, Claude Organ, a giant among American surgical leaders, stated in 2003: "Unfortunately, though, the technology that research has created too often becomes a substitute for good surgery. This is the fault of surgeons, not of technology. We have spawned a generation of surgeons who are the high priests and priestesses of laboratory and radiographic triage."[11] In a word, young surgeons rely on X-rays and other imaging methods rather than their hands, eyes, noses, and ears to make a diagnosis.

In a parallel universe, minimally invasive laparoscopic operations have limited the modern surgical resident's exposure to open operations (cases performed through a traditional incision). Open surgery skills of trainees have declined, as many of us who are ardent surgical educators have observed in the operating room. Surgical residents spend a majority of their operative experience performing (or watching their attending surgeon perform) laparoscopic operations. They wield the knife less often and with less skill. Minimally invasive surgery is good for patients but not so good for surgical residents who have diminished skills with a scalpel. Hinging on this reality of reduced training experience is the present confusion over the role of hospital volume and surgeon volume with respect to outcomes (best results, fewest complications) and the role of specialized, high-volume surgical centers.[12]

The First Attempts at Endoscopy—A Very Brief Historical Note

It was a lost moment in history.

No one knows exactly when the first inquisitive premodern doctor attempted to discover where disease hid within living tubes or where pain originated deep in the cavities of the human body. Certainly, at some point in the past, an ancient healer peeked inside a natural orifice with spread fingers seeking answers. And at some point these early healers devised a crude scope to probe further into the body's natural openings. And it is profoundly ironic that the most cutting-edge surgical technology today has bent its cognitive brilliance like a beam of light around the human form and has come back to the use of NOTES (natural orifices transluminal endoscopic surgery).

The Hippocratic corpus of writing describes a rectal speculum similar to those we use today. And about 62–79 CE, in the ruins of Pompeii, archaeologists found a speculum among other surgical instruments in Region VI in the House of the Surgeon. To this day a speculum with three or more blades is used to hold back the tissues or walls of natural orifices such as the nostrils, ears, mouth, vagina, and anus.[13] Also, in Spain Abu al-Qasim (936–1013 CE) used several endoscope-like instruments to examine the throat and the urethra (tube leading to the urinary bladder). These early efforts scratched the surface of a colossal medical mystery: What lies inside the human body?

As I mentioned earlier in the chapter, the first true scope generally recognized by medical historians was made in 1806 by Philipp Bozzini in Frankfurt. He cobbled together a system of mirrors to reflect candlelight into the body. He called it a *Lichtleiter* or light conductor. But it was in 1877 in Berlin when Max Nitze introduced the first modern cystoscope that endoscopy began in earnest.[14] Nitze's cystoscope incorporated the idea of a rigid optical system with special lenses and a light source, the scope that figures heavily in the origins of laparoscopy. It was Georg Kelling who used it as what we now call a laparoscope to look inside the abdomens of dogs. Working on the problem of bleeding into the abdominal cavity, Kelling inserted Nitze's cystoscope directly into dogs' belly cavities to observe the effect of high-pressure insufflation on the abdominal contents. Thereafter, the technology sat balanced on the verge of discovery as a tool for human use. But Kelling abandoned his efforts and moved on to other areas of research. Fortunately, very soon thereafter a covey of investigators unfamiliar with Kelling's work nudged the frontier of indirect endoscopic abdominal examination toward its 20th-century fate.

The Revolution Begins

I could tell you it started suddenly. But you will discover that the winds of change had been blowing steadily in our faces for some time. We turned our backs on the emerging technological trend. We huddled down against the gusts of the revolution. Eventually, when we looked over our shoulders, what we saw stunned us. There in the forefront stood the public waving placards begging us for less traumatic operations. In a heartbeat, surgeons were no longer in control of their own destiny. Nor were the internists who had come to believe they could steal the gallbladder from the surgeons by dissolving gallstones with pills or smashing them with lithotripsy.

The race to refine minimally invasive operations began in the United States in 1988 when a gynecologist and a general surgeon with urology training laparoscopically removed the first gallbladder in North America in Marietta, Georgia. As some surgeons began to seriously consider less traumatic operations in 1990, it remained a time when real honest-to-goodness general surgeons looked with disdain on the laparoscopic antics of mere gynecologists. Cooperation was unheard of until Barry McKernan and William Saye collaborated and shared their operative skills in designing a new laparoscopic gallbladder operation. As I mentioned earlier, they weren't aware of similar work across the Atlantic Ocean. But in 1988 this duo joined their German and French colleagues in a revolutionary redirection of surgical care in the United States toward less invasive trends.

In 1990, general surgeons (and every subspecialty thereafter) ceased ridiculing their innovative gynecologic colleagues about doing Mickey Mouse surgery and joined the field of laparoscopic surgery. In the preceding 1970s and 1980s, the mantra went, "Small surgeons use small incisions." I recall dismissing an article on laparoscopic gallbladder removal in *Time* magazine that a patient brought to my office. I insisted, "It'll never work."

Many of my colleagues reminded me that they, too, had belittled the less invasive operations with invective and vulgar put-downs.

Then, the laparoscopic revolution quickly ran over us with unstoppable force.

In a mad dash to catch up, general surgeons plunged into this exciting era of surgical innovation. Other new operations using the laparoscope were born. The true surgical innovators of laparoscopic general surgery led a determined charge into the teeth of what was a harsh and verbally abusive pushback by aggressive academic surgical leaders who initially saw little value in the use of the laparoscope. Fortunately, early private-practice adopters followed the true innovators, who willingly showed us how to maneuver the strange new instruments inside a pig's belly.

In time I along with many other surgical teachers would discover that the impact of laparoscopy wasn't just on the practice of surgery. The revolution also had a profound influence on the practical and philosophical foundations of surgical education. Eventually, the adoption of less invasive operations would become a major reason for overhauling our flawed notions of what constituted safe surgery and appropriate surgical education techniques.

Before adopting the new gallbladder operation, staid senior surgeons balked at the idea and spoke derisively about the dangers of less visibility and the inability to directly handle tissue. It wasn't right to *not* use an incision. It was downright unsafe, they preened. Yet despite early resistance from academic and community surgeons alike, the laparoscopic stallions sprinted out of the starting gate.

Some members of the media were quick to identify the uncertainty associated with laparoscopic surgery. Lawrence K. Altman wrote in an August 14, 1990, Science Desk piece for the *New York Times*: "But medical experts are concerned that too many surgeons are being trained too fast in courses that vary in length and quality. . . . In some courses surgeons practice on pigs whose gallbladder anatomy most closely resembles that of humans. In other courses, no animal work is done. . . . In the rush, surgeons have rejected suggestions that the procedure be confined to specialized medical centers until its track record is established."[15] We rejected the suggestion because of pressure from the public, who demanded the less invasive operation *right now*, and because surgeons had made a business decision without expressing much interest in scientific deliberation.

Two years after the first gallbladder had been removed laparoscopically in Germany and a year before the first gallbladder operation would be performed laparoscopically in the United States, an editorial in the *British Medical Journal* by J. E. A. Wickam, director of the Department of

Minimally Invasive Surgery, Institute of Urology, London, wrote: "Surgeons applaud large incisions and denigrate 'keyhole surgery.' Patients, in contrast, want the smallest wound possible, and we at Britain's first department of minimally invasive surgery are convinced that patients are right."[16]

Of course, our technical skills lagged at first. The Wild West character of the early days of laparoscopic surgery are best described by Dr. Alfred Cuschieri of Dundee, Scotland, who said, "The early post-LC (laparoscopic gallbladder removal) years witnessed an uncontrolled expansion of surgical endoscopic practice, at times not far short of abuse, which amounted to the biggest unaudited free-for-all in the history of surgery."[17] *Not far short of abuse? The biggest unaudited free-for-all in the history of surgery!*

Sadly, Dr. Cuschieri's remark confirmed that in the early 1990s, patients were exposed to marginal laparoscopic competence in the hands of some poorly prepared general surgeons. There were few sheriffs in the early frontier days of minimally invasive gallbladder removal. In his 1990 book, *Laparoscopic Biliary Surgery*, Dr. Cuschieri noted, "In the early days of this procedure a number of ill-conceived courses were launched with training on inappropriate animal species. This did not provide any constructive education for the course participants."[18]

Patient safety wasn't an issue *because no one talked about it.*

Surgeons pushed ahead. The average patient with gallstones knew nothing of this initial level of laparoscopic incompetence. In fact, 10 years after the introduction of laparoscopic gallbladder removal, two British surgeons wrote regarding the operation, "The latter was introduced in an inappropriate manner, which has led to the evolution of teaching of technical skills away from an apprenticeship-based activity towards more formal skill-based training programmes."[19] This 2000 statement focuses the paradox of modern surgical care: the mess we made training to learn less invasive laparoscopic operations led to enormous improvements in surgical education, but not before surgeons stumbled along their learning curves with little documentation of their results.

By the end of the last decade of the 20th century—against all odds and despite resistance from an entrenched culture of surgeons—minimally invasive (laparoscopic or MIS) surgery had become a reality. The smell of blood evaporated in our operating rooms as the overhead lights were dimmed and TV screens, laparoscopic suction equipment, and novel energy instruments abutted the operating table. In the 1990s, the OR morphed into something unrecognizable. Performing an operation without an incision, we lost our bearings. We lost our finely honed sense of touch. We lost tactile contact with human tissue. Gone was the customary 3-D visual field, now degraded to 2-D via a video camera and skinny scope with images projected onto a TV screen. We lost depth perception, lost our balance staring up at TV monitors in the dark instead of down into the belly under brilliant lights.

Mostly, we lost the necessary reassurance that we could reach into the belly and fix whatever might have become injured or incorrectly dissected. The operating room was now crowded with flickering TV screens and draped tables laden with unfamiliar long instruments. We stood alone outside of the abdominal temple, perplexed. What no one saw coming was the surgical profession's abject inability to safely learn and then teach both traditional open operations and minimally invasive procedures in a five-year surgical residency training program. We quickly learned that the old unsupervised apprentice model wouldn't work as a stand-alone method of instruction in laparoscopic surgery.

Surgeons are agile, confident souls. Surgeons adapt. As has often been said, surgeons are sometimes wrong but never in doubt. Driven by public demand, general surgeons quickly learned to place those skinny trocar tubes through the abdominal wall.

We didn't like it. A puny telescope? A chopstick for a dissector? It didn't feel right, didn't sit well with our self-image as trauma titans, as cancer warriors, as scalpel scions.

But we did it anyway.

CHAPTER THREE

Disorientation: My First Waltz with a Laparoscope

The pace of technological, medical, and social change is almost breathtaking; it is difficult to say with certainly what laparoscopy and general surgery will look like in fifteen to twenty years.

G. Litynski, *Highlights in the History of Laparoscopy*, 1996

The current health care system falls terribly short in its ability to ensure that new technology is introduced safely and effectively and to translate the evidence generated by research into practice.

T. R. Russell, MD, executive director, American College of Surgeons, 2003

A Personal Side of the Revolution

In the early 1980s, my chairman at Baystate Medical Center, Paul Friedmann, MD, FACS, agreed with my idea of setting up a small technical skills lab in my office in the Department of Surgery. It would be a place for medical students and possibly residents to practice suturing and knot tying. No patient would be harmed. Mistakes, stumbles, and awkward moves would be expected and remediated one-on-one. I would keep surgical instruments and suture material available in my office for planned or impromptu teaching sessions.

In 1970, I began my surgical training at Baystate Medical Center under the chairmanship of Dr. Dominic A. DeLaurentis from Temple University, a hard-nosed leader in the old-school style of resident education. Dr. Friedmann joined him in 1968, and when DeLaurentis returned to Philadelphia in 1971, Paul Friedmann became my second chairman. I didn't realize at the time how active both surgeons were in the Whipple Society, which would dissolve and be replaced by the Association of Program Directors in Surgery (APDS). After much discussion among national surgical leaders, the APDS was born and held its first meeting and annual forum on

October 14, 1981, in San Francisco. Among the topics discussed were the legal implications of dismissing a resident, the pyramid system (lots of interns on the bottom, only one or two chief residents graduating on top), and to our interest here, endoscopy. In his talk, Dr. Stephen F. Hedberg stated, "It is my perception that endoscopy will not achieve its rightful place in gastrointestinal surgery until more surgeons have a vested interest in the procedures, the findings, the equipment, the space, and the training of endoscopists. . . . I believe that gastrointestinal surgery will suffer irreparable damage unless we can find ways immediately to train surgeons in endoscopic surgery."[1] At the time, this prediction of "irreparable damage" to general surgery almost came true as a majority of general surgeons expressed little or no interest in endoscopy and subsequently in its cousin, laparoscopy.

Dr. Friedmann had been instrumental in forging our relationship with Tufts University School of Medicine a few years earlier. We became the school's Western Campus and one of the medical school's major teaching sites. That year marked the beginning of my personal growth as a surgical educator while still a surgical resident. The skills lab idea arose from my background in physical education. When I was the clerkship director in surgery at Baystate, the notion of getting third-year medical students and residents to practice surgical skills in my small skills lab rather than in the operating room on real patients made sense. After all, I had coached for years, and you don't learn to swim butterfly for the first time in a competitive swim meet. A few residents tried practicing knot tying at one station and suturing whatever I had on the low shelf at a second station in my office. But there was little interest at the time in practicing technical skills outside the OR—other than tying suture material to chairs in the operating room lounge.

Jock to Doc

I was a physical-education major during my first four years of college. As my passion for anatomy and kinesiology (the study of human movement) grew and as my cross hairs inevitably focused on a surgical career, I became reluctant to talk about my "jock" training. After all, most premed students in my college class assumed phys-ed majors were a less intelligent species (ironically, in my sixth year of college as a teaching fellow in comparative anatomy and embryology, I taught the premed students). To pay my bills, I coached swimming at Suffield Academy in the Connecticut private school league and knew how coaches thought and taught (interestingly, coaching is currently a hot topic among surgical educators). So, for me one-on-one teaching of motor skills grew as a professional passion. Teaching technical skills to medical students and surgical residents on inanimate models seemed a no-brainer. But without faculty support or resident interest, my technical skills lab idea faded.

Yet the idea itself eventually emerged from a murky sports background and flittered about in the minds of other surgical educators as the rise of less invasive operations made mastering laparoscopic skills *before* going to the operating room considerably more urgent than learning open skills. No one talked about deliberate practice back then. No one talked about how many hours of practice might be involved in the training of a capable surgeon, a chess player, a musician, or a general surgeon: 10,000 hours for the musicians and chess players, as it turns out. Obviously, this is more than a residency program can provide. But it takes fewer hours to train a competent surgeon, especially when intraoperative training is preceded with skills laboratory instruction. As our understanding of deliberate practice improves with immediate, high-quality feedback given to the learners about their surgical technique during protected skills lab teaching, the time available to residents for mastering a variety of operations is used more effectively.

In fact, a surgeon from the United Kingdom, Hedley Atkins, in his 1965 book *The Surgeon's Craft* wrote, "The manual dexterity of the pianist, the violinist and the juggler are of an altogether different degree of complexity from that required of the surgeon. Thus the executant musician must spend many hours a day 'practicing' in order to maintain the quality of his technique. Surgeons never need to do this."[2] This is a difficult passage to interpret. Was he saying surgery is easy to learn? Or was the implication that surgeons are so uniquely and innately qualified to perform their art that they would not be expected to improve with the benefit of daily practice? To a kinesiologist and coach, this statement carries the faint accent of professional airs.

The mind-set of surgeons from the very outset of modern open surgery in the late 1880s never included the notion of practicing or warming up before a case. From the beginning, surgeons seldom paid attention to other experts. For decades few novel ideas were introduced into the arena of surgical training. All of this changed as laparoscopy found its way into the surgeon's skill set. Suddenly, we were helpless without expert input into our anemic laparoscopic programs.

My skills laboratory project withered because surgeons in our institution and elsewhere believed you learned surgery in the operating room doing surgery. Typical of the surgical personality, they were absolute about it. Trainees learned to operate in the OR on real patients. *Period*. Even though virtually none of these dogmatic surgeons had formal training as educators, the silliness of "See one, do one, teach one" reigned for decades. This absolutism only reversed itself as a few academic surgeons returned to the classroom and became expert educators, a movement that eventually led to the formation of the Association for Surgical Education. That organization, along with the APDS, mentioned at the beginning of the chapter, and the Division of Education of the American College of Surgeons (ACS), led by the country's foremost surgical educator, Dr. Ajit K. Sachdeva, spawned the current explosion of research on how to develop reliable methods of training and assessing surgeons in the modern era. Much of this research focuses on training techniques used in the skills lab, although such issues as how, when, and why to ask questions in the operating room are currently hot surgical education topics.

Surgeons Discover Coaching

Ironically, many surgeons are former athletes.

They grew up learning how to throw a football in practice, for example, not during a game. Many surgeons are accomplished musicians. Clearly, outside the operating room surgeons practiced motor skills—golf swings, tennis, bicycling, piano, violin, and so forth—and no doubt taught their children sports activities and went to their kids' school practices and insisted they take music lessons. And yet a profound disconnect remained in the minds of surgeons between surgical skills teaching and intraoperative performance. There was no thought of teaching surgical skills to trainees *before* their first awkward attempts to sew and dissect on a real patient. This profound historical lack of insight has not, as far as I know, ever been discussed in surgical circles.

As an undergraduate physical-education student, I was taught how to teach motor skills as parts as well as a whole skill. Concepts regarding serial tasks and repetitive tasks also have universal application. We routinely broke down complex movements into smaller skill sets and had learners practice the subset move before combining them into a more complex motor activity. This method of teaching sports skills was often difficult for the really talented student-athletes (I wasn't one of them!). They were so innately skilled that when asked to instruct others, they would often teach moves going from *A* to *B* to *D*, forgetting move *C* because they had performed it in sequence automatically so many times they were unaware of its role in the overall skill.

Similarly, talented surgeons who otherwise had no formal skills training other than their own experience with "See one, do one, teach one" fell short as educators. Having studied theories of skills acquisition, I had been surprised that this knowledge was not used in the early 1970s during my own surgical residency. It seemed illogical to me to think you could learn to play the violin for the first time sitting in the orchestra on opening night—and every major surgical operation is an opening night. Back in the day when I failed to perform a particular surgical skill properly on a patient, the learning experience frequently degraded into an explosion of malignant anger and frustration by the surgeon who completed the case. Of course, I dutifully recorded the case in my log book despite the profound lack of learning during the operative experience. Sadly, there are still many surgeons who believe the real learning goes on only in the operating room.

Fast forward to 2015 and an article entitled "Surgical Coaching for Individual Performance Improvement,"[3] in which the Wisconsin Surgical Coaching Program outlined the basic principles that physical-education majors had been learning for decades. I was delighted to see the promotion of these time-tested ideas: the impact of preperformance rehearsal, self-reflection, and instant feedback on skills acquisition. I would add to these important concepts from my own coaching education the role of mindfulness about *conscious proprioception* (muscle sense or "memory") and *conscious motor control* as they apply to individual performance.[4,5] The Wisconsin group interviewed sports coaches and reviewed many excellent contributions to the field. Only one reference predated the year 2000. (I was among a group of swimming coaches who used the terms *conscious proprioception* and *conscious motor control* as far back as 1963.)

Similarly, another sentinel report in the *New England Journal of Medicine* (*NEJM*)[6] failed to identify the early historical origins of innovators in the field of motor skills learning as compared with the delayed adoption of these concepts by surgical educators. From a perusal of the available reports from the 1960s through the 1990s, it seems about 40 years passed before surgeons became familiar with, talked about, and utilized motor skills theory with some regularity. There appears to be a reluctance to admit the large gap of time between the contributions made 40 years ago by coaches and physical educators and the *NEJM* authors' awareness of this specialty knowledge. These respected surgical educators stated in 2006 in reference to a classic 1967 textbook on motor skills learning that the "three-stage theory of motor skills acquisition is widely accepted in both motor skills literature and the surgical literature."[7] In the surgical literature? This is where a credibility problem arises for me because even today some academic surgeons still avoid pretraining surgical residents in the skills lab.

When I trained as a surgical resident in the early 1970s, no one discussed any theoretical basis for motor skills acquisition. Our surgical literature was silent on the topic. In fact, the only other published reference cited by the authors of the *NEJM* article quoted above (which provided as evidence that Posner and Fitts's 1968 three-stage motor skills learning theory[8] was known to surgical educators) was a 1971 report in an orthopedics journal.[9] Remarkable insight was revealed by a prescient orthopedic educator ahead of his time whose references were all from the basic motor skills and kinesiologic literature of the 1960s. But it would be sliding down a Mount Fuji of truth into a murky forest of implied understanding to suggest that a solitary article published in an orthopedics journal was read by general surgical educators.

Let's face it. Surgical educators came to kinesiology class late.

The paucity of references to the coaching literature of decades past speaks to the catch-up game surgical educators found themselves confronted with as the demands of less invasive operations made a purely apprenticeship model of skills learning obsolete. I certainly never encountered in my own teachers an awareness of kinesiology and coaching theory and practice. No reports were available as far as I can determine. I don't recall grand rounds presentations on coaching, kinesiology, or sports psychology. The truth is that only when we were forced into a corner by the new demands of the laparoscopic revolution with guns to our heads did surgical educators begin to learn from other experts, including sports coaches and human factors scientists, and from several branches of psychology. Until recently, the notion of "See one, do one, teach one," a methodology barren of any foundational educational theory, stood in for the motor skills learning concepts established by and fostered through the activities of jocks.

However, let it also be said that surgical educators not only discovered the principles of coaching and skills teaching but plunged into surgical educational research with energy and insight. Dr. Richard Reznick's critical research on an improved method of teaching and objectively testing technical skills as early as 1993 marked the beginning of true assessment of surgical skills.[10] What has emerged since then is a strong body of knowledge from Resnick's University of Toronto and other research groups that has transformed surgical training into an outcomes-based endeavor. And although the final methodology has yet to find its form, surgical education is currently on sound scientific footing as a consequence of the strong leadership provided by the Association for Surgical Education, the Association of Program Directors in Surgery, and the American College of Surgeons Division of Education.

I'll reflect on four representative reports from 2012 and 2015 as examples of how surgical educators have jumped on the coaching bandwagon with enthusiasm. An editorial in the *American Journal of Surgery* in 2012 discussed "lessons learned from sport," concluding, "Sports is another human endeavor in which a long learning period of skill acquisition leads its practitioner to the point in which putting such skills into practice is expected with the highest possible level of expertise."[11] An exquisite description of surgical residency! Similarly, in the same year Dr. Mark L. Friedell in a presidential address discussed such great basketball coaches as John Wooden, Mike Krzyzewski, Pat Summitt, and Bobby Knight and the way they handled teaching and guiding their players. Wooden, as an example directly applicable to residency training, taught the four Ps: planning, preparation, practice, performance.[12] Friedell noted, "All the coaches stressed the importance of direct, honest, timely feedback to the players so that they could reach their full potential both on the court and later in life. They did not walk away from difficult performance conversations."[13] His presentation was entitled "The Carrot and the Stick," referring to a philosophy of kind encouragement versus hard-nosed, in-your-face criticism. Fortunately, we have sailed from the rocky shores lined with surgeons banishing heavy clubs to beaches with educators holding up encouraging signs. However, I will admit a few more sticks today might redirect some of our millennials more quickly.

Two studies published in 2015 revealed the difficulty involved in learning how to coach. One determined that faculty overrated their coaching skills in nontechnical areas such as communication.[14] The other report proved the value of video-based coaching on laparoscopic skills.[15] Just as feedback is an important component of coaching, a study demonstrated that video-based peer feedback through social networking using a robotic simulation improved performance as well.[16]

Another Good Idea

Reviewing my notes (written in the 1980s) describing how I planned to set up a more complete skills lab, I marvel at how close I had come to engaging in a process that would eventually transform surgical education over two decades later. I noted Kopta's 1971 report in the orthopedic journal on the development of motor skills because it was alone in the surgical world, as far as I could determine, in acknowledging the field. But I missed the opportunity. Perhaps this was because I somehow thought (or had become convinced) that the motor skills learning theory I had been exposed to as an undergraduate didn't apply to the remarkable surgeons from whom I would learn my craft. I admit I was intimidated into "doing in Rome" what the rest of the residents in our program were doing.

Although my surgical skills lab project lapsed, another idea handed to me by Dr. Friedmann caught my imagination. And although I didn't see it coming at the time, these two ideas—the creation of skills labs for surgical training and the introduction of the laparoscope into clinical practice—would coalesce and transform our profession of general surgery. I wish I could tell you I saw it coming, but I didn't. And as far as I can tell, no one else glimpsed the revolution brewing over the horizon.

Looking back, I feel privileged to have acquired a background in coaching, despite being embarrassed to reveal my anemic academic beginnings ("Really, you were a jock?"), as well as to have been introduced to *diagnostic* laparoscopy. A professional stage had been set for me by well-meaning people who could not have foreseen their impact on me and on other surgeons. I didn't appreciate my good fortune; I didn't see the future of it. Yet these two vectors—a background in coaching and early exposure to diagnostic laparoscopy—would foster my career and contribute to my minor role in our local history of laparoscopy.

And so it was that about the time when my skills lab idea got torpedoed that Dr. Friedmann introduced me to a novel piece of diagnostic equipment. He handed me a five-millimeter needle scope with a tiny eyepiece and a skinny body smaller than a drinking straw. He explained that the laparoscope was being used in some surgical practices to assess the inside of the abdominal cavity without making a huge, painful incision (to avoid a so-called exploratory operation). Staging cancer and identifying blunt abdominal trauma injuries were two uses of the laparoscope. We toyed with the laparoscope one afternoon and surveyed the interior of an abdomen. Later, Dr. Friedmann encouraged me to take a course in diagnostic laparoscopy.

What I Didn't Know about the Coming Revolution

A lot of general surgeons I've talked to agree that almost none of us saw the potential of laparoscopy's role in our practices, not even those of us playing around with diagnostic laparoscopy. At the time (the early 1980s), there wasn't a hint of anyone actually *operating* through such a scope. Well, not general surgeons at any rate. A 1991 report concluded in this regard that "no technologic advance in recent memory has engendered the amount of widespread interest and debate as has laparoscopic cholecystectomy. Since its introduction less than 2 years ago, numerous postgraduate courses, some excellent but some hurriedly and incompletely organized, have been offered and quickly filled."[17]

As it turned out, the gynecologists whom we had derided for struggling with their laparoscopes in darkened operating rooms were light-years ahead of us. For example, Dr. Max Borten wrote a textbook, *Laparoscopic Complications: Prevention and Management*, published in 1986 at about the time when a few of us (general surgeons) around the country were attempting diagnostic laparoscopy.[18] Unaccustomed to reading gynecology texts when I began doing diagnostic laparoscopy, I never sought out the extensive information in Borten's book, which included a vast chapter on diagnostic laparoscopy for gynecologic disorders. I suspect that most other general surgeons beginning to perform diagnostic laparoscopy at the time were not aware of the book either. The 1991 report mentioned above agreed, stating, "Diagnostic laparoscopy is unfamiliar to most general surgeons who until now had found little use for it in their practices."[19]

In the 1980s, I knew almost nothing about the skinny laparoscope I was poking into the abdominal cavity. I knew nothing about a gynecologist named Kurt Semm. Having developed the field of modern pelviscopy (gynecologic laparoscopy), Semm had already performed the world's first laparoscopic appendectomy in 1980 in Germany. I did not know he would suffer the derision of academic surgeons everywhere rather than receive the accolades he so richly deserved.

I did not know that Kurt Semm would personally influence a German surgeon named Erich Muhe, modern general surgery's forgotten (laparoscopic) hero.[20] I didn't know, as I fumbled with the five-millimeter laparoscope diagnosing cirrhosis of the liver and other intra-abdominal conditions, that Muhe had launched a revolution, becoming the first surgeon to perform the original laparoscopic gallbladder removal in the world. I did not appreciate that I had the privilege of participating in a very small way at our medical center in the beginning of a surgical revolution.

Nonetheless, I became the only surgeon at Baystate to poke the needle laparoscope through tiny stab incisions in order to access selected patients' abdominal cavity for clues to their diagnosis. At first, there were no TV screens, no video cameras. I simply leaned over the patient's (sterile) draped belly and squinted into the tiny eyepiece. Searching for life in the inner space of the abdominal galaxy, I cautiously slid the scope in and out in order to survey strange anatomy. I'd never seen the liver or small intestine or colon from the laparoscopic perspective. I didn't know that, at about the same time in 1987, a French surgeon with considerably more advanced laparoscopic skills than mine was also awkwardly draping himself over his patient's body, peering into a thin scope while removing her gallbladder. The conceptual journey for me (and for any general surgeon who thought about it) from making a laparoscopic diagnosis to removing a gallbladder through the same instrument was immeasurable.

Although the popularity of laparoscopic removal of the gallbladder was driven by patients, the industry quickly jumped on board. Instrument manufacturers saw gold in the yet undeveloped world of laparoscopic equipment that would proliferate and revolutionize the future of surgery. It is one significant reason that health care costs continue to soar into the stratosphere today. Laparoscopy was indeed a disruptive technology. It changed everything we thought about and did in the operating room. And this was exceptionally valuable.

Commercial surgical-instrument vendors invaded operating rooms to assist general surgeons in the early 1990s, even though by then our gynecologic colleagues had made pelvic laparoscopy or pelviscopy a safe, daily event. Surgeons, who for their entire careers had run the OR with an iron hand while clutching the scalpel, were now compelled to ask nonphysician equipment sales reps for assistance. Similarly, it wasn't long before the atmosphere at national surgical meetings changed dramatically. Huge halls reserved for vendors echoed like subterranean caves; vast wastelands of floor space became chopped up into sections strewn with commercial booths. Row upon row of sales personnel hawked chopstick-like instruments with "pistol-grip" handles and video systems with ever-improving optics. Surgeons were beginning to sense the inevitability of the public's acceptance of less invasive operations. In no time their enthusiasm for less invasive operations flourished, and virtually every area of surgery fell to the innovative attempts of general surgeons.

But the public remained ignorant of the flimsy underpinnings of the stage on which the laparoscopic revolution was being played out. Many patients did well and benefited from less invasive operations. As advanced procedures were developed in academic centers, more control was exercised over training for these complex operations. The quality of surgical care improved. But in some hospitals the implementation of less invasive operations did not always go well. Behind drawn hospital curtains in the early 1990s lay injured and dead patients. Victims of avarice and greed, these patients were not brought to the public's attention. But our profession was becoming aware of a significant increase in the numbers of such complications as bile duct injuries.

Granting Privileges: Who Should Do the Laparoscopic Gallbladder Operation?

The issue of granting privileges at hospitals was addressed in 1991 by Dr. Thomas L. Dent, who outlined an acceptable approach to credentialing:

> Adequate training for surgeons already experienced in abdominal and biliary tract surgery can be acquired through a preceptorship in diagnostic

laparoscopy, attending a course in laparoscopic surgery that includes both didactic instruction and live animal experience, assisting with the procedure in humans, and being proctored and certified as competent by an experienced general surgeon. . . . Since laparoscopic surgical procedures involve techniques that are unfamiliar to most general surgeons, surgical leaders have a responsibility to determine what constitutes adequate training for their safe performance and to recommend the criteria necessary for the granting of hospital privileges in laparoscopic surgery.[21]

The notion of difficult learning curves and other special training challenges of the less invasive surgical operations took on a life of its own. Specialty surgical organizations were born. For example, the Society of American Gastrointestinal and Endoscopic Surgeons (SAGES) is a nonprofit professional organization that had its first independent meeting in 1986. The society has grown into the premier organization for minimally invasive surgeons throughout the world. SAGES's mission statement reads, "To provide leadership in surgery, particularly gastrointestinal and endoscopic surgery, to optimize patient care through education, research and innovation."[22] In addition to its newsletter *SCOPE*, SAGES provides guidelines on all aspects of laparoscopic, robotic, and endoscopic surgery. Since the mid-1980s, new journals dedicated to surgical endoscopy have proliferated. And an incendiary explosion of new knowledge disrupted the well-being of established surgeons and trainees alike. In 1990, SAGES established guidelines for the training and credentialing of general surgeons in laparoscopy.[23] Thus, according to Grzegorz Litynski, SAGES accomplished three important steps:

- SAGES acknowledged that laparoscopy was more than just a fashion or a fad.
- SAGES guidelines were the first published and served as a model for many hospitals in the United States.
- SAGES gave laparoscopy its stamp of approval.[24]

It has been said that an optimal professional development format—a standardized protocol for teaching and introducing new operations into practice—has *still* not been established for surgeons. Perhaps the following historical comment will shed light on the chronic nature of the problem of assuring surgical capability. In his 1935 presidential address to the ACS, Dr. Edward Archibald said, "Fellowship in the American College of Surgeons did not assure sufficient mastery of both the art and science of surgery."[25] Today fellowship in the ACS remains a helpful and necessary step in the process of assuring basic technical, knowledge-based, and ethical competence. But competence in *all* domains of general surgery is not a certainty; it's virtually impossible to obtain by any single practitioner in the 21st century.

Surgeons have always known that their various certificates cannot hide an irreducible level of incompetence. The word carries a sting, an indictment bordering on moral lapse. *Incompetence.* We avoid the idea. We are repelled by it. We deny it in the face of overwhelming evidence, as we did at the beginning of our dance with laparoscopic cholecystectomy. And yet ineptitude wallows in the shallow waters of early adoption of complex new surgical operations.

One of the key issues for a hospital board in determining whether separate privileges are needed by practitioners is whether the new procedure is sufficiently different to require additional training. Dr. Dent summarized the main issues chiefs of clinical services or credentialing committees should consider in deciding whether granting new privileges is necessary:

- Advise the board if they feel separate privileges are required.
- Consider separate privileges for risky, controversial, or high-visibility procedures.
- Create a statement of criteria for granting such privileges.
- Define minimum amounts and types of additional training required.
- Determine whether proctoring (assistance in the OR from an expert) is required.
- Determine the specific methods of assessing the surgeon's capability.
- Acquire, as appropriate, specialty society statements of criteria, and so forth.
- Review documents for bias favoring a particular specialty.[26]

Early Missteps Introducing Laparoscopic Gallbladder Removal

Early in the 1990s a few professors of surgery (including urology and thoracic surgery) worked on pigs to learn how to use the laparoscope. Caution was called for by academic surgeons. In 1989, internationally respected laparoscopic leader Dr. Alfred Cuschieri stated in an article anticipating the introduction of laparoscopic cholecystectomy in the United Kingdom entitled "The Laparoscopic Revolution—Walk Carefully before We Run," "There is a genuine concern that this procedure will be taken up by surgeons without proper training in laparoscopy and laparoscopic surgical techniques."[27] However, as mentioned before, both in the United Kingdom and especially in the United States, many general surgeons plowed ahead and introduced laparoscopic gallbladder removal into their practices with little training and less than optimal help from experienced laparoscopic colleagues. Many hospitals established their own methods of granting privileges and of certifying surgeons in laparoscopic cholecystectomy. Dr. Cuschieri, in a moment of clarity, added, "There is currently an explosion of laparoscopic cholecystectomy in North America where surgeons have established hasty cooperative teams with gynecologists to perform this operation and some using NdYAG lasers to dissect the gallbladder from the liver bed—a notably unnecessary step but a money spinner to the technologically minded patient hoodwinked by the term 'laser cholecystectomy.' "[28] It was Eddie Joe Reddick who, because of his experience with the laser performing hemorrhoidectomies, had pushed for the use of the laser energy source for laparoscopic gallbladder removal. The method quickly fell out of use.

Nonetheless, "money spinning" was an integral part of the introduction of general surgery laparoscopy. Immediately, less invasive operations and the subsequent demand for novel instruments became snarled in capitalism's web. Dr. Cuschieri also pleaded for prospective randomized control trials of the new operation. They never occurred.

In our institution, three board-certified surgeons scrubbed on each laparoscopic cholecystectomy—regardless of who represented the surgeon of record. We thus rotated who did the operation, who held the camera, and who assisted with gallbladder retraction and other helpful maneuvers. After ten cases, we went to two surgeons—the operator and the camera holder-assistant. Then, after 10 more cases, we let the surgical residents assist us.

There was no established way of accounting for the early results of the new laparoscopic operation. Complications were occurring. A report stated, "Rumors of a steep learning curve, common bile duct injuries, massive hemorrhage, and even deaths following laparoscopic surgery are rife."[29] Some reached public recognition. As an example, in a 1992 letter in the *Washington Post*, a patient described her unfortunate postoperative ordeal when her surgeon had cut her common bile duct and failed to recognize his mistake.[30] Thus, the issue in the early 1990s was (and remains today) just how effective short courses are in training surgeons in the use of complex technology. So remember my repeated cautionary remarks; robotic surgery presents the same basic challenges today that the introduction of the laparoscope offered in 1990.

Does operating on a few pigs over a weekend constitute training that produces clinical competency? By contemporary standards, this was entirely inadequate training. The surgical leadership knew it but could do little to reign in the public's demands for less invasive operations, not with the snowballing effect of practicing surgeons' commercial interests in minimally invasive operations, and not with the rising financial interests and investments of hospitals.

Thus, by 2000 a consideration of the ethical dimensions of learning and teaching surgery became the elephant in the room. We could no longer skirt the reality that laparoscopic operations were here to stay in our field of general surgery. In those lingering days of the first decade of the laparoscopic revolution, we confronted the need to place the patient's welfare first and foremost and above surgeon self-interest and practice building. We had to be truthful about our results, to foster public trust and document our results. The essence of our task as educators was articulated in 2000 by ophthalmologists Charles Zacks and John Hoepner, who declared, "As with other technical knowledge, it is reasonable to assume that achieving competence in surgery is not instantaneous but incremental and that inexperience confers additional risks to patients that are expected to diminish with greater experience."[31] That was key. While the revolution occurred spasmodically all in a rush, individual surgeon capability required slow, progressive baby steps of skills acquisition.

An odd thing happened at the beginning of the struggle to learn laparoscopic cholecystectomy. It initially involved a denial of a role in our practices for less invasive operations and therefore a blind spot for what constitutes a capable modern general surgeon. At the time, for example, a dismissive posture about the value of less invasive operations was taken by Professor Alan Johnson of the University of Sheffield in the United Kingdom. In 1997 he insisted that "laparoscopic surgery has been a fascinating technical development for surgeons, but in terms of patient outcomes and overall management of abdominal disease it has been a very small advance, after a huge financial investment."[32]

A Very Small Advance?

Or was the introduction of laparoscopy into general surgery in fact transformative? Surgeons still argue about whether the dramatic adoption of less invasive laparoscopic operations was an evolution or a true revolution. Most agree that the early history of endoscopy (gastroscopy, colonoscopy, cystoscopy, etc.) was cautious and pedestrian in character as compared with the explosive introduction of laparoscopic cholecystectomy into the field of general surgery. Just as Kurt Semm's work in the 1970s and 1980s fired off a laparoscopic revolution in gynecology, the new laparoscopic gallbladder operation first performed in the United States in 1988 transformed general surgery on an even larger stage in the United States and around the world.

So, the information we had available about laparoscopic surgery in the early 1990s was inconsistent. First, a 1992 National Institutes of Health report stated that laparoscopic gallbladder removal is a safe operation requiring little formal training.[33] Belatedly, the increased numbers of catastrophic common bile duct injuries resulting from poor laparoscopic training were revealed to the public. Then, from across the pond in the United Kingdom, the message came that the benefits of laparoscopy for patients are trivial, that minimally invasive surgery is a small advance. Yet within a few years of the index laparoscopic gallbladder operation in Germany, academic surgeons and private practitioners begin to devise even more complex laparoscopic operations.

This bipolar posturing—laparoscopic surgery is very safe, but on the other hand a very small advance—only makes sense when you understand that we were all incision-bound practitioners with rigid surgical personalities. We were incapable of appreciating the new technology emerging before our eyes. And as history has taught us, this very small advance turned out to be the greatest technical accomplishment in the history of modern medicine, ranking, as mentioned, easily with the discovery of anesthesia and the discovery of sterile surgical technique (asepsis). The magnitude of this misreading of the revolutionary advances in less invasive surgical technology highlights the many miscues that hide in the shadows of the early history of laparoscopic surgery.

A larger philosophical (as well as practical) question no one asked at the time soon blossomed: Would the public have subjected themselves to laparoscopic cholecystectomy if they had known of the increased risks of complications because of the minimal levels of surgeon training in those early years? If the patient-safety programs of today had been in place in 1990, would the uncontrolled spread of the less invasive gallbladder operation have occurred at all? Or would it have been shut down?

Once again, gynecologists were miles ahead of us. Kurt Semm in his 1987 book, *Operative Manual for Endoscopic Abdominal Surgery*, described the use of a pelviscopy trainer outside the operating room.[34] In a laboratory setting in the hospital far from patients, this "box" device allowed novice surgeons to practice intricate maneuvers that made up crucial steps in a laparoscopic operation. They could repeat the maneuvers over and over using plastic models or dead tissue, such as a chicken breast. And there was no risk to the patient. Kurt Semm had set the table for a future of virtual reality trainers, box trainers, and other high- and low-fidelity laboratory learning devices, including robotic trainers. As the public's awareness of safety violations grew, so did the surgical profession's commitment to improved technical education.

The Origins of a True Patient-Safety Initiative

Patient safety was nudged onto the national scene in the 1980s and early 1990s at the same time that the laparoscopic revolution hit its stride. The number of patients who were injured or who died during hospitalization whether following major surgery or during complicated medical treatment was alarming, according to major studies that focused on patient safety. What I find remarkable in researching these two evolving movements is the parallel compilation of scientific studies (a) on poor hospital performance in general regarding patient-safety measures published during the same years as (b) the early warnings challenging the safety of minimally invasive surgery. It seems that no significant connection between the two issues was ever clearly established. And while many features of hospitalization were identified as being dangerous for inpatients, early on laparoscopic surgery was not specifically pinpointed as a factor causing surgical complications.

Dr. Lucien Leape, among many others, led the safety-awareness charge. He wrote in 1994: "When patients enter a hospital, they reasonably assume that their treatments will make them better, or, at least, not make them worse. But modern hospital medical care is complex, involving many human interactions between patients and nurses, doctors, pharmacists, technicians, and others. Each encounter, indeed, each treatment or diagnostic maneuver, presents an opportunity for error. And errors inevitably occur."[35] Prior to making that statement, Dr. Leape and his colleagues (in the 1991 Harvard Medical Practice Study of patients hospitalized in 1984 in New York State hospitals) described an adverse event (AE) as "an unintended injury caused by treatment that resulted in prolongation of hospital stay or measurable disability at the time of discharge."[36] The study revealed that

- almost 4 percent of all hospitalized patients suffered an AE.
- 7 percent of disabilities from an AE were prolonged or permanent, and 14 percent of patients died of their injuries.
- more than 70 percent of AEs were preventable.
- 20 percent of AEs were judged to be due to negligence.
- 87 percent of technical complications during surgery were preventable.[37]

That was data from the 1980s *before* surgeons began attempting to learn the strange and awkward new laparoscopic gallbladder operation. It was at about this time that medical errors became national news. Simultaneously, a laundry list of new, minimally invasive laparoscopic operations was released to a public who remained unaware of the questionable credentialing practices of many hospitals.

Have we improved our safety record since 1984?

In fact, the estimated annual in-hospital death rate, which had stunned health care professionals in 1984 (44,000 to 98,000 deaths per year),[38] was estimated to exceed 400,000 in 2012.[39] Few of these deaths today are related to laparoscopic surgery. Yet many risks to hospitalized patients clearly persist, and surgical patients must be diligent in finding a capable surgeon who works in a reliable hospital. For example, a 2010 report on 10 North Carolina hospitals confirmed that there was little evidence of patient-care improvements that would reduce harm to patients.[40] The authors conclude, "Our findings validate concern raised by patient-safety experts in the United States and Europe that harm resulting from medical care remains very common . . . the penetration of evidence-based safety practices has been quite modest."[41] Modest improvements in patient safety can partly be related to health care workers' attitudes about safety.

In her book *Human Error in Medicine*, editor Marilyn Sue Bogner stated succinctly, "Human error is a fact of life. . . . For those providing medical care, the consequences of an error may be serious injury or death for the very individuals they intend to help."[42] Bogner nailed the essence of every surgeon's daily concern: Will I hurt someone today? Will I cause a serious complication? Will I make my patient better or worse? In the same volume edited by Bogner, Joshua A. Perper lists many of the adverse characteristics of some health care providers involved in treatment misadventures in which mistakes are made. These behaviors and attributes seem particularly bothersome if they are witnessed in surgeons (see Chapter 10):

- Inexperience or ignorance (shorter training hours)
- A reckless practitioner or a risk taker (arrogance)
- Absentmindedness
- Deafness to communication or argument (self-satisfied about skills and knowledge)
- Impatient (or distracted)
- Incompetent slowpoke (too old with age-related skills deterioration, poorly trained)
- Procrastinator (indecisive under stress)
- Fatigued (30–40 percent of surgeons are burned out)
- Substance abuser
- Reluctant to seek advice (self-centered, overconfident)[43]

Scattered reports published at about the same time regarding some of the worst results of laparoscopic gallbladder removal included Dr. Lawrence K. Altman's 1992 article in the *New York Times*. He wrote: "Alarmed about rising numbers of deaths and serious injuries from a new method of gallbladder surgery, in which surgeons use miniature video cameras and instruments inserted through tiny incisions, the New York State Health Department has demanded tighter regulations. . . . New York's action is forcing doctors and health officials elsewhere to begin to deal with a fundamental issue they have long failed to address: the learning curve."[44]

Learning curves will always define capability. We will never be able to avoid the need to learn new technology and difficult surgical techniques. The quicksand of innate talent will torture us with its lack of specificity and its enticement to train harder. Or, for the self-certain surgeon comfortable with his or her skills, the uncertainty of innate ability must be dealt with, not swept under a rug of hopeful professional pieties.

In the past it was not unusual for surgical trainees to work 110 or more hours per week. We learned the traditional open operations by repetition. We did lots of them. And we chuckled at the darkened rooms where gynecologists poked telescopes into their patients and dug around in the pelvis like pigs after acorns. As this was occurring, medical specialists were eyeing our specialty of general surgery and quietly planning an assault on our sacred halls.

At first, we missed the signals spelling our demise.

PART 2

Radical Surgery Reigns: The Calm before the Storm

CHAPTER FOUR

The Capable Surgeon: Surgical Competence and the Patient-Safety Movement

While it should be the goal of the training program to finish the chief resident, who is able to practice independently, it is highly unlikely that a trainee will reach the "expert" level by the end of the residency or fellowship training.

Joel T. Allison, Ronald C. Jones, and George H. Terrazzos, *Archives of Surgery*, 2005

The current health care system falls terribly short in its ability to ensure that new technology is introduced safely and effectively and to translate the evidence generated by research into practice.

T. R. Russell, MD, executive director, American College of Surgeons, 2003

Surgical Competence—The Challenge

What every patient wants is an expert surgeon. You want a master practitioner with the knowledge, skills, and appropriate attitude of a qualified member of his or her particular specialty. You want the best in the field.

Fortunately, almost every large and small community in the United States has a lot of surgical talent. Surgical patients in smaller towns will be faced with a lack of choice because of geography; many rural areas of the United States don't have any general surgeons. Some patients are restricted because of insurance issues. And the shortage of surgeons may force general surgeons to attempt more complex operations with which they may not have adequate experience.

Still, a smoldering question quietly tugs at the heartstrings of all surgical patients: *On any given day will my surgeon be at the top of her game?*

Obviously, along with many other factors at the core of this query is the issue of the *technical capability* of the surgeon. But should patients view a surgeon's capability as primarily technical in nature? Or is it safer to recognize other elements of true competence?

Roughly 10 million general surgery cases are performed in the United States every year at a cost of about one billion dollars. Roughly 13 percent of these patients develop complications, and 2 percent die as a consequence of their operation. Two thirds of the complications occur during surgery, and 65 percent of them are technical errors.[1] These numbers reflect all risk factors, especially such comorbid or patient health–related issues as diabetes, high blood pressure, and kidney disease. Certainly, some of these patients are deathly sick. And there are other aspects of surgical outcomes, such as hospital personnel, surgical equipment, anesthetic capabilities, and staffing patterns (e.g., ratio of nurses to patients), to mention a few.

But some surgeons are not well trained in certain operative procedures. For example, a recent study of 20 bariatric (weight loss) surgeons used a peer-review process. This means that at least 10 other similar surgeons (their peers) reviewed a representative video of the surgeon doing a laparoscopic gastric bypass operation on a patient. Involving over 10,000 patients, the research showed that the bottom quartile of surgeons (with poorer surgical skills as compared with the top quartile) was associated with higher complication rates, longer operative times, and higher reoperation and readmission rates.[2] It is well known from this and other studies that outcomes for complex surgical operations vary across hospitals as well as among individual surgeons.

By comparison with the training of general surgeons, it takes 10,000 hours of deliberate practice for a professional musician, chess master, or athlete to reach an expert level of performance, as previously mentioned.[3] Yet surgeons in training spend fewer than 3,000 hours actually learning in the operating room or skills lab. This represents about 6 percent of their total training time when they are directly engaged in learning technical skills.[4] This data aligns with my primary theme with regard to technical training and the overall capability of trainees and practicing surgeons in the modern era: no single surgeon can master the entire modern field of general surgery. Again, although surgical educators don't need 10,000 hours to train a surgical resident in the basics of common operations, additional time is now required to bring trainees closer to full capability in performing *both* open and minimally invasive procedures. And a definition of competence is as elusive as is the task of determining the appropriate length of surgical training.

Surgical Capability—Attempts at Definition

Tension cinched the consciences of our national surgical leaders as the revolutionary changes brought about by the introduction of less invasive operations disrupted our broad-based general surgery specialty. Moral as well as practical questions dribbled out of the uncertain souls of practitioners and national leaders alike. Who should be doing this particular laparoscopic operation? How should surgeons be trained? How can we assure that this surgeon really knows how to perform this particular operation? And a query not asked often enough: How can we explain our varying levels of competence to our patients?

In this regard, discussions about a surgeon's capability often devolve into a patient insisting, "I don't care about her bedside manner. I just want the best technical surgeon available." Of course, this attitude ignores many of the skills a surgeon must possess beyond eye-hand coordination and visual-spatial capability. What patients who focus solely on a surgeon's skills ignore is the potential for confusion and miscommunication during preoperative informed-consent discussions and postoperative follow-up, especially if the outcome is less than perfect.

Most medical litigation arises from unmet expectations. So, if you have an operation by the best in the field and it turns sour and a major complication occurs, you will find yourself stewing in the acid broth of unfulfilled expectations. If your surgeon is not particularly compassionate, not particularly articulate, or indifferent—or, heaven forbid, a malignant narcissist—you may wish you had engaged a truly compleat surgeon.

Thus, among other qualifications a capable surgeon must have are well-honed communication skills. In the past, as anyone who has ever tried to talk at length with a surgeon will attest, surgeons did precious little explaining. Surgeons felt they had the authority to decide rather than to explain to their patients their operative choices. Informed consent was often skimpy, paternalism rampant. We now know that there is a proven relationship between nontechnical skills (communication, empathy, situational awareness, etc.) and the masterful technical completion of an operation. Who the surgeon is (regarding the surgical personality, see Chapter Ten) is inseparable from how he or she performs the actual operation.[5] Or, as stated in a report on "a performance-based conception of capability," "Competence reflects situational relationships among doctors, their patients, and the systems in which they perform and, thus, is only partly dependent on the attributes of individual actors."[6] Hence, in the modern era there is an emphasis on teamwork in all aspects of hospital care. Back in the day, as studies have shown, surgeons often worked in what was traditionally a self-induced vacuum.[7] Today, surgeons share their expertise, doubts, and quandaries with each other both formally during conferences and one-on-one through various venues. Although this communication isn't entirely new, it is more open and honest than in the past. Refined communication skills, then, are one of the most important components of a surgeon's capability.

Among the many other influences that have repercussions on what makes up a capable practitioner and safe practice environment are innate talent, the amount and quality of training, board certification, actual experience in practice, surgical personality, local and national medical politics, hospital credentialing, professional oversight, third-party oversight, and some uncontrollable aspects of the current practice environment. Also, there are potential risks when dealing with surgeons of less than desired competence because they are at one or the other end of the age spectrum. Younger surgeons may be expert with many minimally invasive operations but may lack experience with both complex laparoscopic and open procedures.[8] Older surgeons may not have the stamina to do long, complex operations but may be better than their younger counterparts with other operations.[9]

Arguably, the most compelling query about a surgeon's competence is *What do the surgeon's credentials have to do with his or her actual capability?*

What Does "Board-Certified Surgeon" Mean?

The imprecise meaning of board certification must be addressed because the idea of certification, although important, is not an absolute guarantee of practitioner competence. This, no doubt, will cause you considerable discomfort. One might reasonably expect board certification to mean that the certified surgeon is technically capable of performing a broad spectrum of operations and is ethically grounded. For the most part this is absolutely true. Board-certified surgeons have undergone a rigorous process of training and evaluation. Make no mistake as I discuss the difficulties with board certification: the process is vital to your safety.

What is particularly remarkable is that the relationship between certification by the American Board of Surgery (ABS) and actual practitioner competence has a long and complicated history. The problem of the meaning of board certification shines a spotlight on the bobbing head of a central reality about modern surgical practice: your surgeon may be really good overall (e.g., board certified) but may lack experience and training with the specific operation you need. This is not a blanket criticism of surgeons or their training. My position is that we are dealing with evolving new surgical techniques, complex technology, and an uncontrolled and ever-expanding knowledge overload. What is odd about regulatory efforts to protect you, the surgical patient, is that in some instances they are less than stringent.

For example, do all health plans require that their doctors be board certified? Are surgeons listed on various health care plans from which you must choose equal in skill and knowledge? One study revealed that 60 percent of the health plans surveyed did *not* require surgical specialists, general surgeons, or nonsurgeon subspecialists to be board certified to contract with the plan. And the study also noted that half of the plans made exceptions to their board-certification policies depending on the geography or network needs.[10] Does this mean that depending on where in the country you seek surgical care many plans hire surgeons with unproven qualifications? It may. An unsolved predicament for rural areas is the need for general surgeons who are willing to live in smaller communities while being pressured to refer complex cases to regional centers of excellence. A long trail of recrimination leads back and forth between rural and academic surgeons regarding volume (of cases performed) for technical competence. The reality is that many rural surgeons are technically better than many of their urban medical-center counterparts in performing a wide variety of procedures.

The same researchers mentioned above also studied the role of board certification and recertification as it applies to hospital privileging. They concluded, "Most hospitals do not consistently use board-certification to ensure physician competence at their institutions."[11] From my perspective this observation speaks volumes about the documented surgeon shortage around the United States. Presumably, in the minds of hospital administrators, an uncertified surgeon is better than no surgeon. These reports confirm the importance of having potential surgical patients ask their surgeon about his or her board-certification status and *experience with a particular operation.*

In addition to the issue of what it means to be board certified, the argument that general surgeons can offer the traditional wide range of operations performed both openly and laparoscopically (with the consistent skill levels and outcomes the public expects) is inconsistent with the data available. The truth is that this uneven distribution of skill involves both surgeons in practice as well as surgeons in training.[12,13,14] As you will discover, the training and evaluation of general surgeons remains an enduring headache for surgical educators working in the trenches, as well as for our national surgical leadership. Nonetheless, an enormous amount of energy and research continues to be dedicated to the task of assuring competence in all surgical practitioners.

A Brief History of Attempts to Define and Measure Surgical Capability

At the beginning of the last century, the American College of Surgeons (ACS) came into existence in 1913 (vigorously opposed by the powerful American Medical Association [AMA]), followed by the establishment of the American Board of Surgery (ABS) in 1937. The results of very early attempts to document the results of surgical operations were marginal, if not deplorable. Mostly, these initial records of outcomes—whether or not the patient survived, died, or developed major complications—were ignored. As Dr. Loyal Davis wrote in *Fellowship of Surgeons: A History of the American College of Surgeons*, "The question of the education of the public about the training of surgeons, the nature of operations and the results which might be accomplished was revolutionary."[15] In the second decade of the 20th century, the AMA attacked the idea of educating the public as well as the suggested methods of doing so. Loyal continued, referring to the opinion of the leadership of the AMA, "'Treat the patient and tell them nothing' was their motto."[16]

In fact, within the body of his introduction to the classic 1910 Flexner report on the deplorable condition of American medical schools, Dr. Henry S. Pritchett, then president of the Carnegie Foundation, wrote, "One of the problems of the future is to educate the public itself to appreciate the fact that very seldom, under existing conditions, does a patient receive the best aid which it is possible to give him in the present state of medicine, and that this is due mainly to the fact that a vast army of men is admitted to the profession and quite without a sufficient experience with disease."[17] As with the surgical profession's refusal to publicly apologize for the sloppy introduction of laparoscopic cholecystectomy, the AMA has never acknowledged its original philosophy: to keep the public in the dark about medical outcomes.

When Ernest A. Codman took on the medical establishment in 1915 and recommended that surgeons keep track of their results, he unleashed on himself a tumult of ridicule and criticism. At the Clinical Congress of the Surgeons of North America (a precursor of the ACS) in 1912, the first committee on hospital care standardization was formed. It served as the precursor of virtually all the current regulatory organizations. The ACS forced the hand of all specialty organizations and has been the most influential of these governing bodies to document surgical results.

Doctors Edward Passaro and Claude H. Organ described the original results of that committee in a 1999 article entitled "Ernest A. Codman: The Improper Bostonian," published in the *Bulletin of the American College of Surgeons*: "It quickly became apparent that the records varied widely both in content and quality from hospital to hospital. Ascertaining what operations an applicant had done was arduous. Most hospital records were useless."[18] Recognizing Codman's outstanding contributions to measuring surgical results long before it became fashionable, Passaro and Organ also wrote about Codman's impact on patient safety: "Increasingly, the evaluation of surgery is based on Codman's end results approach, relying on patient's assessments in contrast to that of the surgeon. Every hospital now engages in quality improvement activities and many select or promote surgeons on the basis of end results."[19] It was Codman's persistence that produced the beginning of true oversight of surgical outcomes and has blossomed into today's emphasis on patient-centered care.

Surgical Capability at the Beginning of the Laparoscopic Revolution

In 1996, in a presidential address to the Society for Surgery of the Alimentary Tract titled "General Surgery in Evolution: Technology and Competence," Dr. Lawrence Way reviewed the results of a survey of 80 surgeons who were asked to predict the future of general surgery. Relative to my primary concern regarding a modern surgeon's capability, Way wrote, "The inability of General Surgery to reconcile a publically expressed broad definition of itself with the development of full-fledged competence throughout its breath was of paramount concern."[20] Here, halfway through the decade that witnessed the introduction of laparoscopic surgery, surgeons clearly felt uncomfortable selling themselves as generalists capable of doing all the operations now collected under the umbrella of general surgery. That was *before* the flood of complex laparoscopic operations that was introduced to the public! Dr. Way also identified the failure of leadership, the failure to "fend off attacks" on general surgery's domain, and failures to ensure that surgical residents were sufficiently trained.[21] Clearly, from this and other similar reports we can conclude that the issue of questioning individual surgeons' capability arose long before the beginning of the 21st century. Now, as in the past, we are struggling with our variable levels of practitioner competence under a dark cloud of public silence.

Dr. Way summarized the impression at the time regarding the impact of new technology, stating, "In retrospect, we now realize that decreased invasiveness stemming from the application of new devices has been a dominant theme affecting the care of our patients throughout these last two decades."[22] Thus, acknowledging the sensational rise of laparoscopic surgery, he pinpointed the plights facing general surgery in 1996:

- Criticism of a profession centers on the difference between the *actual performance of a practitioner* and the *ideological claims of the profession* or reasonable expectations of the public.
- The cardinal ethic of medicine is competence, defined as the possession and use of the requisite knowledge, technical skill, and humanism.
- General-surgery residencies did not at the time produce full competence in general surgery.
- General surgery has historically displayed ambivalence about new technology and—until the introduction of laparoscopy—the instruments surgeons were using were the same as those used in World War II.
- General surgery was squandering precious training opportunities on residents who would practice in other fields of surgery while graduating incompletely trained general surgeons.

Dr. Way concluded that general surgery residencies were falling short of providing adequate training.[23]

Thus, halfway through the first hectic decade of the laparoscopic general surgery revolution, surgical leaders had identified the crucial message of this book: because of the rapid and relatively uncontrolled rise of technological advances, there were too many operations to learn by a single practitioner in the course of a five-year training program. This was also *before* the reduction in duty hours. I will summarize the ongoing debates by our surgical leaders on the evolving idea of surgical capability. Specific dates are listed to orient you to the discussions as they relate to the beginning of the laparoscopic revolution in 1990. Although the first laparoscopic cholecystectomy was performed in the United States in 1988, most of us dived into the rising tsunami of minimally invasive surgery in the early 1990s.

The Year Was 1999

Two articles published at 10-year intervals address an ongoing capability conundrum for physicians of all stripes. The issue is that of individual versus systems causes of medical errors. For surgeons it's an issue that won't go away; what I do technically depends on my knowledge, skills, and training. That is, if the needed instruments are in good repair, cooperative OR support staff, focused anesthesiologists, and other systems factors don't fail.

In a 1999 article in *Academic Medicine*, entitled "Systems Errors versus Physicians' Errors: Finding the Balance in Medical Education,"[24] doctors Casarett and Helms describe the best features of a systems approach to errors as a way of looking beyond the proximate cause (the individuals who appear responsible) to the work environment, fatigue, discontinuity of care, and other reasons for latent errors. Individual reasons for errors include incomplete knowledge, flawed reasoning, inadequate attention to detail, poor communication, and excessive workload. Addressing the risks of a systems approach to errors in medical education, the authors stated: "When they search for external causes of their errors, house officers (residents) are employing deep-seated defense mechanisms that have been well described. . . . Externalizing the responsibility for medical mistakes may be an attractive way to cope with one's errors. . . . In fact, it is reasonable to suppose that physicians who ascribe adverse outcomes to factors beyond their control are less likely to examine their own reasoning and action."[25]

Similarly, 10 years later Dr. Anthony D. Whittemore insisted in an article in *Annals of Surgery* in 2009, entitled "The Competent Surgeon: Individual Accountability in the Era of 'Systems' Failure," that the current examination process involving written and oral tests, continuing-education requirements, recertification exams, and the maintenance-of-certification process "still fails to provide ongoing evaluation of sustained clinical competence. . . . The process still falls short of any consistent real time assessment of a physician's specialty-specific skills, as it is routine, for instance, in the airline industry with regard to pilot competency."[26] And he makes a particularly sobering statement regarding an individual surgeon's capability when concluding, "Irrespective of certification by the American Board of Surgery, actual credentialing and privileging remains within the domain of the local institution through processes that are neither standardized nor particularly rigorous."[27] Thus, all patients must ask appropriate questions regarding a surgeon's experience with a particular operation and in a particular hospital.

The Year Was 2000

The reality of variable capability of general surgeons poses a nearly insoluble problem for patients seeking surgical care in hospitals clawing their way toward financial viability. For example, boasting about their robotic surgery programs, as well as the availability of other complex technology, hospitals may pressure their surgeons into doing procedures with which they have little training. This forces the practitioner to perform operations while early in his or her learning curve when more mistakes and complications occur. In this regard, it is important to note the shifting patterns of surgical-trainee operative experience.

For example, between 1991 and 1997, surgical residents increased the number of carotid artery (neck) operations they performed for arteriosclerosis but decreased the number of open gallbladder procedures.[28] Carotid surgery is done by vascular surgeons, whereas open gallbladder operations remain part of general surgery. Of the 10 most frequently performed operations between 1991 and 1997, laparoscopic cholecystectomy replaced open gallbladder surgery at number one (in 1997, open cholecystectomy was number 10); groin hernia remained number two; modified radical mastectomy disappeared from the top 10 list of 1997; carotid endarterectomy appeared on the 1997 list for the first time; and breast biopsy drifted from number three in 1991 to number five in 1997.

The training of general surgeons was becoming less appropriate with respect to trainees actually being taught how to do the operations they would perform in practice. However, the main issue in these shifting operative experience numbers for trainees is that, for example, thyroid removals increased from 12 to 14.3, while parathyroidectomies (small neck glands controlling calcium metabolism) rose from 4.1 to 6.2.[29] But neither of these increased operative experiences is robust enough to meet minimal case numbers to assure practice-based capability, regardless of how innately talented the resident is. This reality also applies to many of the other essential general surgery operations.

Thus, since the outset of the laparoscopic revolution in 1990, the numbers of operations performed by surgical residents in most categories aren't adequate to ensure that a trainee is minimally proficient in independently doing these operations. My discussion now begins to reflect the earnest reconsideration of the impact of what happened to general surgery over the last decade. Beginning in 2000, approximately 10 years after the first laparoscopic cholecystectomy was performed in the United States, the American Board of Medical Specialties (ABMS)—the umbrella organization that oversees its 24 member boards—struggled mightily to define competency.

In a 2000 article in the *Bulletin of the American College of Surgeons*, Dr. David Nahrwold, regent of the ACS and vice president of the ABMS at the time, stated, "The ABMS and its member boards recognize that board-certification does not warrant that a diplomat practices competently, and that the public has begun to understand that as well."[30] Then, referring to the newly formed ABMS Task Force on Competence, he quoted the ABMS's *Description of the Competent Physician*: "The competent physician should possess the medical knowledge, judgment, professionalism, and clinical and communication skills to provide high-quality patient care. Patient care encompasses the promotion of health, prevention of disease, and diagnosis, treatment and management of medical conditions with compassion and respect for patients and their families. Maintenance of competence should be demonstrated throughout the physician's career of lifelong learning and ongoing improvement of practice."[31]

This comprehensive 2000 summary articulates in clear, unambiguous language all the elements we now understand to be an integral part of capable physicians, including practicing surgeons. The issue, therefore, is not about understanding our goal. The problem lies in the *implementation* of proper training and the measurement of competence in both novice surgeons and seasoned practitioners attempting to assimilate new skills. For the first time, six general competencies outlined by the Accreditation Council for Graduate Medical Education (ACGME) aligned with the ABMS's Task Force on Competence. These six competencies guide our educational efforts today in all specialties (Box 4.1).

Box 4.1 The Six ACGME General Competencies

- *Patient care*—trainees must provide comprehensive, compassionate, and effective care in treating disease and promoting overall health.
- *Medical knowledge*—medical students and residents must be able to demonstrate knowledge about anatomical, biochemical, clinical, epidemiological, and social-behavioral sciences as applied to patient care.
- *Practice-based learning and improvement*—residents must be able to evaluate their own practices (successes and mistakes) and appraise and assimilate scientific evidence and improve their individual practices through self-reflection.
- *Interpersonal and communication skills*—students and training residents must demonstrate interpersonal and communication skills as well as teamwork involving patients and their families and with their professional associates.
- *Professionalism*—students and residents must demonstrate a commitment to ethical behavior that is empathetic, globally aware of the practice environment, and sensitive to diverse patient populations.
- *System-based practice*—trainees must be sensitive to the larger system of health care and be able to employ all resources offered by the system.

The Year Was 2001

A year later, Dr. Wallace Ritchie, then executive director of the ABS, wrote a report on the status of the competence movement in an article in the *Bulletin of the American College of Surgeons* entitled "The Measurement of Competence: Current Plans and Future Initiatives of the American Board of Surgery." Referring to the traditional role of medical boards as merely certifying doctors, he wrote: "That stance is no longer tenable and the reason is simple: the pressure is on the boards to link possession of a certificate to competent performance in practice. . . . Now they must prove certification and competence are related."[32] Dr. Ritchie referred to the development of a "maintenance of certificate" concept (now a reality) as well as to the six competencies established at the time as guidelines. This maintenance-of-certificate concept would require surgeons not only to report evidence of professional standing but also to undergo lifelong learning and periodic self-assessment and recertification. In his words, "The goal is to ensure that the certificate is and always will be closely linked to competent performance."[33]

There had to be a solid link between certification and actual clinical capability. Dr. Ritchie also identified a particularly nefarious issue facing efforts to ensure a surgeon's competence. It is the very problem driving my arguments regarding how to find a competent surgical practitioner: the extraordinarily heterogeneous nature of various general surgery practices. Although we have a core of operations all general surgeons perform (hernias, gallbladders, appendectomies, etc.), there also exists a mixture of operations that some surgeons do and some don't. That general surgeons do many different operations in their practices makes the evaluation of specific technical skills difficult. Dr. Ritchie stated, "General surgery in particular poses an especially troublesome difficulty for the board: the development of universally applicable outcomes analysis for a major constituency of the board whose practice profile is incredibly varied."[34] The competence initiative, he insisted, was aimed at providing specific practice feedback to individual practitioners for the sole purpose of practice improvement. At the time, the ABS contacted the various surgical boards, including those for vascular, pediatric, and oncologic surgery, to address the issues of "Which outcomes? Which endpoints? What methodology? And how can improvement be measured?"[35]

That year, 2001, other groups also addressed the competency predicament. Referring to the "weakest aspect of assessment in surgical training," U.K. surgical education experts Darzi and Mackay discussed the evaluation of surgical skills in the operating room.[36] Although recognizing the contribution of organizational and systems failures to surgical errors, the authors nonetheless stated: "Concerns about the assessment of technical competencies (which have been difficult) have given rise to an increasing interest in the objective scientific measurement of technical performance. . . . However, if we limit discussion of the surgical skills and competencies to the defining clinical and practical ones, it becomes clear that the necessary skills remain multiple and complex."[37] The authors comment on newer methods of evaluating technical skills, including (a) the Objective Structured Assessment of Technical Skills examination (OSATS; "Show me that you can actually *do* and not just describe these intricate maneuvers"), (b) hand-motion analysis ("Are your movements clean and precise, without extra jerky, uncontrolled motions?"), and (c) virtual-reality testing technology ("Show me that you can remove this virtual gallbladder on the TV screen with few errors"). Not mentioned is a new method involving eye-tracking technology. In 2001, these authors concluded, "Technical skills are the least well assessed component of the clinical process because assessment techniques currently in use are highly subjective and are poorly standardized and validated."[38]

The Year Was 2002

The next year, the stellar cast of doctors Richard Satava, Anthony Gallagher, and Carlos Pellegrini (to become the president of the ACS in 2014) defined clear terminology for definitions, taxonomy, and the metrics (measurements) of surgical competence. In their report published in the *Journal of the American College of Surgeons* in 2003, the authors described *surgical competence* as "a global term composed of the six component competencies."[39] These six components of a capable surgeon are listed in Box 4.1. By comparison, *surgical proficiency* is defined as "the level of performance in each of the specific components of competence, and as such, is an attribute of the evaluation of overall surgical competence. . . . It is the sum of all levels of proficiency that determines global competence."[40]

The goal of surgical education, therefore, centers on using measurements (metrics) that test funds of knowledge, recall of information, analytic thinking, decision making, and overall judgment. Not long ago, we (surgical educators) were doing poorly in implementing changes based on clinical performance data. For example, regretting a lack of performance analysis, in 2004 Dr. Robert W. Beart, a colorectal surgeon from the University of Southern California, commented on over 30 articles published on the quality of surgical care in his field. In an article entitled "We Are Not All the Same—What Are We Going to Do about It?" he stated, "In virtually every article and by every measure, surgeons with more specific training and greater operative volumes perform better. Yet, we as a profession have not embraced these findings."[41]

The argument for further specialization and for developing regional centers of excellence and hospital and surgeon volume standards stumbles along today without resolution.

Doctors Ronald Epstein and Edward Hundert presented a list of the "Dimensions of Professional Competence" in a report in the January 9, 2002, issue of the *Journal of the American Medical Association*. Of note, they declared, "However, there is no agreed-upon definition of competence that encompasses all important domains of professional medical practice."[42] Again, we encounter the reality that over a decade ago medical educators struggled to define the essence of their profession. The authors added, "Competence depends on habits of mind, including attentiveness, critical curiosity, self-awareness, and presence. Professional competence is developmental, impermanent, and context-dependent."[43] *Context-dependent* means that the surgeon's capability must be appropriate for the particular circumstance doing a specific operation (e.g., a rapidly evolving abdominal emergency).

The Year Was 2009

In a report entitled "What Makes a Competent Surgeon? Experts and Trainees' Perceptions of the Roles of a Surgeon," the authors, respected surgical educators from the Imperial College, London, continue our journey through the briar patch of surgeon capability by addressing the Canadian (CanMEDS) definitions of surgical competence in the form of seven roles: medical expert, communicator, collaborator, manager, health advocate, scholar, and professional.[44] They echo the previous lament of ambiguity by stating, "The surgical literature remains 'imprecise and nonspecific' in defining what constitutes a competent surgeon."[45] They performed a survey of surgical attendings (faculty) and trainees and compared each group's opinion of the importance of each of the seven roles for surgeons. Junior trainees attributed lower importance to the roles of manager, communicator, collaborator, and professional. Trainees failed to see the value of leadership and managing a clinical team, and appreciated the need for good communication, collaboration, and patient advocacy. The authors stated that their survey highlights the gap between what educators think they are delivering and what trainees feel they are actually accomplishing.[46] Interestingly, not a single surgeon claimed to have achieved competency in all the CanMEDS roles!

In summary, the characteristics that define a capable surgeon must be considered to be more than just an assumed or expected professional stance of technical competence. There is more to the art of providing comprehensive surgical care than simply tying knots, dissecting tissue, and reconstructing anatomy—whether done open or laparoscopically. Today, a surgeon's level of competence is tracked through several mechanisms, including the ABS's Maintenance of Certification process. But even the current oversight pressed on surgeons isn't enough to ensure that all practitioners are equally capable. Certainly, our assessment of surgeons in training today is far better than what was done as recently as two decades ago. Assessment of surgeons in practice remains in its infancy.

The myth that every surgeon is a master technician of all general surgery operations evaporated in the early days of laparoscopic gallbladder removal. We thought that picking up a laparoscope would be as easy as wielding a scalpel. Many practicing surgeons believed that they could do just about any operation they chose to do because of their extensive experience with other procedures.

Sadly, as we picked up the laparoscope we were all innately superstars in our own minds. We were wrong. And almost certainly the discussion of individual surgeon capability isn't over.

Romancing the Stone: A Specialty in Decline and How General Surgeons Almost Lost the Gallbladder

In the early years of the last decade it looked as though surgeons were about to lose a substantial piece of their gastrointestinal territory with the inroads being made by alternative treatments for gallstones, notably dissolution therapy and extracorporeal shock wave lithotripsy.

S. Banting and D. C. Carter, *Surgical Laparoscopy*

Urologists and radiologists are becoming more aggressive in performing extraction of gallstones after dilating the percutaneous tract. . . . Gallbladder calculi can also be dissolved rapidly after percutaneous cholecystostomy with direct application of cholesterol solvents, such as methyl-tert-butyl ether.

Nathaniel J. Soper, *Surgery*, 1991

Her gallbladder stuck out black and white on ultrasound, a pear-shaped pouch packed with little rocks, the bile bag's wall thickened with scar tissue. Daily, it inflicted waves of nausea and right upper abdominal pain. She was the wife of a good friend. I wanted her surgery to be safe with as little surgical trauma as possible. Assisted by a superb surgeon, I created a small upper abdominal midline incision no longer than a Band-Aid. Using long forceps and scissors, as well as an extension on the cautery, we struggled to remove her gallbladder with a mini-incision perhaps eight centimeters in length. She recovered swiftly. Her scar was remarkably cosmetic for a gallbladder operation.

My mini modification of the traditional gallbladder incision seemed to hold promise for at least some of my patients. At the time, I wasn't entirely aware that many surgeons who were dissatisfied with the prolonged recovery time for an open gallbladder operation were exploring the use of smaller, less painful incisions:[1,2] short incisions and using long, skinny traditional handheld instruments as focused overhead lights aimed deep in the belly at the target organ, the gallbladder. You might conclude that performing a minilaparotomy (small open abdominal incision) was a logical step heading toward even less invasive laparoscopic surgery.

Actually, we got the steps out of order.

What's fascinating about this early trend toward using less painful incisions is that in the 1980s interest in minilaparotomy was a vision pursued as an end in and of itself. No one using small incisions had thought about laparoscopy. We were still anchored in scalpel thinking. Laparoscope thinking was a few years away. That surgical miniaturization would evolve and become the hallmark of the new laparoscopic surgery revolution was a Himalayan paradigm shift away. This exploratory step toward minimally invasive operations using minilaparotomy served as a blindfold. Downsizing our belly cuts maintained our collective indifference to what other specialists had already accomplished with the laparoscope. Mini incisions kept us entrenched in our scalpel mind-set.

What we call *biliary tract diseases* are the pathological conditions of the gallbladder, bile ducts, liver, and pancreas. They begin with excess cholesterol in the bile ("supersaturation") that produces cholesterol stones, or forms of calcium-containing stones called pigmented stones. In other words, gallstones form when chemicals in solution (dissolved in bile) settle out as solids. With time, the wall of the gallbladder becomes abnormal and diseased. Acute gallbladder infection (acute cholecystitis) and symptomatic gallstones, which cause crampy pain (biliary colic), affect more than 20 million Americans annually. The cost of caring for these patients exceeds $6.2 billion a year. Roughly 700,000 to 800,000 gallbladder removals occur each year in the United States.[3] In fact, between 1990 and 1993 there was a 28 percent increase in the total number of gallbladder removals performed in the United States.[4] Other diseases such as colon cancer, groin hernias, gastroesophageal reflux disease, and appendicitis also knelt cautiously before the laparoscope.

Nonetheless, no other disease process presents as dramatically as an infected, pus-filled gallbladder with a thickened, inflamed wall and packed with stones. No other pathology seemed more indisputably surgical in nature. And yet with what seemed to surgeons (at least to some degree) like magical thinking, the biliary tract became fair game for the interventions of gastroenterologists, urologists, and internists—all nonsurgeons who had never held a sick gallbladder in their hands.

Even the ethics of other specialists taking on the treatment of complications of gallstones was confused at the time by the alchemy of avarice and ego. In their minds these nonsurgeons approached the diseased gallbladder properly and with caution. For example, in their seminal report, urologists Kellett, Wickham, and Russell wrote, "We believe strongly that it is unethical to treat patients with gallstone lithotripsy without having a percutaneous method of drainage and stone retrieval to avert severe obstruction or cholangitis."[5] From the perspective of general surgeons, immediate problems arise with this seemingly reasonable statement. First, draining the gallbladder does not treat cholangitis. Cholangitis is a severe infection of the entire biliary tree both inside and outside the liver and has little to do with the gallbladder per se. Often life threatening, pus in the main bile ducts (cholangitis) is most commonly treated by removing a stone in the distal common bile duct (by a gastroenterologist using an endoscope), by surgically placing a T-tube in the duct, or by draining the biliary tree with a catheter placed through the liver, a process done by an interventional radiologist. Rarely can infected bile ducts be drained through the gallbladder and its cystic duct. Only an experienced general surgeon is able to handle the severe challenges of acute cholangitis surgically. So, was it ethical for urologists to approach a disease (gallstones) with which they had no residency training and no clinical experience? And only because they had a toolbox that contained *one* of the many tools necessary to treat the plethora of gallstone-associated diseases?

Where Was General Surgery at the Beginning of the Laparoscopic Revolution?

I discovered a fascinating piece of the laparoscopic surgery story hidden in the compressed pages of an old surgical journal. In this historic 1989 document lay the seeds of professional uncertainty woven into a broad outline of the future of general surgery. A variety of experts reported on how general surgery would look in the near future. Of note, it also contained opinions about what many experts thought would *not* be part of the future of general surgery. The failure of these experts to identify the revolution perched on their doorstep is another example of how none of us saw the laparoscopic revolution rushing at us. In a sense the report showed an enduring lack of respect for what gynecologists and urologists had already accomplished. In other words, the report was in keeping with the overall rejection of laparoscopic surgery at the time by virtually everyone except gynecologists and urologists themselves.

Nonetheless, the report by the AMA's Council on Long-range Planning and Development[6] underscores how medical professionals everywhere missed the ramping up going on around them leading to an explosion of minimally invasive operations. Despite the AMA's otherwise reliable projections for general surgery, the single most spectacular technological advance in modern surgical history—that of the rise of laparoscopic surgery—was never mentioned in the 1989 report.

In 1986, according to the report, about 32,000 physicians defined themselves as general surgeons. Half of the approximately 1,000 surgical residents training at the time would graduate and complete further training in a subspecialty such as orthopedics, ophthalmology, neurosurgery, and so forth; the other half would enter the broadly defined field of general surgical practice. The scope of practice—what surgeons actually do in their practices—was expected to change significantly in the next decade (the 1990s), according to the AMA report. Many of the changes the report predicted have, in fact, occurred. Interventional radiologists have learned to stick catheters (small tubes) into abscesses with CT guidance and drain them rather than subject the patient to a painful operation. X-ray-guided core breast biopsies using tiny puncture wounds replaced ugly, painful breast biopsy incisions. And high-powered drugs had shut down stomach acid and effectively ended the era of gastric surgery for peptic ulcer disease.

The AMA report, however, was at odds with the plot of the laparoscope's growing story line. Referring to the use of shockwaves to destroy gallstones, the report states, "This, and the development of other noninvasive therapies, will undoubtedly redefine the scope of practice of general surgeons."[7] The report echoed the prevalent belief that such nonsurgical approaches as smashing gallstones with shock waves (lithotripsy) or dissolving gallstones with bile salt pills would shrink the general surgeon's workload. In fact, in our own literature, the death of general surgery had been predicted and bemoaned more than once.[8,9]

Luckily, everyone got it wrong.

Surgical innovation in a fading wisp of time gave birth to an entirely different story. Fortunately, it left general surgeons to do their work without scalpels. Nonetheless, for an agonizing moment in our recent surgical history, the gastrointestinal, urological, and radiological wolves were drooling at the general surgeon's door.

A switch to medical treatments for gallbladder disease, as the AMA report predicted, would have significantly emptied our surgical wallets. To our collective sigh of relief, the laparoscope's story veered off in a different narrative direction. Although we didn't deserve our eventual reward, laparoscopy in general surgery emerged triumphant. And so, ironically, the irate surgeons who fought the development of less invasive operations ultimately were saved by them. The surgeons who ridiculed the laparoscope as an instrument associated with gynecology's darkened operating-room witchcraft fell back in disbelief as the unstoppable forces of change overwhelmed their resistance to minimally invasive operations. In the end, the technology we belittled saved our bacon.

In the meantime, off the radar of many practicing surgeons was the significant effort by internists, urologists, and gastroenterologists to attack gallstones without a knife. These nonsurgical, noninvasive medical technologies arose during the last two decades of the 20th century. I'll now review what these physicians were doing just before Erich Muhe stabbed and deflated their nonsurgical gallstone balloon with a laparoscope.

Briefly, the first wave of treatments using bile salt pills to dissolve gallstones began in the 1970s. In 1985, shock waves (lithotripsy) mimicked the treatment of kidney stones; and, in the process of smashing bile rocks, a hysteria known as "lithotripsymania" swept the medical profession. One author stated, "The most popular topic for conference panels and lectures was 'The treatment of gallbladder lithiasis (stones): what is left for the surgeon?'"[10] In 1986, a prominent researcher in the field of gastroenterology made a remarkable statement regarding the future of the treatment of gallstone disease. It was made a year *after* Erich Muhe performed the first laparoscopic cholecystectomy in the world and a mere two years *before* the first laparoscopic cholecystectomy would be performed in the United States. The gastroenterologist, unaware of the emerging new operation for gallstones, commented, "Thus, the treatment of gallstone disease was gradually taken over by physicians. Rapid development over only 15 years has enabled us to remove gallstones from deep inside the patient without even scratching the skin. And there is no prospect of an end to this development."[11]

No prospect of an end to nonsurgical approaches to gallstones. And without even scratching the skin!

Without scratching the skin was, of course, a less than oblique statement alluding to the aggressive abdominal incisions surgeons inflicted on their patients. The gastroenterologists had a point. General surgeons had not really accepted minilaparotomy to reduce painful incisions and prolonged recovery from open cholecystectomy. However, within a few brief years this unrealistic proclamation would crash into the energized proponents of a Wild West that characterized the beginning of the laparoscopic surgery revolution. Note that the tone of unchecked hubris of the statement by a gastroenterologist ironically matched the occasional arrogant proclamations surgeons often used to deride gynecologists.

The conviction by medical practitioners that gallstones were no longer a surgical problem denied the existence of innovative surgeons clamoring in loud voices outside the gastroenterologists' door. Resolute, gastroenterologists, urologists, and radiologists huddled inside their professional bastions serving up the gallstone-dissolving potions with which they had fallen in love. The din of gallstone-smashing lithotripsy machines joined the loud impacts of huge machines smashing kidney stones down the hall in the urology suites. Outside their doors huddled a cadre of hopeful general surgeons. These were the innocents. Still denying the impending arrival of the laparoscope, these general surgeons looked longingly to the gastroenterologists to be thrown an occasional referral bone for an open cholecystectomy.

What seems odd in retrospect is that gastroenterologists around the world knew very well that their nonsurgical gallstone treatments were only successful a third of the time. Surgeons still operated on their failures, on the really sick patients, those with complications of gallstone disease. Some patients staggered from the gastrointestinal (GI) and urology suites to the operating room when lithotripsy failed and the natural history of gallbladder disease played out its predictable course.

A fundamental pathological process (disease-causing body malfunctioning) about which the various nonsurgeons were in denial was alluded to in a symposium in 1990 during which alternative methods of treating gallstones were discussed: "The objective common to some of these newer approaches has been directed at achieving gallstone clearance while leaving the gallbladder in situ."[12]

That is, the gallstone-producing factory and its walls were left standing.

How Gastroenterologists, Urologists, and Radiologists Attempted to Steal the Gallbladder from General Surgeons

Stones of different compositions may form in the gallbladder (the major source of gallstones) as well as in the bile ducts. The complex biochemical pathways leading to stone formation are fascinating but beyond the needs of my story. Basically, when there is an imbalance among the concentrations of bile salts and other chemicals, stones form. Small gallbladder stones may tumble into the common bile duct, or common duct stones may actually form in the bile ducts themselves. Approximately 5 to 10 percent of stones in the gallbladder migrate through the cystic duct into the common bile duct. When discovered, common bile duct stones require special techniques for their removal.

To give a better sense of the historical timing of the laparoscopic revolution, it's worthwhile to briefly review how the gallbladder and its cache of stones almost became a surgical orphan. What seems remarkable in retrospect is the amount of effort that went into designing nonoperative therapies for symptomatic gallstones.

Trials Using Chemicals to Dissolve Gallstones

Less invasive methods that were designed to get rid of gallstones flourished in the 1970s. The therapeutic ball got rolling in 1972 when a report describing the dissolution of gallstones appeared in the *New England Journal of Medicine*, inciting enthusiasm for nonsurgical treatment of bile stones.[13] Other methods quickly emerged.

One technique struck me as ultraradical, if not patently dangerous. The technology speaks volumes about the gastroenterologist/radiologist team's desperation to exclude surgeons from the gallbladder's playing field. First, with this technique the volume of the gallbladder was determined using X-ray contrast dye, and then by injecting exactly that volume of a corrosive chemical called methyl tert-butyl ether (MTBE), the gallbladder was distended until it was full. The chemical was injected through a catheter snaked through the nose, down past the stomach, into the common bile duct, and finally into the gallbladder. The tube was removed after irrigation with the corrosive chemical was repeated four to six times an hour and until the stones were gone; that is, until the stones were no longer seen on X-ray (some were less than completely dissolved). The chemical MTBE is explosive. It can cause anemia and destroy gallbladder tissue if left in too long. It also causes kidney failure.[14] So, the technique fell into disfavor as complications grew. Some physicians also considered the magical destruction of the gallbladder by other toxic agents a "chemical cholecystectomy."[15]

The most popular method for getting rid of gallstones, carried out under controlled clinical trials at the time, involved dissolving the rocks using tablets of bile salts taken by mouth. Bile salts included a brain-numbing drug called chenodeoxycholic acid, which only works on cholesterol stones. Another similar drug called ursochenodeoxycholic acid was an improvement on its sibling salt, but the results of these trials were relatively dismal. The technique required a functioning gallbladder and compliance by the patient (regularly taking the pills). Complications of its toxicity included diarrhea, abnormal liver function, and elevations of cholesterol. Bile salts produced an average success rate of only 38 percent.[16,17] After five or more years, over 50 percent of patients so treated experienced a return of their stones. Dismal results led to recommendations to combine the two drugs.[18]

In the 1980s, a big study called the National Cooperative Gallstone Study revealed that it took two years to get only a 19 percent complete dissolution rate (meaning that stones disappeared completely).[19] And there was other bad news. Was the absence of stones in the gallbladder on an X-ray a reliable sign they had been completely dissolved? Or did it mean that they were smaller but still present and not detectable because of the dye the X-ray study used—stones that would regrow?

A Very Short Story—Smashing Gallbladder Stones

Smashing gallbladder stones is called lithotripsy, and the technique is alive and well today in the field of urology. Kidney stones may be shattered with shock waves transmitted to the stones hiding in the ureters. Ureters are the long living tubes running from the kidney to the urinary bladder. Lithotripsy also smashes stones that are stuck in the kidney's upper (urine) collecting system. Small stone fragments are then washed out in the urine through the ureters into the bladder and out of the body.

Ureters are larger and more anatomically consistent drainage tubes, and they more easily permit the passage of kidney stone fragments, certainly more than do the variable and smaller cystic bile duct. Sometimes urologists place stents (hollow tubes) in the ureters to help stone fragments pass into the bladder. Urologists also *extract* stones (and stone fragments after lithotripsy) from the kidney itself by inserting a tube into the kidney through the flank skin and then washing out the stones through the sheath.

In the 1980s, a few academic urologists decided that they could operate in a similar way on the gallbladder. However, there are many cautionary aspects to this portion of the gallbladder's tale. First, when applied to gallstones, lithotripsy was less effective because of the anatomy and location of the gallbladder, as just described. The cystic duct leading from the gallbladder to the main or common bile duct is quite variable in size and length, unlike the ureters, and has valves where stone fragments get stuck. Also, the success rate for lithotripsy shocking of gallstones depends on the size and number of stones in the gallbladder. Even the idea of removing gallstones through the sheath pushed through the right upper abdominal wall (as with the kidney) fell dead in its tracks.

Urologists Attack the Gallbladder—How Did They Get into the Gallstone Game?

Trouble starts with the opening sentence of the classic article by British urologists Kellett, Wickham, and Russell entitled "Percutaneous

Cholecystolithotomy" (or "how to extract gallstones from the gallbladder the way we do with kidney stones, by poking a rigid tube through the skin and into the gallbladder"). They wrote, "A percutaneous method was used to remove stones from otherwise normal gallbladders, as assessed by cholecystography and ultrasonography."[20] Normal gallbladders? The error these urologists make, of course, is that a gallbladder that harbors stones is a *pathological* gallbladder. The composition of the bile is critical to stone formation as well. Urologists never made the leap to cholecystectomy—-*because they were never trained in biliary tract surgery*. The authors ended their discussion with the tired suggestion—rejected by surgeons since Carl Langenbuch performed the first open gallbladder removal in the world—that perhaps the diseased gallbladder could be left in the body and magically would not again form stones. Unfortunately, their involvement in gallbladder disease reflects just how completely general surgeons abjured any association with less invasive methods of treating such a common disease. Our failure to study laparoscopy in the 1980s led the way for others to intervene and fill the void of public demand.

As with all technical surgery, the accrual of a delicate touch, an appreciation for tissue quality, tissue planes, and skill with delicate tissue dissection, and avoidance of damage to vital structures only comes with training and experience. One could argue that urologists should never have invaded the general surgeon's territory to begin with because they lacked appropriate knowledge, skills, and basic training to handle such operative emergencies as a patient bleeding to death from a liver injury. Put differently, how would urologists have reacted if general surgeons had begun performing nephrectomies (kidney removal) in response to the urologists' attempts to steal the gallbladder?

Thus, in June 1990, to confront the misguided attempts by nongeneral surgeons to treat gallstones surgically, the American College of Surgeons published its "Statement on Laparoscopic Cholecystectomy" in the ACS bulletin, stating, "For optimal quality patient care, laparoscopic cholecystectomy should be performed by surgeons who are qualified to perform open cholecystectomy. Only such surgeons possess the skills to perform biliary tract surgical procedures; such surgeons are able to determine the best method of cholecystectomy; and only such surgeons can treat complications consequent to laparoscopic cholecystectomy."[21] The ACS made it clear that little support (read: in medico-legal cases) would be available to nonsurgeons who developed complications by overstepping the boundary of their specialty. Parenthetically, this statement also curbed any enthusiasm by gynecologists to turn their laparoscopes north toward the gallbladder.

In the 1980s, as nonsurgeons chased creative ways to rid the body of gallstones without huge surgical incisions, general surgeons, fearful that lithotripsy and bile salt therapies would become *the* new gallbladder treatments, began experimenting with less aggressive operations. But before arguments about the best therapy for gallstones became moot by the introduction of laparoscopic cholecystectomy, an intermediate treatment stage entered the fray. I mentioned it earlier. It sounded attractive at the time.

Mini Incisions—Moving in the Right Direction

The transitional phase in the tale of laparoscopy in general surgery occurred when some surgeons began thinking small. My shift to smaller incisions mentioned at the beginning of the chapter was misdirected. As it turned out, at first none of us were thinking small enough. It was that magical year of 1990 when the notion of considering surgery's painful consequences *from the patient's point of view* slowly squeezed its way into the minds of a few surgeons. Back then patients who had their gallbladders removed stayed in the hospital five to seven days. Lying in bed, they flirted with life-threatening complications, sprouted plastic nasogastric (NG) tubes from their nostrils, and lay restrained with IVs stuck in their arms and, in some cases, with catheters in their urinary bladders. These patients truly were in agony with ugly incisions a foot in length, slanted gashes under the right rib cage.

Back in the day, I shifted to short midline incisions (rather than under the rib cage) and sent my patients home in two to three days. Part of my routine was to feed the patients through a special tube immediately in the recovery room.[22] Minilaparoscopic surgery cut my patients' pain experience and hospital stay in half. But it turned out that not even a short incision could compete with the laparoscope.

This discussion of small incisions leaves a final fascinating point to ponder. Erich Muhe's ingenious 1985 innovation was his "galloscope," followed by his open tube design of a laparoscope with a circular light. The tantalizing issue is this: the diameter of Muhe's open tube was 4.5 centimeters.[23] That, of course, was almost the same size as the incisions used by the minicholecystectomy surgeons. The difference was that Erich Muhe used Kurt Semm's laparoscopic instruments, whereas the minilaparoscopists used traditional surgical instruments. So, was Erich Muhe's very first laparoscopic cholecystectomy a true laparoscopic operation? Or was it a minicholecystectomy performed through a tube? From my perspective, because Muhe used laparoscopic instruments and followed the principles of minimally invasive surgery, his procedure was a truly laparoscopic operation.

Another Loss for General Surgery, a Huge Gain for Patients—Common Bile Duct Stone Removal by Gastroenterologists

In about 8 to 10 percent of cases when surgeons used a traditional incision, we opened the common bile duct to remove stones at the time of removing the gallbladder. Patients walked around with a rubber tube hanging from their belly for weeks. An X-ray through the tube was then done to prove that no further stones were present, at which time the T-tube was removed: all in all, a rather annoying and sometimes complicated postoperative course to endure.

Then, in 1970, for the first time the murky distal end of the common bile duct was visualized with an endoscope. Two Germans (working in Erich Muhe's former academic medical center in Erlangen, before he moved to Boblingen) and Japanese researchers were the first groups to refine this way of looking at the common bile duct and its little controlling circular muscle, the sphincter of Oddi. The intervention is called endoscopic retrograde pancreaticoduodenostomy (ERCP), and the papillotomy is the cutting of the muscular ring around the end of the common bile duct, a papilla or small nipple-like structure that pokes into the duodenum, the first part of the small intestine. The stones in the common bile duct tumble into the small intestine and are passed in the stool.

This major accomplishment performed by innovative gastroenterologists employed a new endoscope and newly designed instruments. Thus, gastroenterology specialists boldly opened the era of nonsurgical treatment of common bile duct stones. In 1998 a report noted, "By 1977, more than 1,500 papillotomies had been performed in ten West German centers, with an overall success rate of 93 percent. . . . Many surgeons were sharply critical of internists' entrance into classical fields of surgery."[24] And another general surgery operation—open exploration of the common bile duct through an abdominal incision—found its popularity wane as the procedure headed toward the dustbins of history. In all these minimally invasive improvements, one can hear the faint echo of lost financial opportunities, framed as an ethical objection to change by general surgeons.

The retirement of the classic general surgery operation (open exploration of the common bile duct) was a direct consequence of the laparoscopic revolution. Our current graduates have virtually no experience with this operation should ERCP fail. Thus, as the example of ERCP demonstrates, the treatment for gallstones and bile duct disease quickly became a shared endeavor for surgeons and their specialized medical colleagues. That symbiosis continues today for the benefit of our patients. Less pain and suffering and shorter hospital stays have become the standard across the laparoscopic landscape.

But these advancements didn't come easily.

CHAPTER SIX

The Gallbladder's Tale: The Chaotic Birth of Laparoscopic General Surgery

The primacy of an idea, the paternity of a discovery is not always evident. The claim is often difficult because victory has many fathers, while defeat is an orphan.

Robert Bendavid, MD, *Hernia*, 2005

We may discover in retrospect that laparoscopic surgery was principally a "transition" form of surgery on the way to telepresence surgery, much the same way that the slider rule was a transition in computational mathematics from traditional mathematical "look-up tables" to the now ubiquitous electronic calculator.

Richard M. Satava and Shaun B. Jones, *Cybersurgery: Advanced Technologies for Surgical Practice*, 1998

Labor Pains

From the very start it was all about the gallbladder. During the closing years of the 1980s, smashing and dissolving gallstones remained on the internist's and gastroenterologist's menu of daily specials. Fewer than a hundred laparoscopic gallbladder removals had been performed by the summer of 1989. Nonetheless, significant curiosity about the new operation had been piqued. As interest grew in Germany, France, and the United States, national surgical leaders gathered that summer at Cedars-Sinai Medical Center in Los Angeles to discuss how to structure proper courses to teach the emerging new gallbladder operation.[1] The challenge was that few legitimate introductory laparoscopic technique courses were available to the thousands of general surgeons suddenly clamoring for skills training.

Aggravating what might have been a safe trajectory for practitioners to learn the minimal-access gallbladder operation was enthusiastic media coverage as multiple outlets quickly caught wind of the keyhole operation. Soon thereafter biliary colic (gallbladder pain) patients started asking their doctors for the new procedure. But in a reflective report on medicine and the media in 1998, Dr. Timothy Johnson identified the issues surrounding surgical innovation in general, which applied directly to laparoscopic gallbladder removal. He wrote in the *New England Journal of Medicine*, "Whereas science traditionally emphasized collective data over individual anecdotes and getting it right over getting it first, representatives of the world of medical science often felt pressure to release early clinical research prematurely to the public."[2] In the same article, recognizing the relentless pressure to report dramatic new scientific and medical discoveries, Johnson added, "There are similar competitive pressures on the medical establishment, a world where medical centers, researchers, biotechnology firms, and individual practitioners increasingly use the techniques of the business world—press conferences, press releases, video mailings, and Wall Street briefings—to gain or maintain market share or to increase the chances of receiving funding for research."[3] Eight years earlier these business trends were creeping into the spread of laparoscopic gallbladder surgery.

Although we didn't know it at the time, laparoscopic cholecystectomy would lead to ill effects as well as excellent results because of the blatant commercial interests of some surgeons. But how did the revolution get started? Who was involved? Were mistakes made? And if so, by whom? And why?

The answers to these questions about the process of how the revolution began are important today because minimally invasive surgery is a transition technology. We're in the middle of technological change that will lead to more change. And change means surgeons must negotiate new learning curves. We know that patient safety flounders during a surgeon's first dozen or so laparoscopic gallbladder cases. Of course, no one had any real laparoscopic experience going into the game, and so there was little or no helping each other. Also, there were few organizations monitoring our training methods or overseeing the credentialing of individual surgeons and their variably refined laparoscopic skills.

Most hospitals followed the early privileging guidelines loosely. The challenges forcing hospital administrators responsible for credentialing surgeons (stating we were adequately trained to do laparoscopic gallbladder surgery) were aggravated by the desire to attract business to their hospital. Credentialing committees had struggled to define the capability of broadly trained general surgeons *before* the arrival of less aggressive operations. The dilemma for them in 1990 was about to become a lot worse.

To reiterate, to patients the gallbladder's tale serves as a cautionary story because robotic surgery and other complex surgical technology continue to search for a role in modern patient care. German surgeon Hans Troidl's observation in 1994 regarding laparoscopy is just as important, if not more so, today. He stated, "We have a new hammer and are actively looking for something to pound."[4] Surgeons are constantly searching for new minimally invasive targets to pound. And as the "hammer" (laparoscope) became a technical tour de force, those targets kept getting more complex. Thus, the introduction of more and more surgical technology each year presents challenges for patients as innovation gallops like a young stallion just ahead of the cart of technical mastery.

Before the Revolution—Gallstones through the Millennia

What is remarkable in today's connected world with instant distribution of information is a persistent theme that meanders through the laparoscope's story: virtually every surgeon or group of surgeons who became involved in designing the gallbladder operation—surgeons who practiced laparoscopic skills in the animal lab and ultimately those who performed laparoscopic cholecystectomy on a patient—thought they were the first surgeon in the world to do so.

Gallstones have ancient origins.

Gallstones and the mischievous diseases they precipitate aren't a consequence of our modern diet, as you might reasonably assume. Gallstones were discovered in 3,000-year-old mummies. Distended gallbladders blocked by stones were frequently confused with ovarian tumors and cysts by surgeons sneaking up on the notion of opening the abdomen with a scalpel. Beginning in the early 19th century, surgeons used small cuts over the gallbladder in the right upper abdomen to empty the hollow, pear-shaped organ of its rock collection. The natural history of gallstone disease involves the inflamed bile bag sticking to the belly wall inside the right upper quadrant of the abdomen. The hollow gallbladder seals itself off from the rest of the belly cavity. Inflammation breaks down the layers of the belly wall, and pus and stone debris from the gallbladder pour out of the abdomen through the path created by nature. Physicians who discovered this process elected to help it along by cutting through the abdominal wall and into the gallbladder, expediting the draining process. Because they created a hole rather than removing the organ, it was called a cholecystos-tomy (*ostomy*=hole; cholecyst*ectomy*=removal or excision).

It was in 1867 that John Bobbs in Indiana performed the first cholecystostomy in the United States. He found a huge distended gallbladder filled with stones, rather than the ovarian cyst he had expected. He removed the stones and emptied the gallbladder, and the patient survived.[5] Others around the world performed a similar operation with variable success. Lawson Tait, a gynecologist in Scotland, championed drainage of the gallbladder in the 1880s.[6] When Carl Langenbuch performed the first open cholecystectomy on July 15, 1882—that is, a complete surgical excision of the gallbladder through an abdominal incision—Tait openly opposed Langenbuch's operation. He did so with derogatory language, calling the procedure "absurd" despite the emerging sensibleness of the operation.[7] Langenbuch had refined his surgical technique on both animals and cadavers, working out how he would control the blood supply (cystic artery) and tie off the cystic duct. Tait kept up his vitriolic opposition to cholecystectomy until his death.

The argument about whether cholecystostomy (simply draining the gallbladder) or complete removal (cholecystectomy) was a better operation would prove resistant to a permanent solution for decades. As Langenbuch himself declared, you have to get rid of the *cause* of gallstones. As I noted in Chapter 5, all the medical therapies described for the treatment of gallstones involved simply getting rid of the stones, but not the stone factory— the gallbladder itself. The very nearly magical ends to which intelligent physicians went to try to wrestle gallstones from the hands of surgeons is a narrative of a quest that reflects human ingenuity in the face of futility. The battle by general surgeons to repossess the gallbladder is the tale of this stubborn reality: the gallbladder must be removed to cure symptomatic gallstone disease. And as Leon Morgenstern wrote in 1992 regarding laparoscopic cholecystectomy, "If Langenbuch himself could somehow be witness to this revolutionary modification of his technique, would his reactions be incredulous or laudatory? We suspect he would smile favorably, admiring the first modification of his century-old technique."[8]

The first open cholecystectomy in America was performed on September 24, 1886, by Dr. Justus Ohage in St. Joseph's Hospital in Saint Paul, Minnesota. The gallbladder was obstructed by a large stone owned by a 35-year-old woman with three years of symptoms. One hundred and thirty-five stones were eventually found in the gallbladder on pathological examination. It would be 102 years later before the technique he used evolved into the minimally invasive operation we routinely perform today.[9]

Ohage was one of nine medical students in 1880 to graduate in medicine from the University of Missouri. Ohage subsequently went on to study in Gottingen, Germany, and at the University of Kiel, where 100 years later

Kurt Semm would be the first in the world to remove the appendix using a laparoscope. In an address before the Ramsey County Medical Society of Saint Paul in 1887, Ohage presciently concluded, "The diseases of the gallbladder belong to the surgeon and only through him can speedy and permanent relief be obtained."[10] Physicians around the world forgot this basic idea while flirting with bile salt pills and washing out the gallbladder with harsh chemicals and inflicting patients with repetitive shock waves—until the laparoscope deflated their aspirations.

Not only did Missouri produce Dr. Ohage. It can be proud of a second development in the cure of gallbladder disease: cholecystography or contrast X-ray examination of the gallbladder (replaced in the 1970s by ultrasound). Further, the father of Charles H. Mayo and of his brother William was an admirer of Ohage and encouraged his sons to observe Ohage operate. This experience no doubt encouraged the Mayo brothers to become surgeons. And that decision in time led to the development of the idea for what became the Mayo Clinic.[11]

How the Laparoscope Challenged the Scalpel—Erich Muhe, the Forgotten Hero

The Year Was 1985

A German surgeon fathered the general surgery laparoscopic revolution on September 12, 1985, by performing the first laparoscopic gallbladder removal in the world.[12] Despite this remarkable achievement, Erich Muhe was ignored by his German colleagues. His reputation was plunged into ignominy when one of his gallbladder patients developed a complication and died after undergoing the untested procedure.

Until that defining moment, Muhe had enjoyed a respectable if not spectacular academic career in Erlangen, Germany. But, it was only when he moved away from his professors to the small town of Boblingen that Muhe originated the technique of laparoscopic cholecystectomy (LC; minimally invasive gallbladder removal). After performing only a few cases, Muhe was stunned by the rapid recovery of his patients. When he attempted to present his work at the German Surgical Society Congress in 1986, he was rebuffed. The *American Journal of Surgery* also rejected Muhe's manuscript in which he described his original work—the creative operation that would radically transform modern surgery. The American editor, a giant in the field, insisted that the German surgeon's English was poor and that the sole purpose of the paper was for Muhe to promote himself.[13]

Shortly after Erich Muhe had performed over 95 laparoscopic cholecystectomies, he was blamed for the demise of a patient who developed a lethal complication. His laparoscopic surgery patient was originally deemed to have died as a direct result of the new operation. Muhe was placed under house arrest. He was convicted of manslaughter, and his medical license was taken away.[14] The innovative surgeon who had started the third-greatest revolution in the history of surgery was labeled a criminal.

A Creative Surgeon and His Bicycle

Erich Muhe loved his racing bicycle. Muscular and compact, he was a well-conditioned and skilled cyclist, and he loved to complete in races against other doctors. Eventually, he beat them all. And yet no one in the surgical field, not even Muhe himself, would have believed that a chunk of his bicycle frame would change the world of surgery forever. While in Erlanger, Germany, early in his career, Muhe produced a respectable body of work. This included a "bed-bike" that patients lying on their backs in bed "rode," a contraption designed to prevent postoperative blood clots in the calves. Muhe penned more than 300 scientific publications before moving to a small hospital in Boblingen in 1982, where, according to Litynski, Muhe admitted, "Very quickly I had a feeling of professional stagnation."[15]

Working with a senior gynecologist in Boblingen in 1983, Muhe learned how to use laparoscopic instruments in the pelvis. At one point during a case, the gynecologist turned the laparoscope away from the pelvis and pointed it up toward the liver. He zoomed in on the gallbladder. Muhe stated in retrospect, "But at that point I had only the concept. I still needed to develop the proper technique."[16] (When Barry McKernan began working with a gynecologist in Marietta, Georgia, in 1988, he followed this same mental path when a gynecologist pointed his laparoscope toward the liver and helped McKernan realize that the gallbladder could be removed via a laparoscope.) Litynski quotes Muhe as saying, at about the same time, "I was convinced that if we passed up this chance like endoscopic cholecystectomy (gallbladder removal), internists and gynecologists would again take away a piece of our competence."[17]

Muhe designed a unique laparoscope. Fashioned from a bike frame, he called it the "galloscope"; it had side-view optics, a light conductor, and valves and a tube for creating a pneumoperitoneum (abdominal cavity inflated with carbon dioxide). Soon, he found the perfect patient on whom to try his new operation. She was thin, young, and had no additional medical conditions. On September 12, 1985, Erich Muhe performed the first laparoscopic cholecystectomy in the world. It took him about two hours. He was stunned by the patient's rapid recovery. Her pain level was minimal, and she ate dinner that same night and was discharged home early the next morning. Not done with innovation, Muhe switched over to a gasless approach and invented an open-tube laparoscope made from the down tube of one of his racing bikes. By March 1987, he had performed 97 laparoscopic cholecystectomies using that technique.

Only much later would he be exonerated of the criminal charges filed against him. It would be too late to save his reputation and his practice. Later, it was discovered that the anesthesiologists who ran the intensive care unit where Muhe's patient had died were responsible for the adverse outcome.[18] Ironically, and tragically, Muhe died in a bicycle-related accident.

I found Muhe's story heartbreaking. It was and continues to be virtually ignored by many academic journals that have published articles on the history of laparoscopy in general surgery. Muhe's story reflects the latent jealousies and malignant personalities that exist in so many academic departments of medicine and surgery around the world. Did German academic surgeons ignore the potential value of Erich Muhe's idea because he was no longer practicing at an academic center? Was this a distillation of the German surgical professors' unfiltered contempt (like their American surgeon counterparts' at the time) for small operations?

Certainly, Kurt Semm's seminal work in laparoscopic gynecology had originally been derided in a tempest of scholarly scorn, despite Semm's numerous contributions to the techniques and instrumentation of laparoscopic gynecology. But as history has noted, so it would be that Erich Muhe's innovative laparoscopic work would also be engulfed in the black hole of professional arrogance and surgical leadership self-certainty. At the Congress of the German Surgical Society in 1986, Muhe used 42 slides, 23 of which were on his open-tube laparoscopic technique. The audience seemed more amused than motivated to seek more answers regarding his innovation.[19]

Nonetheless, there can be no doubt that Erich Muhe's creativity launched the most dramatic chapter in the history of modern surgery. Litynski documents the reception of Muhe's remarkable work at the 1986 German Surgical Society meeting: it was considered "Mickey Mouse" surgery, "small brain-small incision" surgery, and downright dangerous.[20] Some German surgeons outwardly scorned Muhe. And instead of being published as a full paper in the society's booklet, Muhe's work appeared as an abstract. Litynski properly attributes the failure of Muhe's work to surgeons' preoccupation with complex operations performed through big incisions. Thus, up to this juncture the surgical world had successfully insulated itself from taking advantage of the contributions of laparoscopic surgery.

Grzegorz Litynski leaves us with a thought that reflects a fundamental point made years later by Malcolm Gladwell in his book *Outliers*. Litynski remarks about Muhe, "He weighed the achievements of the internists and gynecologists and apprehended the ramifications of their work for his own interests in endoscopic cholecystectomy."[21] Erich Muhe dared to mix with and learn from the gynecologists in his institution. He worked diligently to refine his skills in less invasive procedures and as a consequence was an outlier general surgeon whose perspective led to laparoscopic cholecystectomy. Gladwell makes the point that success usually has a personal precedent, perhaps akin to luck favoring the prepared mind. Regarding the capricious nature of success, he states, "It was the story of how the outliers in a particular field reached their lofty status through a combination of ability, opportunity, and utterly arbitrary advantage."[22] Similarly, the French and American general surgeons who subsequently believed that they had invented laparoscopic cholecystectomy had also learned urological techniques and rubbed elbows with gynecologists and urologists to make laparoscopic history.

Erich Muhe would have to wait until 1992 before the German Surgical Society would acknowledge his incontrovertible reshaping of modern surgery. But the biggest shock to the general surgery ego arrived in 1980. It was delivered by Kurt Semm, the creative gynecologist who first plucked out the appendix using a laparoscope. And one suspects, given his dedication to making surgery less invasive, that Semm knew he had set what was at the time an impossibly high technical bar for general surgeons.

Stealing the Appendix—A Lead-Up to the Gallbladder's Tale

To begin with, the appendix "belonged" to us, to general surgeons. And make no mistake about it, in the 1980s, as I have suggested, a lot of surgeons viewed gynecologists as second-class technicians. Ours was a recalcitrant professional hubris that was not altogether unearned. Back in the day we bailed out many gynecologists who created complications for themselves and their patients during their early laparoscopic attempts, burning holes in the intestines and creating bloody misadventures. So, in a surgical world where bits and pieces of general surgery were being chipped off by subspecialists, Semm's theft of the appendix was intolerable.

Once again, Litynski's extensive personal trove of recorded conversations and letters from major contributors to laparoscopic research and publications in German helps our understanding of the fervor that erupted over Semm's laparoscopic appendectomy. Litynski translates a journalist's summary of criticism directed at Kurt Semm:

> The danger of expanding the endoscopic appendectomy, which only
> seems to be easier and less dangerous to perform than conventional

methods, is that still more unnecessary appendectomies will be performed than have been to date. We thus face the following fundamental question: Do the advantages of endoscopic operations—avoidance of laparotomy (incision), diminishing the pain of the incision, early mobilization, and avoidance of post-operative adhesions—outweigh the disadvantages—greater expenditure on technology and more complicated methods of operating?[23]

Although the obvious tone of the editorial was to deny laparoscopic appendectomy its place in the surgeon's armamentarium, history has proven the opposite to be true. It seems odd that having access to a less invasive operation would be considered a reason to increase the rates of appendix removal when the primary indication for appendectomy has always been acute abdominal pain. General surgeons decried the minimally invasive appendix operation as too dangerous. After all, why substitute a misguided, complicated new procedure for a simple open operation? Had competent surgeons not performed hundreds of thousands of open appendectomies over the last hundred years? These surgeons had a valid point. But they had used the same argument to discredit laparoscopic cholecystectomy.

Litynski reduces the problem to its essence when he writes, "A gynecologist teaching a surgeon how to perform an operation was simply unthinkable. . . . Psychologically the gap between surgeons and gynecologists was immense. Many surgeons believed that gynecologists had 'operation envy', that 'real' operations were exclusively the domain of surgeons not gynecologists."[24] This comment cuts to the core of general surgeons' beliefs about their abilities as compared with gynecologists. Addressing the resistance offered by general surgeons to the use of laparoscopy, George Berci wrote, "The surgeon may resent infringements on his territory by the laparoscopist, particularly if the endoscopist is an internist. One way to avoid this unpleasantness would be for the surgeon to evaluate laparoscopy and become more familiar with it."[25]

In 1981, the Society of American Gastrointestinal and Endoscopic Surgeons (SAGES) was born. Major players in the early going were Gerald Marks, George Berci, Alfred Cuschieri, Fredrick L. Green, Leon Morgenstern, Kenneth A. Forde, Jeffrey Ponsky, James A. Lind, Thomas L. Dent, John A. Collar, Lee E. Smith, Theodor R. Schrock, Carol Scott-Conner, and many others. Berci was the leader, and because of his fluency in foreign languages, he engaged Europeans and Americans in a discussion of the role of laparoscopy in gastrointestinal surgery. A German organization also arose at this time. Both organizations focused more on flexible endoscopic assessment of gastrointestinal disease than on less aggressive operative treatments.

They paid relatively little attention to laparoscopy. That oversight would not last for long.

Three Innovative Frenchmen

Outliers—Surgeons with Something Extra: The Year Was 1987

While Erich Muhe went about the business of removing gallbladders with his novel laparoscope, in 1987 three Frenchmen were about to meet each other and puzzle over their own techniques for gallbladder removal. Unlike Muhe, these surgeons used the new electronic laparoscope with an improved light source and the Hopkins optical system for better visualization. The first Frenchman to perform a laparoscopic cholecystectomy was Philippe Mouret of Lyon, a private practitioner with few publications and no significant research interests.[26] What Mouret had was a tight affiliation with a gynecologist in his practice. He scrubbed on GYN cases and became familiar with their laparoscopic equipment. And so in 1983 with little fanfare and almost unnoticed, he performed a laparoscopic appendectomy. Thematically in line with this story, Mouret was unaware of Semm's 1980 laparoscopic appendectomy success. In March 1987 he operated on a woman with both gynecologic problems and a sick gallbladder. He removed her gallbladder and performed the needed GYN surgery at the same time.[27]

In 1990 another creative Frenchman, Francois Dubois, and his associates published the result of their first 36 laparoscopic gallbladder removals and described their technique. The results were excellent.[28] Dubois's story is unique in that at the time of hearing about laparoscopic cholecystectomy, he prided himself on the small size of his minilaparotomy (open) incisions. Asking a circulating nurse (whom he did not know had worked with Mouret) if she had ever seen a smaller gallbladder incision than his minilaparotomy, she told him that she was familiar with an even smaller incision method. Dubois, annoyed with the nurse's response, replied somewhat angrily, "Laparoscopic cholecystectomy is not possible!"[29] Then, Dubois contacted Mouret and subsequently met him at the Paris Hilton and studied two videos of Mouret's laparoscopic technique. He said little to Mouret and returned home. He studied Semm's textbook and borrowed instruments from local gynecologists. At first he had to open the abdomen through a larger incision to finish his cases. But at the end of April 1988, he performed his first laparoscopic cholecystectomy.

The third Frenchman to get involved with laparoscopic gallbladder removal, Jacques Perissat from Bordeaux, had been interested in smashing stones with lithotripsy for a long time. He possessed considerable experience and had refined a method of breaking up gallstones with an ultrasonic lithotripter inserted into the gallbladder through a five-millimeter trocar. In October 1988 he laparoscopically removed a collapsed, empty gallbladder and thus joined Mouret and Dubois in a creative geographic triangle to place France in the vanguard of laparoscopic gallstone treatment.[30] The important facts about the three surgeons in the "French connection" are (a) an association with gynecologists and familiarity with their laparoscopic techniques, (b) a drive to learn a new procedure, and (c) prior knowledge of a technique that contributed to success (Mouret, gynecology; Dubois, expert biliary surgeon; Perissat, gallbladder lithotripsy).

Then, as Litynski observed, "Personal contact and exchange provided the catalyst to the spread of LC in France. . . . News of the French work in LC soon swept beyond the country's borders. It reached Cuschieri in Scotland, Katkhouda in southern France, Klaiber in Switzerland, Phillips in Los Angeles, Troidl in Germany and others."[31] Two important events followed when Perissat presented a video of his laparoscopic gallbladder removal technique at the April 1989 SAGES meeting in Louisville and then three weeks later Dubois's paper appeared in the *Annals of Surgery.*

The First Gallbladder Falls to the Laparoscope in the United States

The Year Was 1988

On June 22, 1988, the first laparoscopic cholecystectomy was performed in the United States.[32] It was this tenuous innovative step that started American surgeons down the path that today is a congested laparoscopic interstate highway. It was also an era of rapid growth of diagnostic technology: CT scans, MRIs, ultrasound, PET scans, angiography, and so forth. Endoscopy was another extremely busy clinical activity being used by gastroenterologists and chest surgeons, and as a diagnostic tool by a few general surgeons. Hard on the heels of laparoscopic cholecystectomy were improvements in the laparoscopic instruments needed for a growing number of more complex minimally invasive operations.

J. Barry McKernan was an outlier.

William Saye was a talented laparoscopic surgeon, a gynecologist. McKernan's and Saye's personal arcs—linked through special knowledge and skills with a laparoscope—connected to make surgical history. McKernan followed an eclectic drummer who led him into areas of study unfamiliar to a majority of general surgeons. In 1999, McKernan wrote in the *World Journal of Surgery,* "During the period of training that followed my internship I went back to school to get a PhD in pharmacology. During this time I developed a relationship with the department of urology, pharmacology, and internal medicine; and I learned to perform urological procedures, mainly cystoscopy and endoscopy, so my familiarity with endoscopes was developed."[33] In other words, McKernan sought to learn and refine what would become his laparoscopic skills at a time when few surgeons had even a fleeting knowledge of minimally invasive operations.

McKernan moved to a small town in Alabama following his training, just as Erich Muhe had moved to a small German town with a small community hospital. There, McKernan completed his Berry Plan military obligation. Also, in Alabama he began doing gastroscopy, endoscopy, and laparoscopy—mostly tubal ligations and culdoscopy (entering the belly cavity through the vagina—a procedure that in 2009 became a form of natural orifices transluminal endoscopic surgery [NOTES]). McKernan describes working on laparoscopic appendectomy in 1978, two years before Kurt Semm performed the first "lap appy." McKernan admits, "I was working on laparoscopic appendectomy in 1978 but was persuaded by my partners to stop because they quite honestly thought we would incur medical/legal problems. I did not revisit laparoscopy for a long time after that."[34] McKernan bided his time, doing as many laparoscopic cases as possible.

This pattern of dedicated practice defines outliers.

When McKernan moved to Atlanta in 1983, he was the only general surgeon performing laparoscopy. William Saye, chief of obstetrics and gynecology at Kennestone Hospital in Marietta, Georgia, at the time, began working with the accomplished gynecologist James Daniel in Nashville. Saye brought patients to Nashville to learn more about advanced "pelviscopy,"[35] the term gynecologist Kurt Semm had used to rename laparoscopy. Barry McKernan went along with Saye to Nashville and operated with the two gynecologists. This was particularly remarkable because, as I have suggested, a majority of general surgeons in the 1980s didn't think of gynecologists or urologists as real surgeons.

The lightbulb flashed in McKernan's mind in April 1988 in Nashville. It was during a case in which Dr. Daniel was cutting and removing scar tissue around the liver. McKernan spied the nearby gallbladder. It was a moment of overwhelming significance because he was *prepared* for it. "The idea of removing a gallbladder by that technique came to my mind for the first time," McKernan recalled.

He said to Daniel, "We can remove a gallbladder."

Daniel replied, "Why not?"[36]

This sequence of events experienced by a surgeon working with gynecologists, learning their laparoscopic moves, peering from the pelvis up north to the liver—and noticing a familiar green bag—occurred, it seems, to these Americans just as it had to Erich Muhe when working with a gyne-cologist in 1985. McKernan and Saye returned to Georgia from Nashville. They fell into the routine of their customary clinical work. Perhaps the two would have left it at that, were it not for another act of serendipity. They discovered that Kurt Semm was giving a gynecology seminar at Johns Hopkins in Baltimore. McKernan and Saye decided to attend. There, they beamed at videos of advanced laparoscopy, including one of a laparoscopic appendectomy.

Immediately, they knew they could remove a gallbladder laparoscopically.

But they had no instruments. So they bought them from Semm. McK-ernan remembered, "Since in those days endoscopic instruments were in very short supply in our hospital . . . we decided to buy our own instru-ments at our own cost. Semm took us over and we wrote him a check, at that point it was $20,000.00."[37] They modified the instruments to work with a laser. Why use a laser? One reason was that gynecologists had been extensively sued for accidents involving burning the bowel using cautery.

In the meantime, May 1988 arrived, and McKernan and Saye performed a laparoscopic appendix removal, the first in the United States. The two were rising to prominence in their respective fields. But not without criti-cism. Appendectomy through an incision was a safe operation. Why make it complicated? Why the gimmick of a scope? It was the sheer force of their creative personalities that ignited the final scene in the story of surgical laparoscopy in the United States.

That same year, at another gynecology seminar in Augusta, Georgia, Saye was teaching laparoscopy. Barry McKernan was there as well. And, as serendipity would have it once again, lining up as one of the soon-to-be brilliant stars in the newly created universe of minimally invasive general surgery, Eddie Joe Reddick was at the conference teaching laser hemor-rhoid treatment.[38]

The three excited laser and laparoscopy enthusiasts met.

They talked. Reddick was looking for other applications of laser tech-nology. As McKernan writes, "We exchanged our experiences and when I told him we had done a laparoscopic appendectomy and that I was going to remove a gallbladder laparoscopically, he became excited. He immedi-ately went to the lab where the laparoscopy was done on rabbits and spent the rest of the day learning laparoscopy."[39] At dinner one night at the con-ference McKernan, Reddick, and Saye drew pictures of gallbladders on napkins and devised an original way to take out the globular gallbladder and its stones.[40]

Historically, barbers and surgeons had a common interest, and in the 1700s this mutual alignment resulted in the formation of the Company of Barbers and Surgeons under Henry VIII's reign. The familiar red and white barber pole was the icon of this relationship until surgeons broke away and formed their own association. In an odd parody of medical history, it was in a barber shop that Bill Saye encountered a woman who bemoaned her crampy, intermittent abdominal pains. Saye recognized her symptoms as those caused by gallstones. He saw opportunity in her distress. And after describing a new operation he was planning to perform on the appropriate patient, she insisted on being the first to undergo the procedure, exclaiming, "I want to have it now!"[41]

On June 22, 1988, Barry McKernan and Bill Saye performed the first laparoscopic gallbladder removal in North America. They did so in Marietta, Georgia. Rather than in a prestigious academic medical center, they performed the operation across the street in a community hospital, a political act that would be repeated throughout the country in the ensuing years. The operation took three hours. They did not have a clip applicator and had to suture the duct and artery. Although routine today, it was very cumbersome then to control the cystic artery and duct in this fashion without clips.

Eddie Joe Reddick became obsessed with the idea of laparoscopic gallbladder removal. He dedicated himself to working to become an expert laparoscopic surgeon. He decided to solve the duct- and artery-control problem by inventing a clip applicator and worked on the new instrumentation with the U.S. Surgical Company. He and Doug Olsen performed their first *laser* laparoscopic gallbladder removal in September 1988. And like Dubois a year before, Reddick had to convert his first laparoscopic attempt to an open operation. He and Olsen were successful on their second try.[42] The next morning, when Reddick walked into her room to make rounds, the woman stood fully dressed waiting to go home. Not in four or five days. But the *next* day. With almost no pain.

Clearly, as Erich Muhe had discovered in 1985, something special was happening with the less invasive gallbladder operation. Doug Olsen commented on their perceived originality in believing they had been first with laparoscopic cholecystectomy as quoted by Litynski: "At the time that we initiated our attempts, we were unaware of any successful laparoscopic cholecystectomy having been performed. Therefore in September of 1988 when a patient of mine was taken to the operating room as the first laparoscopic cholecystectomy, she was told she would be the first patient in the world to undergo this procedure."[43]

The Year Was 1989

The Berlin Wall fell, and the number of surgeons interested in lasers and laparoscopy grew rapidly. I will continue to rely on Litynski's rich trove of historical data to sketch out this crowded year in the laparoscope's story. Virtually none of this material is available in print or other form. Litynski cleverly tape-recorded the pioneers' recollections and had the wisdom to record them in his remarkable book, from which I am borrowing with gratitude.

Jonathan Sackier, a surgeon in London, traveled to the United States in late 1988 and eventually joined Berci's group at Cedars-Sinai Medical Center in Los Angeles. Ed Phillips from Cedars-Sinai at the time was on his way to Paris to learn about the new laparoscopic gallbladder operation from Dubois. Then, in early 1989, after visiting Nashville, Berci and Phillips returned to Los Angeles to work on what they had learned from Reddick and Olsen. And with Brendan J. Carroll they experimented on dogs and then moved on to patients.[44] In early summer of 1989 another rising star, Robert J. Fitzgibbons Jr., went to Nashville to observe Reddick and Olsen before returning to Creighton University, where he spent six months working out laparoscopic cholecystectomy. At about the same time, Joseph B. Petelin from Kansas, who was interested in laser applications for general surgery, heard about Reddick's course and traveled to Houston to take the course from Reddick and Saye.[45] And in St. Louis, Nat Soper was working on pigs to determine whether cautery was as safe as the laser when used to dissect the gallbladder off of the liver.

At the SAGES meeting in Louisville in 1989, Jacques Perissat showed his soon-to-be famous video of his method of laparoscopic cholecystectomy. Little interest ensued. According to Fredrick Greene, "I do not think Perissat impressed and convinced people about laparoscopy. . . . There was really very little interest in laparoscopy in SAGES at that time."[46]

In Chicago, surgeon Sung-Tao Ko, who already had experience with transanal endoscopic microsurgery, having studied with Gerhard Buess in Tubingen, Germany, also took Semm's course on pelviscopy, operating on pigs. Ko became yet another surgeon who believed that laparoscopic gallbladder removal was possible (unaware that it had already been done). He, like the others before him, ordered instruments from Semm and studied his textbook. Then, Dr. Mohan Airan, then head of surgery at Chicago's Mount Sinai Hospital, caught Ko's enthusiasm and went to Kiev to observe Kurt Semm at work. Returning, Airan and Ko performed a few laparoscopic cholecystectomies, believing they were the first in the world. When they contacted Berci, according to Litynski, Airan stated, "We learned that Olsen and Reddick had performed twenty laparoscopic cholecystectomies at the time. We, Berci and Phillips, had performed three each."[47]

But it was at the 1989 annual meeting of the ACS that Reddick and Olsen showed their dramatic video of laparoscopic cholecystectomy to a stunned audience of general surgeons. Rather than applying for a slot in the scientific

program, they demonstrated their video at the Storz and U.S. Surgical industry booths on the massive exhibition floor. Crowds of muttering surgeons
gathered around the video presentation. The two innovators alternated in
describing what was on the screen. In Olsen's words, "We had literally hundreds of surgeons mesmerized, fixed to the video screen."[48] And although
Nat Soper had agreed regarding the seminal impact of the Reddick-Olsen
video, Litynski recorded Soper's somewhat different take on the overall
reaction of surgeons who viewed the video: "Hundreds of surgeons viewed
this movie, most of whom left the area muttering and shaking their heads
saying it would never work, whereas the remaining few rushed head-on
to try to buy instruments and sign up for courses."[49]

Perhaps the concluding sense of forward motion of the laparoscopic revolution should be accorded to Dr. Carol Scott-Conner, who performed a
literature search at the time while at the University of Mississippi. She
found no publications for two reasons: the journals in which Reddick and
Olsen had originally published were not on MEDLINE, the database Scott-
Conner used (the laparoscopic cholecystectomy articles were in laser
journals). And second, Dubois first published only in French. Litynski
summarizes Carol Scott-Conner's predicament in learning laparoscopic
cholecystectomy as her experience reflects what was happening all over
the country. Litynski revealed, "Scott-Conner's account calls attention to
a unique feature of the introduction of laparoscopy into surgical practice:
a professor of surgery, head of a university clinic, waited to take a course
taught by a former resident—and private surgeon to boot."[50]

Litynski offers concrete reasons why the Reddick-Olsen video was a
milestone in the development of laparoscopy in general surgery: (a) they
established organized courses in place of one-on-one teaching, (b) they
brought laparoscopic technology from subspecialist to general surgeons,
(c) they took training out of the universities, (d) they popularized use of the
laser, and (e) they inaugurated outpatient laparoscopic cholecystectomy.[51]

Thereafter, laparoscopic cholecystectomy ran rampant throughout the
country and around the world. The chaos that resulted from the uncontrolled spread of laparoscopic cholecystectomy resisted what few controls
existed and flared in popularity with only loosely organized credentialing
in many hospitals. The greatest social change was that now the demand
for less aggressive operations was coming from patients. General surgeons
weren't advertising their new wares; the instrument and telescope indus-
tries were doing it for us. Nonetheless, soon we were racing to be the first
kid on the block with a shiny new laparoscope.

A final comment highlights how tenuous laparoscopic cholecystectomy's
role was in the practices of most surgeons. As Barry McKernan remembers

the events, their first video camera was from a company called Wolfe. But when the president of Wolfe watched them operate one day, he demurred that the procedure would never be accepted. Also, the first clip applier was made by a company called Weck. Their open division produced clip applicators for traditional open surgery. The Weck laparoscopic division refused to make clip applicators for minimally invasive surgery. In a moment of flawed judgment, these two manufacturing giants ignored the biggest emerging surgical instrument market since the production of scalpels.[52]

The Year Was 1990

The year 1990 in American surgical circles bubbled over with the frenzied activity of general surgeons racing across the country in search of weekend courses to learn the basic elements of laparoscopic gallbladder surgery. Approximately 25,000 general surgeons struggled to master the new minimally invasive gallbladder removal technique. It was the year I took the Reddick-Saye course in Marietta. Some of the courses were less than appropriate—one might reasonably say unethical—because they offered no hands-on operative experience with animals. Those surgeons with no hands-on experience placed their patients in the position of being their guinea pigs.

Early in 1990, the wormy appendix fell to the laparoscope. Then, groin hernias were approached through the televised wizardry of the laparoscope and repaired from inside the belly cavity. Less invasive but more complicated groin hernia operations spawned a debate regarding what the best overall hernia repair might be—a dialogue that continues to rage in surgical circles today. Spleens, stomachs, colons—even the secretive adrenal glands perched atop the kidneys and buried in fat—were soon displayed on TV monitors.

For aggressive, knife-wielding surgeons, the switch to indirect surgery wasn't easy. In many respects, the laparoscopic revolution didn't feel like a success at first. In the early 1990s, disagreements arose between the private community and academic surgeons regarding who should do laparoscopic gallbladder surgery. Credentialing issues arose. Surgical educators today still have only rough guidelines on how many operations a trainee or established practitioner should perform to become a capable laparoscopic surgeon.

Nonetheless, the emergence of uneven surgical expertise from the chaos of the early days of the laparoscopic revolution still haunts our profession today and no doubt will for decades to come.

PART 3

Telescopes Replace Scalpels: The Struggle to Maintain Surgical Competence Begins

Innovative Surgeons, New Laparoscopic Operations, and the Dilemma of Patient Safety

It's a pickle of a paradox: As our knowledge and expertise increase, our creativity and ability to innovate tend to taper off.

Janet Rae-Dupree, *New York Times*, December 30, 2007

When innovative surgeons who take unaccredited courses return with uncertified skills to introduce nonvalidated treatments in trusting patients, we have a recipe for disaster.

Martin F. McKneally, MD, PhD, *World Journal of Surgery*, 1999

A Dubious Sales Pitch

In an October 20, 2008, *U.S. News and World Report* article, a patient's photograph revealed complete recovery after he underwent a no-incision NOTES (natural orifices transluminal endoscopic surgery, done through the mouth or any other natural opening, such as the vagina, ear, or anus) removal of his appendix. The operation, according to the report, opened the way to allow the patient to "drive across country to grad school."[1]

The problems with this report highlight major issues surrounding the introduction of new and innovative technology into surgical practice. Of most concern is the idea of definitions: What exactly is innovation as compared with the modification of an operation? When do significant alterations in an operation become experimental? For a potential patient, it's a matter of deciding whether the operation you are offered is an established, standard procedure or is *nonvalidated*—it has not been subjected to scientific scrutiny.[2] Somewhere between these two positions are operations that may require a minor alteration to an existing procedure.

In the case of the NOTES (no incision) appendectomy described above, the informed-consent discussion provided by the surgeon would have involved revealing the experimental nature of the operation. In the article the author states it took two weeks for the patient to convince his mother that the NOTES appendectomy operation was safe. That is an issue because acute appendicitis is usually an emergency requiring surgery within hours, not weeks—assuming the patient isn't being treated solely with antibiotics. More important, if this patient had undergone a laparoscopic appendectomy, or for that matter, a traditional open appendectomy, he could have driven cross country a week or two later.

One of the experts quoted in the article stated that it would take two to three years for through-the-mouth no-incision NOTES appendectomy to become mainstream. That was 2008. It hasn't happened. Chances are reasonably good that it won't occur for years, if ever.[3] We're not training surgical residents how to do intricate robotic appendectomies, let alone the technically challenging and experimental NOTES procedures. Thus, in general surgical practice both open and laparoscopic appendectomies are the safest *established* operations.

This is an example of an untested innovation pounced on by the media. It represents good reading by a public breastfed on high-technology medicine. The reality is that NOTES in many applications may never fly. This is not to discredit innovative surgeons working on NOTES projects. I'm confirming that our trainees are not being taught this approach in any significant way because of its technical challenges. However, the media has established an unreasonable expectation. Besides, there is probably a technology we still haven't developed that may replace the idea of poking holes through perfectly normal organs like the stomach (which is what NOTES requires) in order to remove another organ (e.g., the appendix).

A discussion of surgical innovation is critical because of the time-honored tradition of constantly working toward better cures with less pain and suffering for patients. Recently, a report stated, "The dominance of innovation in surgery is hardly surprising, as most surgeons innovate on a daily basis, tailoring therapies and operations to the intrinsic uniqueness of every patient and their disease. Surgeons currently have in their armamentarium in excess of 2500 different procedures; the focus of recent advances in surgery is less on adding to the sheer number of procedures, but rather to ensure improving success of the available treatments."[4] In truth, you face both the constant addition of new less invasive operations as well as the modification of those procedures. This is why understanding the role of innovation is crucial to your preparation for a major operation.

The Disequilibrating Effect of New Procedures on Surgical Competence

Think of disequilibrating as setting up an imbalance, a loss of balance as if tottering on one foot, a loss of equilibrium.[5] Something unsettling occurs when the surgeon tries a new operation. Uncertainty sets in. The overall level of competence the surgeon possesses shifts when he or she tries to do an unfamiliar procedure. Looming in the picture is the need to negotiate yet another steep learning curve, where the most mistakes occur in the early cases. Surviving in clinical practice is about maintaining capability. The best surgeons do the same operations repetitively and thus maintain their skills.

Competence requires training, repetition, and experience. Board certification, although not perfect, establishes a level of documented capability, but it does *not* include ongoing assessment of new skills as complex technology is introduced into a surgeon's practice. Recertification is supposed to ensure competence with new techniques. But as one author wrote in 1999, "The rapid expansion of new surgical technology creates moral hazard for surgeons forced to learn challenging and dangerous new techniques such as endoscopic cardiac valve replacement or gastric fundoplication."[6] The last operation mentioned (fundoplication) involves wrapping the stomach around the lower end of the gullet to prevent stomach acid from washing into the esophagus, causing heartburn. Performing the operation laparoscopically requires major changes in the technical aspects of the procedure as compared with the skills used doing the procedure open (through an incision). Some surgeons believe they can do the operation well laparoscopically because they did it well through an incision. As a consequence, failure rates for laparoscopic fundoplication can be unacceptably high.[7]

Of course, there was no mention in the upbeat NOTES appendectomy article about how surgeons might learn to safely perform such a technically advanced operation. Nor was there any suggestion that multidisciplinary surgical teams are required, not just the skills of a single surgeon—a requirement not achievable in many smaller hospitals. No mention was made of the horrible NOTES disasters that will inevitably result if the trend toward inadequate training in new surgical technology continues as the reality of the day. Yes, rock-filled gallbladders have been removed without an incision using NOTES technology. In one report, it took seven refusals to finally find a patient who wanted the new NOTES cholecystectomy.[8]

The dilemma facing surgeons and our surgical leadership regarding the best method of introducing complex technology and new operations has a long track record. For our purposes it encompasses the decades of the laparoscopic revolution and began when gynecologists first attempted to use the laparoscope to treat pelvic diseases. As I have done previously, I will divide our discussion into eras to create a framework that will shed light on the difficulty our profession has had defining innovative surgery. This adventure—deciding just what innovative surgery is—reflects light onto the larger issue of overall surgeon capability.

How Does a New Operation Develop?

Innovative surgical operations often have little or no track record when they are offered to patients. Remember, William Saye met the first patient in the United States to have a laparoscopic gallbladder operation in a barbershop! These procedures are performed because a few surgeons learn how to do them and collect small series of cases and report on them. Ideally, the innovative surgeon works on an animal model or cadavers initially, refining the new operation. Then, the surgeon offers the experimental procedure to the first patient. This is not unreasonable if the patient is well informed about the risks of the untested operation—something surgeons have done abysmally in the past, especially with some of the less invasive laparoscopic operations. Of course, moving ahead with innovations in minimally invasive surgery is the ultimate goal. As one observer stated in 2006, "It reminds me of 1989 when the first laparoscopic cholecystectomy videos were being shown. Even if a particular procedure doesn't pan out, the goal of pushing toward even less invasive, or even incisionless, surgery is a valuable journey for the lessons learned and the tools created."[9]

The ideal situation regarding informed consent was spelled out in a 2009 report contrasting surgeons' former minimal information exchange with patients with the modern obligation to provide patients with enough information to make a reasoned decision about surgery. Entitled "Informed Consent and the Surgeon," the report stated, "Armed with the tool of informed consent, surgeons now were expected to have a formal mechanism both to recognize patient autonomy and to address patients as self-determining moral agents."[10] It is critical for surgeons to respect their patients' right to decide what they want for treatment—or to elect no treatment in certain circumstances—and engage the patient in the process. True informed consent is the opposite of paternalism (when the surgeon tells the patient what is going to happen). In dire emergencies, paternalism is mandatory, assuming the patient's family wants all possible treatment to occur. But paternalism has no place in elective surgery.

For the most part, surgeons typically start to do a new operation with coaching from a colleague with extensive experience who scrubs with the surgeon. Or we take a short weekend course—the value and validity of these encounters have been challenged. For really innovative complex operations, such as opening up the scarred distal end of the gullet (esophagus) using an endoscope from the *inside* (rather than the traditional open or laparoscopic outside approach), the procedures cannot be learned alone. My colleague Dr. John Romanelli and his team at Baystate Medical Center traveled to Japan to learn the gullet-opening operation known as per oral endoscopic myotomy (POEM) from the original innovator. Then, they worked as a team to perform their first series of operations here in the United States. However, no-incision or NOTES operations, like laparoscopic gallbladder surgery before them—despite media attention, such as the anecdote that opened this chapter—have sparse data to support their introduction into mainstream surgical practice. These innovative operations should remain in academic centers until proven safe and effective.

What Is Surgical Innovation?

Surgeons modify common operations all the time.

We may not do a standard operation on the next patient exactly the way we did on the last patient. It could be something as routine as a different way of sewing mesh into place in a groin hernia repair. Perhaps the surgeon tries different types of sutures—perhaps absorbable (dissolving) rather than permanent or a different caliber of suture material—or uses tissue glue instead of sutures to fix the mesh. Sometimes we do things differently because the anatomy is abnormal in a particular patient. Occasionally, we discover unsuspected pathology that must be dealt with in a slightly modified way.

Most of these alterations or variations of a standard operation are relatively minor. They are small changes in an otherwise well-designed surgical procedure. There is nothing particularly original in most of the little tricks we teach our residents. In fact, no two surgeons do the same operation in exactly the same way. A surgical educator in the past commented about residents learning bits of technique here and there from different surgeon teachers as if "collecting a posy of other men's flowers." To expand the metaphor, no two surgeons carry the same bouquet. And if we don't pass on our hard-earned surgical skills, then like delicate flowers they die and are lost forever. But they are not truly innovative.

Definitions—What Are We Talking About?

Innovation in general is the act of introducing something new into the world. It may also mean using something like a standard surgical instrument in a completely different way. For surgeons, true innovation means developing an original instrument design or designing a completely new operation, as well as wedding the new instrument to a novel operation. It almost always means building on something that already existed—working with someone else's innovation. A 2016 report stated, "Surgical innovation can be thought of as the introduction of new concepts and ideas or, more specifically, as the practical use of a new technology, technique, or some combination of both."[11]

Consider the agonizing discussions among clinicians and academicians on the characteristics of innovative surgery that have occurred since the 1990s. As one author wrote in a report entitled "Innovation in Surgery: From Imagination to Implementation," "Surgeons perhaps more than any other specialists, recognize the concept of furthering the current state of the art by making conscious changes, whether by tweaking how a surgical procedure is done to push the envelop of minimally invasive techniques, finding novel means of advancing surgical education in the face of work hour restrictions, or advancing quality initiatives in an era of health care reform."[12] The innovative pathway described included four steps: *plan, do, check, act.* The author also noted innovations in surgical education with work-hour restrictions as well as the use of physician extenders to combat the surgical workforce shortages.[13]

Innovative Surgery from the 1990s through 2000

In a 1990 report in *JAMA* entitled "The Case for Reassessment of Health Care Technology," the authors wrote, highlighting obsolete surgical procedures, "Health care technology has a life cycle—it is developed, comes into use, becomes obsolete, and is dropped from use."[14] The authors note that most medical technological advances occur incrementally, noting the increasingly less invasive nature of surgery. The Blue Cross Blue Shield Medical Necessity Project and the American College of Physicians Clinical Efficacy Assessment Project represent attempts to reduce costs as well as unsafe new technology. Laparoscopic cholecystectomy was born in the throes of the 1980s concerns about unnecessary surgery. The report noted that in 1989, "A new Agency for Health Care Policy and Research was established to provide federal leadership in technology assessment."[15] The authors concluded (incorrectly regarding gallstone treatments, as our story of the rise of laparoscopy has demonstrated), "In a time of rapid technologic change, when such technologies as lasers and lithotripsy are replacing conventional surgical therapy, reassessing this field seems particularly important."[16] The same year the *New England Journal of Medicine* published an article that concluded (regarding technology assessment), "In an era when government, insurance companies, and employers insist on cost containment, the new technology assessment can be the most powerful tool physicians have to protect the interests of their patients."[17]

Surgeons initially paid too little attention to the safety implications of the laparoscopic surgery revolution. As stated in an article in *JAMA* in 1991, "Over the course of the last 1 year, laparoscopic cholecystectomy has evolved from being unavailable in most communities to being a commonly used technique for cholecystectomy."[18] In this report, reference to common bile duct injuries and fatal bowel injuries served to temper the enthusiasm for this general surgery innovation at the time. The authors concluded, "We can hope that with the further expansion and application of laparoscopy, critical analysis of *prospective* [original italics] trials on the outcome of such procedures will be accomplished before reliable techniques or procedures of the immediate past are abandoned."[19]

A particularly nasty question remains before us: Can surgeons actually randomize (offer one operation to this patient and another operation to that patient) their patients to do research on new innovations? In other words, can they offer patients one of two or more treatment choices and expect them to understand what is at stake? Can a surgeon adequately describe the risks and benefits of an untested operation? How do you describe your expertise with a new operation if you have virtually no experience doing it? A report published in 1992 at the outset of the laparoscopic revolution in general surgery listed reasons why a randomized controlled study of laparoscopic gallbladder removal was never performed.[20] This is a list of reasons why you must be aware of how true surgical innovation can sneak into surgical practice:

- The only true placebo is a sham operation, which is unethical.
- It isn't possible to blind the operating surgeon or the patient to which procedure is being done.
- How do you measure individual surgeon skill with the new procedure?
- How do you calculate the bias of a surgeon who is wildly enthusiastic about the new operation?
- How do you account for differences in hospitals when doing multi-institutional studies (pooling information from many hospitals involved in the study)?
- What if patients only want the old or the new operation?
- What if the innovative surgeon doesn't want to share his or her innovation in order to keep a corner on the market?

Technology Follies—The Uncritical Acceptance of Medical Innovation

In 1993, Dr. David A. Grimes of the University of California published a prescient report (whose title I have used for this section) that defined many of the mistakes physicians have made over the years when introducing new technologies into the practice of medicine.[21] He explored his own field of obstetrics and gynecology for evidence of poorly conceived treatments and questionable technology. Dr. Grimes documented the ineffectiveness of a number of gynecologic practices, including measuring estrogen products in the urine of pregnant women to monitor the well-being of the fetus, fetal monitoring (causing increased risk of a cesarean or forceps delivery), and using episiotomy, which lacks scientific support. He also documented the uselessness of electricity to speed up bone healing and the failure of bone marrow transplants.[22] He correctly gives credit to the innovation of tubal sterilization, a less invasive operation performed in the outpatient department and used widely throughout the world.

However, Dr. Grimes didn't anticipate the overwhelming replacement of open operations by minimally invasive procedures when he wrote about laparoscopic-assisted vaginal hysterectomy: "Courses to teach this technique to gynecologists are proliferating exponentially, despite the absence of any randomized controlled trials showing that this operation is preferable to standard vaginal hysterectomy."[23] He was correct in that, at first, there were no good studies to support the safety of laparoscopic-assisted vaginal hysterectomy. The use of a morcellator (a tool to laparoscopically "chew up" fibroids for removal through a small trocar sleeve) proved dangerous for unsuspecting patients. But as we now know, laparoscopically assisted vaginal hysterectomy was refined and became standardized. Dr. Grimes pinpointed the unsolved issue of whether or not short courses train physicians to a significant level of competence.

What Dr. Grimes has given us is a clever assessment of why, in 1993, so many barriers existed that served to block the proper evaluation of new technology. He suggested that the following factors were responsible for errors in the critical assessment of medical technology:[24]

- "Seduction by authority"—practitioners do what thought leaders tell them to do without questioning why (see Chapter 10 on the surgical personality).
- "The false idol of technology"—physicians and patients alike love new gadgets; they want them badly enough to subject themselves to untested medical advances without understanding the risks; besides, doctors are paid for doing things to patients (sometimes using untested technology).

- "The inevitable tendency to let sleeping dogmas lie"—or as we often explain lamely, "We've always done it that way" without critical reassessment, or often ignoring the first published studies that prove the dogma to be wrong. The story of laparoscopy—like the stories of antisepsis and anesthesia—are pockmarked with arrogant cannonades of rejection by our professional leaders.

- "Medical education produces 'scientific illiterates' "—medical education (surgical education is a slave to this error) stuffs doctors with useless information that does nothing to teach them how to reason, especially when it comes to evaluating new technology; this deficiency is complicated by poor oversight.

Grimes cautioned, "A double standard in tests and treatments prevails. While new medicines must have rigorous proof of efficacy and safety before clinical use, tests and operations do not. Specifically, *there is no Food and Drug Administration for the surgeon* [my italics]."[25] He adds a final warning that all surgical patients in the 21st century considering a new laparoscopic or robotic operation should keep in mind: "Too little money is spent on comparative trials, and too much is spent on sales and marketing. Powerful advertising forces from industry and economic incentives promote acceptance of new, unproven technologies without critical assessment."[26]

How Are New Operations (Supposed to Be) Evaluated?

There is a proper way to study new drugs, tests, and procedures. Doctors are supposed to get permission to study and use untested technology on real patients. The crucial issue is to decide what represents research on human subjects versus what is a lesser degree of modification of an existing operation. None of what is to follow—the scientific, carefully controlled, and reasonable ways to evaluate new operations—occurred when laparoscopy was introduced into general surgery.

Usually, a physician gets an idea and begins an investigation by publishing a *case report*. Sometimes several cases are reported in a small series. There are no controls. This means there is no information in the report about how the new operation compares with a traditional operation.

The next-best study would *compare the new operation to a control group* who underwent a traditional procedure (lap chole vs. open gallbladder removal). In this method, there is still a problem of selection bias regarding which patients are assigned to what group—do the healthier patients get placed in the new operation study group? Is that why they do better?

Best of all is what researchers call a *prospective double-blind, randomized, placebo-controlled study or trial (RCT)* characterized by investigators collecting data going forward and distributing known and unknown factors (patient health status, surgeon experience, etc.) equally between the study group and the controls. Patients are assigned randomly to the new operation, for example, or the traditional operation. Yet despite a general agreement among physicians that RCTs are the best way to evaluate new technology, as of the year Erich Muhe performed the first laparoscopic cholecystectomy in 1985, only 10–20 percent of all new technology introduced into the practice of surgery in the prior 40 years had been assessed using this rigorous method of evaluation.[27] I'll review some of the ethical issues squirming beneath the surface of 21st-century surgical inventiveness.

The Ethics of Surgical Innovation

By the end of the creative decade of the 1990s, which fostered minimally invasive general surgery operations, a few academic surgeons began questioning the moral obligation surgeons had toward patients to whom they were offering new, less traumatic and invasive procedures. A valuable contribution to the issue of informed consent came from a report by Dr. Martin F. McKneally, who emphasized the term *nonvalidated procedures* as a more honest substitution for the expression we've been using, namely *innovative* surgery.[28] McKneally stresses the implications of the word *innovative* as "a seductive connotation of added value in a progressive society. . . . The term accurately captures the sense of moral hazard that should be attached to their use in vulnerable and trusting patients before they become widely accepted throughout the expert medical community."[29] You would be wise to remember McKneally's admonition that the word *innovation* carries with it an unearned and seductive suggestion of added value, of something that very well may not exist.

Patients trust their surgeon to do the right thing.

The surgeon is guardian of the patient, and that commitment is expressed in such rituals as scrubbing, draping, and approaching the unconscious patient with respect and dignity. The public expects the surgeon to do only what they have agreed on during their exchange of information that constitutes informed consent. The OR staff represent a collective moral force working in the patient's best interest to protect the patient from harm. But, as McKneally writes, "The discipline that provides this protection is under increased pressure as more entrepreneurial and sometimes less patient-centered interests of equipment manufacturers, insurers, and others penetrate the sanctuary of the operating room."[30] This penetration of commercial interests into the sanctity of the operating room is even truer today than in the earlier decades of laparoscopic innovation. As practice expenses grow and payments to hospitals shrink, the least expensive surgical equipment may get the nod.

McKneally's second concern involves the way in which new technology may compromise a surgeon's capability—the ethical dilemma at the center of this book. Surgeons have an obligation to continue to refine their expertise and to not engage in performing operations with which they have little experience. Yet, over a decade ago, McKneally wrote, "Practicing surgeons can rarely return to the sanctuary of residency training to learn under supervision, and university surgeons are no more prepared than community practitioners to learn, develop, or teach nonvalidated new procedures, which may have originated in an entrepreneurial biotechnology company."[31] In this regard, in an article entitled "The Place of Trust in Our Changing Surgical Environment," Dr. F. William Heer wrote, "The primary relationship between the patient and the physician, in which the patient's best interests are the principal ethical obligation and goal of the physician, has been disrupted by a third party whose commercial interests are not necessarily similarly motivated."[32] So the technical challenges of surgical innovation in the United States frequently have a travel companion—financial gain. Similarly, Dr. Kenton C. Bodily eloquently wrote: "Are we to be gladiators in the surgical arena vying to be the first to try some new technology or unproven procedure? Being the first surgeon may provide us with an ego trip, increased peer recognition, a sound byte on the evening news, or improved marketability of our practice, but being the first patient may entail a prolonged procedure, a higher risk of complications, disfigurement, or even death."[33]

Innovative Surgery from the 2000s through 2010

Through the exciting first decade of the 21st century, the issue of defining innovative surgery remained stubbornly unresolved. In a 2002 report entitled "Ethical Regulations for Innovative Surgery: The Last Frontier," the authors remarked, "There are regulations and guidelines for participation of human subjects in biomedical and behavioral research, and there are federal laws pertaining to human testing of drugs and devices, but there are currently no clear federal regulations pertaining to innovative surgical procedures."[34] These authors highlighted reasons for the lack of oversight by noting that in their study, two-thirds of surgeons responding to a survey "stated that government regulations for the protection of human subjects of innovative surgery would not be appropriate."[35] It seems clear from these reports that the problem of determining what is research and what is just a modification of a standard operation centers on surgeons not agreeing with each other. The authors referred to knowledge deficits among surgeons regarding innovation by stating, "There are uncertainties and disagreements among surgeons as to what an acceptable variation on an existing surgical technique is versus what is a new or innovative technique that would ideally warrant IRB (hospital Internal Review Board) evaluation and the patient's specific informed consent for an experimental procedure or a research study."[36] In another survey published three years later in 2005, the same authors reported that surgeons scored lowest on their knowledge of governmental bodies regulating clinical research. In fact, only 50 percent of surgeons surveyed thought that comparing a truly new operation to a standard operation was research.[37]

Many of these surgeons are from the era of the laparoscopic revolution and participated in and witnessed the greatest violation of trust by surgeons in the history of modern surgery. In other words, having recognized in retrospect the failure of appropriate oversight and regulation at the outset of the laparoscopic revolution, now 15 years later some surgeons still believe that they should not be held accountable by a federal regulatory body. The authors quoted above concluded (from further research on surgeons' attitudes about innovation) that "most surgeons do recognize true research activities and respond accordingly, but for certain forms of human subject research (e.g. retrospective reviews, cohort studies), the surgeons demonstrated a lower level of appreciation for the federal rules."[38] Nonetheless, they concluded in their 2005 study that "innovative surgery is not clearly defined, nor is it formally regulated by governing bodies as is the development of new drugs and medical devices."[39]

Thus, numerous reports published midway through a second decade of surgical innovation (following the introduction of laparoscopic general surgery into mainstream practice) have confirmed that there was little agreement on the best method for introducing creative changes in surgery. These reports support the view that surgeons seemed ill-informed about the line between innovation and small changes they could reasonably be expected to make in their surgical techniques. In fairness to all surgeons, as I stated earlier, every operation can fall outside of the framework of that procedure as difficult anatomy or pathology dictate the need to make technical modifications. Thus, you can appreciate a surgeon's reluctance to support federal meddling into what is an operative tweak versus basic research versus a reasonable modification of a standard technique.

A Reiteration of Uncertainty about Surgical Innovation

In 2008, the Society of University Surgeons wrote a position statement on the subject of surgical innovation that begins, "The field of surgery has a unique culture and rich tradition of innovation. Surgeons are trained to perform continuous situational assessment, decision analysis, and improvisation in preparation for the challenges and creativity required by nearly every clinical case."[40] Tailoring treatments, therefore, is a part of virtually every patient encounter in the operating room. And to highlight the driving issue of innovation in surgery, the authors noted: "The surgical innovator has historically been allowed to 'tinker' with procedures, introducing modifications of varying degrees to the point that a procedure could arguably be called new. . . . But there are currently no formal regulations that apply to surgical innovations."[41] The year was 2008, and there still were no formal regulations of innovative surgery.

Looking back to the beginning of the laparoscopic revolution, we see the impact of this impasse regarding a definition of innovative procedures. As the innovator of a new way to operate, Semm's gynecological instrument inventions, however, were *innovative* in the extreme. Before him none of his fellow gynecologists attempted to work deep in the pelvis using long, skinny instruments while looking through a scope or up at a television screen. And so when Erich Muhe used Semm's laparoscopic instruments to remove a gallbladder through a newly designed laparoscope, it was innovative and revolutionary. And even though Kurt Semm's pelviscopy-based procedures were becoming mainstream, laparoscopic gallbladder surgery was anything but a technological baby step.

The Challenges from Industry

More and more shiny new technology was hauled into the public arena of health care untested. But nonvalidated machinery cannot be allowed a place on the instrument table simply because of the crushing power of advertising and promotion by salespeople. The intrusion of business interests into the clinic and operating room isn't new. But special interests are more pervasive today than ever. There's a lot of money to be made in the world of the sick and dying.

In this regard, a report from 2010, "Physician Attitudes toward Industry: A View across Specialties," noted, "Physicians can readily access independent information about drugs, but surgical specialists rely on industry representatives for information about new devices and the training to use them, with industry representatives in the operating room."[42] Confirming this reality in an invited commentary on the report, Dr. Jo Buyske reminded us: "The success of the laparoscopic revolution hinged on the collaboration between surgeons and industry in developing the instruments that made basic and then advanced laparoscopy widely accessible. . . . The baby must not be thrown out with the bathwater. Physician-industry interactions are not all created equal, and it is incumbent on us to be sure that policymakers and patients understand the distinction."[43]

To highlight the unfinished business of defining surgical innovation and the quotations from surgical leaders, here are the titles of three reports from 2015: "Hey, I Just Did a New Operation! Introducing Innovative Procedures and Devices within an Academic Health Center";[44] "Assessing Awareness and Implementation of a Recommendation for Surgical Innovation Committees";[45] "Getting Clearer about Surgical Innovation—A New Definition and a New Tool to Support Responsible Practice."[46]

Thus, the debate regarding the precise nature of innovation is hardly over. For smart patients the essential message is to ask your surgeon about the nature of your operation, the possibility of using new technology, and the possibility of having to modify your operation. This discussion should be included in any conversation about informed consent with a surgeon. So, you might begin the dialogue by asking whether there is any possibility that your procedure might involve a real departure from the standard operation described to you. Consider further qualifying the answer by asking, If there is a possibility of innovation, will it involve a new, innovative *surgical technique*, or will it involve an *innovative device*?

The introduction of a less invasive way to remove the human gallbladder broke many rules of professional conduct *before* big business got into the act. Research and development dollars from industry have done much good, but the threat of uncontrolled innovation for patients remains largely without a public voice. As a surgical patient, you must be aware of the reality that the climate for safe surgical innovation within our hospital walls is still not uniformly oriented toward your personal welfare.

CHAPTER EIGHT

How Surgeons Discovered Learning Curves: Defining the Idea of a Capable Surgeon

This is the uncomfortable truth about teaching. . . . We want perfection without practice. Yet everyone is harmed if no one is trained
for the future. So learning is hidden, behind drapes and anesthesia
and elisions of language. Nor does the dilemma apply just to residents, physicians in training. In fact, the process of learning turns
out to extend longer than most people know.

Atul Gawande, *Complications: A Surgeon's Notes
on an Imperfect Science*, 2002

A Little Disaster Story

It happened in a small New England hospital. The name of the hospital
isn't important. But the disastrous result of a surgeon's incompetence is
another matter. From a number of public reports, we learn that not one,
but both tubes (ureters) draining urine from the kidneys to the bladder
were accidentally cut during a gynecologist's first robotic hysterectomy at
that hospital.[1] The magnitude of this technical misadventure is almost
impossible to imagine. But the case highlights everything you need to know
about learning curves.

Often, surgeons start doing robotic cases on their own in private hospitals after only a few supervised cases. The actual number of repetitions
of a specific case a novice must perform in order to become a minimally
capable robotic surgeon (according to many experts) is more like 35 to
50—or quite possibly for some operations, 200 or more repetitions. As I
have stated several times, this number is subject to many issues, the least
of which is the innate talent of the surgeon. More critical is the amount of

deliberate and repetitive practice the surgeon engages in to learn the new operation. On the other hand, the folks selling robotic systems as well as those peddling laparoscopic instruments state that there is no single training method for surgeons. Learning curves differ from one surgeon to another, according to these entrepreneurs. They insist without proof (without research studies) that there is no particular number of cases a surgeon must do to become a capable practitioner.

The argument hints at innate ability. But the diagonal dodge from reality evaporates quickly under the heat of scientific scrutiny. What is ironic about listening to this flawed line of reasoning from industry is that learning curves originated from industry itself. Modern medical device manufacturers and instrument makers seem not to know (or refuse to acknowledge) their own history. How many of them have heard of a pricing curve? And if they have, how can they deny the reality of performance (learning) curves?

Actually, it was the psychologist Hermann Ebbinghaus who described the learning curve phenomenon in 1885, although he didn't actually use the term.[2] He described aspects of memory and learning in his classic work. It is also known in industry as a cost curve, an efficiency curve, an improvement curve, and a start-up curve, as well as other aliases. In his book *The Learning Curve Deskbook*, Charles J. Teplitz refers to the learning curve: "Having been described as far back as the ninth century, the term learning curve is still the most commonly used term. As defined by experimental psychologists such as L. L. Thurstone, the learning curve is a graphical representation of the learning-by-doing phenomenon observed in people performing manual tasks."[3] Teplitz also noted that in the 1920s Theodore Paul Wright, studying the effect of learning on production costs, gathered manufacturing data from the construction of small aircraft and defined what he called the doubling effect. Teplitz states, "The doubling effect suggests that as the quantity produced doubles, the resources needed will be reduced to a percentage of the original requirements."[4]

Learning curves are complex, and some are mathematically derived to demonstrate a number of different phenomena. I will refer only to the general idea of documenting learning in surgery by looking at such parameters as time to complete a task (operation), number of errors created, number of postoperative complications, length of hospital stay, and so forth. Learning motor skills can also be demonstrated by examining different types of learning curves that reflect varying rates of learning for trainees of different innate skill levels, the impact of coaching and feedback, and final levels of accomplishment.

One stumbling point is the term *steep learning curve*. Figure 8.1 shows a rapid increase in skill level over a short period of time (the dashed line) reflecting the impact of coaching and feedback, and a shallower curve representing slower mastery of a skill (the dotted line) of a solo learner without coaching and feedback. In the use of deliberate practice with immediate feedback and being pushed out of one's comfort zone, the learner quickly ascends the steep part of the curve where rapid learning occurs with expert coaching.

Steep suggests a difficult curve to master. Many errors may be made early in the learner's experience. Metaphorically, you may think of climbing up a Mount Everest of a learning curve as the ultimate psychomotor challenge (for complex laparoscopic operations) in which a lot of the most difficult climbing (learning) is accomplished early in the ascent. If the learner is less innately talented, the curve is more gradual on the vertical axis whether with deliberate practice or not. The learner never reaches the high level of skill mastery of the innately talented student with or without coaching and feedback. In the surgical literature, steep learning curves serve as a warning that considerable training is required up front with careful supervision and skills laboratory training to become capable with a particular

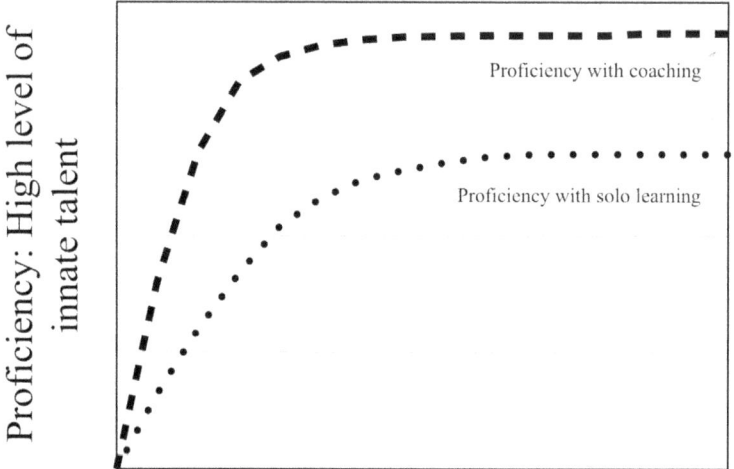

Time or Repetition

Figure 8.1 A Steep Learning Curve Reflecting Rapid Learning with High Innate Talent and Deliberate Practice (Coaching and feedback versus solo learner with high innate talent).

procedure. Also, they mean that more complications occur in the first patients in the surgeon's personal series, the steep part of the curve.

It is worth quoting a study on resident skills testing, which states, "It must be stressed that the term 'learning curve' is, in fact, a misnomer. Learning is a parameter that cannot be measured in itself. It is usually an extrapolation from changes in performance over time."[5] Perhaps this is splitting hairs. The curve reflects improved performance, a performance gain reflected in a curve, a learning curve. Besides, the term is embedded in many aspects of our culture and is well understood to reflect such parameters as reduced surgical errors and reduced operative time, which demonstrate learning.

The good news is that a novice learner can be "trained up" to the level of others with more innate talent.[6] The bad news is that studies have also shown that a significant number of trainees never become proficient at certain motor tasks even with extra training. A report stated that testing on a laparoscopic simulator revealed that "in our study, 20% of the participants had such a low level of innate abilities that they were unable to achieve acceptable performance in our minimal-assess surgery (MAS) simulation."[7] The bothersome idea that some trainees have low innate talent is also observed in practicing surgeons. In another study from 2003 testing experienced surgeons on simulated tasks, 10 percent of those tested performed significantly worse than the group's overall average performance.[8]

Where do these surgeons end up? What happens to trainees who consistently underperform even with remediation? How do we identify these individuals? Can they be remediated? Do they want to be remediated? Do less well trained surgical residents slip through the cracks in the educational process? And, most important, did these underperformers get adequate deliberate practice with a mentor or coach using refined, time-tested teaching methods?

Answers to these questions aren't fully known. But the use of performance or learning curves serves to identify slow learners and underperformers, as well as the superstars in surgical residency programs. Hundreds of studies have refuted the foolish idea that you can master complex technology on the run after just a few repetitions, or at a weekend course. Yet the drive to maximize revenue somehow manages to encourage many salespeople to cling to this fantasy (and hospital administrators too often pressure surgeons into using the robot, for example, so they can advertise their high-tech wares). I wish to emphasize the inescapable reality that training and experience come with time and exposure to the nuances of surgical technique.

There are no shortcuts in surgical education.

A 1997 report entitled "New Surgical Procedures: Can Our Patients Benefit while We Learn?" posed the most vital question at the heart of this book: "What, if anything, does a patient need to know about her surgeon's position on the learning curve?"[9] I submit that patients need to know as much objective information as the surgeon can provide regarding the number of cases the surgeon has performed. Surgeons resist this idea of transparency at the very time when the term *transparency* is spread like goodwill in all sorts of health care reports. Too often, transparency is absent from the informed-consent process. The study also states, "Sales representatives can exert pressure as they tout the usefulness of new products and devices. Industry-sponsored conferences expose gynecologic surgeons to new techniques but may do so in a way that encourages the use of expensive disposable equipment. Generally speaking, these individuals' primary concern is the success of their company's product rather than the health of patients or the economic well-being of a hospital, practice, or managed care organization."[10]

Returning to this chapter's opening robotic case with double ureter damage, the Joint Commission that oversees all things related to hospital safety reviewed the case. The commission felt there was no need for improvement in the robotic surgery program at that hospital. How is this possible? The patient required *four more operations* to fix her damaged ureters. This is all the more tragic when one realizes that between 1988 and 1991 gynecologists reduced their complication rates with other operations by 50 percent.[11] The patient described above was never given proper informed consent. She was not told that the surgeon operating on her was a trainee. She was never told that her rookie surgeon would be working with another surgeon whom the patient had never met. A catastrophe of this magnitude (including two other patients at the hospital with urinary bladder lacerations) is seen as an acceptable incident? Learning curves, specific training methods, and credentialing apparently were not thought to be an issue. This is the same Joint Commission that will shut down a hospital for putting trash in the wrong-colored bag.

I have recited this case not to demonize the hospital or surgeon, but rather to make the point that inadequate training occurs all too often in our world of new, complex operations. We have no national guidelines for robotic training. Individual surgical residency programs are incorporating robotic training on simulators as well as in the operating room, but graduates do more observing than actual operating with the robot. In 2003 in an article entitled "Who Will Help Surgeons Climb the Learning Curve?" Dr. Phillip R. Schauer identified the then-poor numbers of laparoscopic cases performed by trainees in residency, stating, "The traditional surgical residency model has been ineffective in training surgeons in these new procedures. . . . Until training volumes in surgical residency programs increase, we are letting loose surgeons ill-prepared to adopt these new but now mainstream operations."[12] In 2016, robotic surgery training similarly lacks adequate numbers of cases to properly train graduates in this next generation of complex minimally invasive operations.

Some surgeons have a bad habit of not discussing their personal experience regarding specific operations with their patients. I have heard countless stories from patients about how they found out *after the fact* about their surgeon's lack of experience. As you will discover, a newer definition of surgeon capability centers on education in practice, or the lifelong need to polish one's knowledge and skills, to buff up the technical skills actually used in practice. The new definition of competence captures not only the idea of effectiveness in caring for patients but also the bigger picture of efficiency when working with other doctors, nurses, technicians, and the health care system itself. Nonetheless, the idea of comparing one's personal experience when performing a particular task with a *standard measure of expertise* (with that task), as I have indicated, is quite a bit older than the laparoscopic revolution. It's about documenting improvement with what we call deliberate practice, as I will describe in detail in Chapter 13.

In surgery, better performance means you have better results and hurt fewer patients. For a surgical trainee, the learning or performance curve

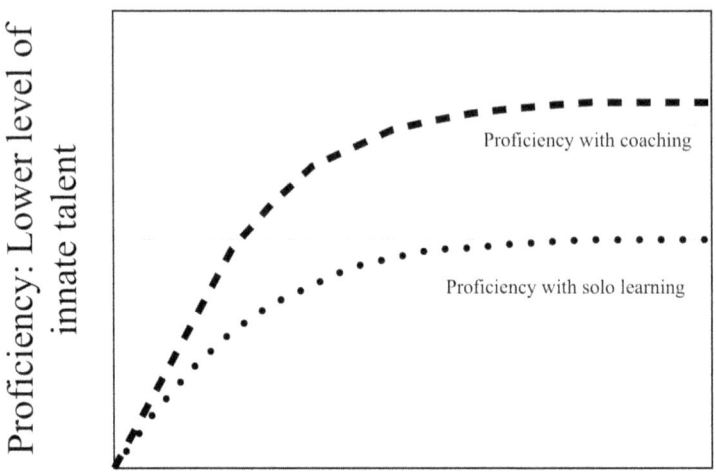

Time or Repetition

Figure 8.2 A Shallow Learning Curve (Deliberate practice versus solo practice with less innately talented learner).

plots the number of repetitions of a skill or surgical operation against the amount of time to complete the operation or the frequency of mistakes (Figures 8.1 and 8.2). It's a record of *experiential learning*—you get better by doing the task over and over. Of course, the assumption is that you will be taught how to do the operation properly the first time and then refine it through practice. Until minimally invasive surgery came along, surgical educators ignored what industry had learned about this valuable method of documenting a worker's performance. Learning curves were not discussed until about the 1970s in surgical education circles. Our past method of determining whether a trainee was technically capable relied heavily on observation—including the influence of the halo effect (that if you feel favorably about a person, you grade him or her higher) and other confounding issues. Until recently we had no objective methods for measuring a trainee's competence in performing core surgical skills or their more complex counterparts.

The New Risks for Patients

Risks of Laparoscopic Education

If an entirely new set of skills was required to manipulate laparoscopic instruments in 1990, then a new method of teaching those skills was imperative as well. Additionally, we had to determine which trainees were capable of performing the skills safely. For several reasons, the new less invasive operations added a dramatic risk to patients in teaching hospitals where surgical training occurred. The dilemma of dealing with a laparoscopic mistake or misadventure (as surgeons are wont to say) would become evident to you if you stood facing a TV monitor in the operating room while observing the crude laparoscopic movements of a novice trainee.

Standing in a dark OR, next to a novice trainee who held the laparoscopic chopsticks outside the belly, I had no control of the case from moment to moment. I could no longer ensure patient safety as the surgical resident poked and prodded poorly visualized tissue to learn on patients. In using tiny incisions with trocars or sleeves, through which we placed our long, skinny instruments as we operated, looking up at a TV screen, it was always possible that the field of vision could easily disappear in an unexpected spray of blood. Thus, attempting to teach laparoscopic surgery in the operating room to trainees with no prior experience with the instruments was by definition unsafe. We had to change our methods of training surgical residents.

Of course, when general surgeons attempted to learn new minimally invasive operations, they subjected their patients to the same added risks.

Additionally, we were often pressured by industry representatives to try new equipment with which we were unfamiliar. In the early 1990s, capitalism had found new opportunities in the operating room.

The Lure of New Technology

Today, the promise of earning big revenues by marketing high-tech operations seduces hospitals into buying robotic and other high-tech equipment. Intrigued by the new toys, surgeons of all stripes try to perform these new operations with which they may have little experience. Remember, true experts in laparoscopic and robotic surgery will gladly give you their statistics, including how many cases they have performed, as well as their outcomes. You need to know this information about individual surgeons' training and experience. Assume that a vague answer to your specific question about the surgeon's case volume is either a sign of lack of experience at the least, or possibly an indication of minimal experience disguised in miscommunication.

It isn't clear how surgeons in practice get their training or how much training most surgeons acquire. Despite one of our local competing hospital's screaming billboards about their possession of the most advanced robotic equipment in the region, we have no idea how their surgeons train or how they assess their results. Are Americans at more risk for robotic surgery complications than patients in other countries? Perhaps so, if you look at the potential threats of this new technology and the potential for inadequate training. It is also a matter of the availability and distribution of new technology. Consider:

- One in four U.S. hospitals has at least one robot.
- 67 percent of all da Vinci robots in the world are in the United States.
- Almost 80 percent of all robotic operations are done in the United States.
- The increased cost per robotic case ranges from $3,000 to $6,000.
- In 2014, 570,000 robotic operations were done in the world.
- In 2015, the newest da Vinci robot cost over $2,000,000, with teaching models more costly.[13]

Can We Measure Expertise in Individual Surgeons?

In order to review learning curves as a way of assessing how skills are acquired, let's broaden the discussion for the moment to a consideration of basic surgical ability. What actually is it? Who has it? Can we measure it? And what happens to trainees who don't have innate ability?

There are many facets to surgical expertise. In particular, when discussing how competent a particular surgeon may be, educators often skirt the issue of *judgment*. This is because teaching and measuring how surgeons make decisions is difficult. However, we are beginning to use the simulation lab to teach, assess, and document our trainees' progress along the slippery and shadowy road to sound clinical judgment. As you know, there are six competencies that must be mastered by a capable surgeon. For the moment, I'm going to focus on the most important aspect of surgeon capability, the one surgical educators often call the seventh competency—technical skill.

Is There Such a Thing as Innate Talent?

There is no doubt that differences exist among surgeons regarding their ability to master and perform complex mechanical skills. Every surgeon is a flawless performer in his or her own mind. However, surgeons have often overemphasized their own slick facility with surgical instruments. We all feel confident that we can master any new procedure. This unflinching certainty in our technical capability is our most effective weapon against the reality that our daily activities are pregnant with uncertainty. In this regard, it is important to remember a 1999 study by Kruger and Dunning from Cornell, which concluded, "People tend to hold overly favorable views of their abilities in many social and intellectual domains."[14] The authors suggest that this overestimation occurs "in part because people who are unskilled in these domains suffer a dual burden: Not only do these people reach erroneous conclusions and make unfortunate choices, but their incompetence robs them of the metacognitive ability to realize it."[15] Fortunately, our virtual reality (VR) machines in the skills lab allow us to construct immediately available learning curves so that trainees are confronted with their incompetence. They must then continue to employ deliberate practice in order to improve.

The surgical personality is constructed out of necessity on a belief in one's ability to perform well in the operating room. But innate ability isn't everything. In fact, it's quite a bit less important than how hard a surgeon trains and how much time a practicing surgeon puts into learning a new operation. Studies have revealed that the performance of trainees with innate talent can be matched by less talented trainees who work hard and engage in concentrated practice. This training up to a higher level of capability is the foundation of modern surgical education. Nonetheless, some studies have proven innate talent to be important. Returning to a study from 2003, the authors divided 30 of their trainees into four groups following

30 simulations over three days and tested them. They documented their findings as follows:

- In Group 1, 16.7 percent had such *high innate psychomotor ability* that they gained little extra improvement with VR training (they were proficient in the task immediately after being taught it).

- Group 2 (*moderate level of innate talent*) *gained improvement* and stability through VR training.

- Group 3 (*moderate level of innate ability*) *gained unstable improvement* through VR training.

- Group 4 (*low level of innate abilities*) *did not gain improvement* through VR training.[16]

In other words, with dedicated practice under proper supervision, trainees who are initially less able to perform surgical skills than some of their peers can, in fact, train themselves up to the level of innately more talented trainees over a period of weeks of deliberate practice. Yet in other studies, although there was collectively (in all participants) an association between the number of cases performed (repetition) and reduction in time and errors, *individually* the correlation doesn't hold up.[17]

Early Reports on Laparoscopic Cholecystectomy Learning Curves

By the end of the 1980s, the first practical reports on laparoscopic cholecystectomy began to trickle into surgical journals. Authors documented their successes as well as their complications—mistakes resulting directly from the technical challenges as well as surgeon inexperience with the new operation. Still, many questions were left unanswered in the early days of the revolution regarding how to evaluate in a meaningful way the difficulty of performing laparoscopic cholecystectomy and other less invasive operations. At the time, surgical educators weren't talking much about learning curves.

The bottom line should have been patient safety. But it wasn't. As Dr. Alfred Cuschieri of Dundee, Scotland—famous for his labeling of the early lap chole years as "not short of abuse . . . the biggest unaudited free-for-all in the history of surgery"—also admitted: "Based on my own personal experience and that of my colleagues, I believe that surgical performance during endoscopic surgery declines after a variable but finite time—on the average four hours. After this, the surgical fatigue syndrome sets in, manifested by mental exhaustion, increased irritability, impaired surgical judgment and reduced dexterity."[18] Also, remember Hans Troidl's warning about having a new hammer (laparoscope) and looking for something (a new organ) to pound. In 1989, innovators Reddick and Olsen reported their highly successful first 25 cases of laparoscopic cholecystectomy.[19] Erich Muhe recorded his five year experience of over 90 cases while others struggled to accumulate smaller numbers.[20] Reddick, Olsen, and others reported on 360 successful laparoscopic cholecystectomy cases with acceptable complication rates by 1991.[21] Perhaps confusion about learning curves is best reflected in a 1990 report on the introduction of laparoscopic cholecystectomy that used the expressions "a rapid learning curve" (suggesting that it was an easy operation to master) and "a significant learning curve" (implying that it was a major technical challenge) all in the same paragraph![22]

Other early reports referred to the learning curve by name and function. For example, in 1993 a study from Hahnemann University Hospital entitled "The 'Learning Curve' in the Performance of Laparoscopic Cholecystectomy" asked the following questions: "First, can Laparoscopic Cholecystectomy be performed as quickly and efficiently as an open procedure? Second, can it be performed safely? Third (and most important), is the 'learning curve' associated with laparoscopic cholecystectomy prohibitively long and drawn out and at what point does that curve 'level out' such that the surgeon is ready to perform the procedure alone?" The Hahnemann report documented an operating time of two hours for the surgeons' first 10 cases. Four of the five cases in the series that had to be converted to an open (incision) operation because of technical difficulty were in the first 10 cases as well. This represents the steep part of their performance curve, where more complications happen and when it takes longer to do the procedure. With more experience, operative time and complications dropped off as the surgeons learned how to do the operation.[23]

A year later, a report entitled "The Learning Curve for Laparoscopic Cholecystectomy" noted, "Most of the complications (75%) occurred in the first 30 cases for all surgeons. . . . We therefore conclude that LC has a definable learning curve and is a safe procedure with proper training."[24] The same year a study looking at injuries from laparoscopic cholecystectomies by the Department of Defense concluded, "The pattern of these injuries supported the generally accepted conclusion that the frequency of complications associated with laparoscopic cholecystectomy, especially bile duct injuries, is related inversely to the experience of the surgeons doing the procedure and that the highest rates of such injuries occur early in a surgeon's experience with the technique, usually during the surgeon's first 10 or 15 cases."[25] Without using the term, this report characterizes the concept of a learning or performance curve perfectly.

The question regarding the length of the tail of the learning curve would only be answered years later. Such complications as cutting the common bile duct would continue to occur along the learning curve to as many as 200 cases.[26] Regarding bile duct injuries, the most dangerous of all laparoscopic cholecystectomy complications, it was estimated as early as 1995 that a surgeon had a 1.7 percent chance of damaging a bile duct in the first case and a 0.17 percent chance of the injury in the 50th case.[27] Operative time also has been measured to document the learning curve effect, in one study dropping from 112 minutes for the first 50 cases to 79 minutes for the next 50 patients.[28]

The argument for better results with high-volume surgeons (more cases, more repetitions) was raised regarding colon surgery, as reported in 1997: "There is a learning curve for laparoscopic-assisted colectomy with respect to intraoperative and postoperative outcomes. As with other laparoscopic procedures, surgeons who perform higher volumes of laparoscopic-assisted colectomy have lower rates of intraoperative and postoperative complications."[29] But experience alone would not ensure safety during minimally invasive operations. With time and diligent study, surgical educators discovered other factors that would make minimally invasive surgery acceptable. They included how the surgeon sees the operative field through a telescope and senses the feel of tissue, of pathology, and the natural variations of the bile duct and other local anatomy. Standardizing minimally invasive operations also reduced failures of antireflux fundoplication ("stomach wrap" to prevent acid from entering the esophagus),[30] as did experienced supervision of that particular operation for 20 cases. This was confirmed in a study that showed the teacher to have the most important impact on the learning curve for fundoplication.[31]

Thus, it seems to me that inquiring about your surgeon's experience—asking about how many repetitions of the operation the surgeon has done and thus locating your case in that surgeon's learning curve—is the most critical information you can obtain during an informed-consent dialogue. Your surgeon may not have his or her exact numbers. But keep in mind the range of 30 to 60 cases a surgeon must complete to attain capability in performing most minimally invasive operations. Some of this training may be done in a skills lab under supervision as a trainee or as deliberate practice of an established surgeon learning a new operation. With deliberate practice, fewer repetitions or actual cases in practice may be needed to improve one's learning curve. This training involves deliberate practice with a knowledgeable mentor or coach using proven teaching techniques.[32]

Surgeons without Scalpels: A Tipping Point Arrives Early for Surgical Laparoscopy

The advent of video-laparoscopic cholecystectomy in 1989 has once again ignited an explosive period of growth not only in the practice of gastrointestinal surgery but also, in all branches of surgery. Thus, we are witnessing one of the six most fertile periods of surgical growth in the last five hundred years.

G. H. Ballantine, P. F. Leahy, I. M. Modlin,
Laparoscopic Surgery, 1994

It happened quickly.

By the cautious standards of our profession it was virtually spontaneous. First, the less invasive gallbladder operation cannibalized our practices and created confusion and grumbling in the operating room. Which instrument on the back table do I need next? Where should the TV screen be located? Who should the screen face? Hold the camera steady, please. Do you see the cystic artery?

Instead of the normal tone of seamless cooperation in the operating room, now there was a sense of foreignness. With the overhead lights off, shadows replaced shiny instruments, and flesh receded from a 3-D presence to a 2-D Hollywood movie. Besides, we required two setups: a full tray of traditional clamps, hemostats, scalpels, probes, and retractors of all sorts in case we needed to open, to make an incision; a second tray was crowded with rows of pistol-grip sticks, laparoscopic instruments with tiny scissors or grabbers on the ends, and sharp sleeves called trocars to poke through the abdominal wall.

Uncertainty replaced certitude. If our laparoscopic efforts failed or caused harm, we dived for the scalpel, switched off the TV sets, turned on the brilliant overhead lights, and opened the belly. Converting to an open operation meant abandoning the less invasive approach. It was, frankly, a hit on our egos to have to admit we couldn't get it done laparoscopically. However, with time and maturity we learned that converting to an open traditional operation required that omniscient, formless, voluble, and essential surgical ingredient—judgment.

The unanswered question in 1990 and 1991 was, Where will it all end?

Two important books written almost 40 years apart explain how minimally invasive surgery caught fire and spread across the civilized world. One, I discovered a dozen or so years ago. Malcolm Gladwell's 2000 best seller *The Tipping Point*[1] caught my imagination when I began thinking about how his ideas about the phenomenon of "tipping" explained what had happened to surgeons exactly a decade before his book was published. The second book describes how, in our instance, the number of surgeons performing laparoscopic gallbladder removal reached a critical mass, as described in Everett M. Rogers's 1962 classic, *Diffusion of Innovation*.[2] Thus, to explain how gallbladder removal using a laparoscope could spread so quickly in mere months, I will turn to these experts and fill in the cracks in the story with surgical research.

Epidemics: How Do They Start and Progress?

Infectious Bugs and Rabid Ideas

How do new ideas catch on? Why do some trends and products spread with dramatic speed while others do not? And who is responsible for the rapid dissemination of ideas, trends, and technology?

Medical history has taught us that disease epidemics spread through various routes. For example, respiratory tract infections easily spread through coughing and sneezing, which sprays bacteria and viruses and rapidly disseminates flu and other respiratory diseases. Bugs can also be carried on objects we use in our everyday lives (pens, books, smartphones, doctors' ties, stethoscopes, hospital sinks, etc.). Epidemics produce huge numbers of victims in a short time span.

Is this a new phenomenon? We tend to think of HIV and avian flu (and the new seasonal flu strains) as modern epidemics. In fact, the epidemics of widespread deaths from puerperal or "childbed" fever in the 19th century ignited vicious battles over whether "animalcules," or what we now call bacteria, actually existed. Puerperal fever was caused by bacteria transported on the hands of doctors rushing unwashed from the autopsy room to the delivery room. Oliver Wendell Holmes wrote of his thoughts of how the deadly disease was transmitted in the 19th century. His idea was ridiculed by many physicians, none less world famous than Boston gynecologist Charles Meigs. Meigs failed to understand the autopsy-to-bedside route of infectious material when he insisted, "Doctors are gentlemen and gentlemen have clean hands."[3] One wonders how many women died unnecessarily because of his and other physicians' misguided beliefs.

The spread of infectious diseases is exponential: imagine how with the flu, for example, one person infects another, who then infects two others and then four others and then sixteen and so on. Some bacteria and viruses have aggressive rates of spread; their genetics are more explosive than others. Some reproduce rapidly, increasing their numbers swiftly; others produce deadly chemicals called toxins.

These highly aggressive organisms are said to be *virulent*.

We also know that virulent ideas can spread from person to person, so-called word-of-mouth transmission. It seems the more rabid the idea, the faster it spreads. Examples of virulent convictions include racism, anti-Semitism, radical Christianity, and radical Islam. And as with quiet coexistence with our neighbors of different belief systems, many bacteria live in and on our bodies that are not harmful, not pathological. Therefore, infectious agents and their method of transmission may be viewed as metaphors for political ideologies that too often destroy the societies that gave birth to them. We would be wise to remember the critical nature of this coexistence of pathogens and people.

But who ever heard of an *epidemic of curing?*

The question encompasses the events of the laparoscopic revolution and the cast of surgeon actors who started and spread the new operations. My own fascination lies in how these innovators individually and in isolation (out of contact with each other) saw something everyone else missed. In *The Tipping Point*, Gladwell describes his book as "the biography of an idea. . . . The best way to understand the emergence of fashion trends . . . the phenomenon of word of mouth . . . is to think of them as epidemics."[4] The tipping point phenomenon refers to the contagious word-of-mouth spread of laparoscopic cholecystectomy, at the time an *untested* and (in the minds of many surgeons) a *detested* new operation. Also, it would be reasonable to conclude that there were two tipping points: the first occurred when laparoscopic gallbladder removal was performed by a critical mass of surgeons in 1990, the second when virtually all specialty areas of surgery fell to a variety of scopes as the decade of the 1990s progressed into the 21st century.

But there is a downside to the transmission of messages.

As you might suspect, messages may become distorted as they are handed off to others. Unsavory aspects of a message—in the case of laparoscopic surgery, poor training and the resultant excessive and serious postoperative complications, including serious bile duct injuries—may be suppressed. Thus, the life-threatening complications seen early with lapa-roscopic cholecystectomy (bleeding, bile duct injuries, bowel punctures resulting in serious infections) were downplayed almost to the point of extinction. Just as rumblings about British military action in 1775 excited revolutionary fervor among the colonists, in the late 1980s a few curious American surgeons became fascinated with reports out of Germany and France about a new way to pluck out a diseased gallbladder. Within weeks the result was the creation of excitement—and not a small uproar of disbelief—among legions of practicing general surgeons. As David Rosin wrote in the preface to his book on minimal-access surgery in 1993: "Lap-aroscopic cholecystectomy exploded onto the general surgical scene like no other procedure before it. Embraced by the public, and promoted by technologic advances, it rejuvenated general surgery. Although there were a few skeptics, the rush to learn minimal access surgical techniques was phenomenal and took surgical trainers by storm."[5]

The Radical Surgical Environment of the 1980s

To grow and mature, new ideas need rich soil. There must be an explicit or implicit sense of a demand for change. Surgeons were embedded in change in the 1970s and 1980s, designing radical cures for a variety of dis-eases, including cancer in its many forms. Neither spoken nor whispered notions of minimally invasive operations were able to seep through the impregnable walls surrounding the radical surgery dogma of the 1970s and 1980s. In parallel with surgery's expanding search for radical cures, the field of anesthesiology had grown into a mature specialty. Anesthesiolo-gists introduced a major patient-safety component into their daily work in the form of *crew resource management* (borrowed from the aviation indus-try). Much later, surgeons followed suit.[6,7] Developing bigger and more complex operations, surgeons worked hand-in-hand with anesthesiologists and pushed their patients' physical boundaries in a search of ever more radical cures for horrible diseases. In parallel with big operations, surgeons and anesthesiologists, together with lung, kidney, and heart specialists, found common ground in treating seriously ill patients. Hospitals soon developed intensive care units, and a new specialty of *critical care medicine* emerged.

Radical surgery, improved anesthesia, and intensive care units (ICUs) became the deep pool, the context Gladwell believes to be important in human affairs, in which laparoscopic surgery found itself wading in 1990.

Litynski noted under the heading "Why Was Muhe's LC Rejected?" (on why Erich Muhe's original and first laparoscopic cholecystectomy in the world failed to catch on): "Many leading abdominal surgeons had focused their attention on organ transplantation and cancer treatment. Abdominal operations were radical and extensive."[8] And Litynski similarly quotes Muhe as remarking regarding his training: "We dreamed of surgeries for extensive removal of tissues and organs. All such operations naturally involved big incisions. Back in those days, the saying was, 'big surgeon—big incision.'"[9] Nowhere in the 1970s and 1980s was there a whiff of the idea of patient-centered care in the realm of general surgery. Patients hid their scars in embarrassment and shame, grateful to be alive. It was nothing if not our ethical imperative to attack aggressive tumors; the war on cancer was on, and military metaphors spewed from our mouths as we rattled our curative sabers.

But disturbing changes were occurring around us.

Quickly, smaller and more efficient video cameras and recording devices were developed. Kurt Semm had proved the plausibility of laparoscopic appendectomy and had invented and produced numerous new instruments for laparoscopic use. A few of us began using the laparoscope in order to make a difficult abdominal diagnosis. At first, treatment was not in our thinking. Defiant, we clutched our dripping scalpels with backs stiffened in rebuke against anything less aggressive.

As I alluded to a moment ago, Malcolm Gladwell emphasized the role of the environment in producing tipping events. He suggests, "Human beings invariably make the mistake of overestimating the importance of fundamental character traits and underestimating the importance of the situation and context."[10] Thus, the shrinking of our specialty of general surgery, in conjunction with the emergence of radical operations, became intolerable. That was an important part of our context. Surgeons were losing little pieces of their specialty, while other, bigger chunks were falling to subspecialization. General surgery was left gasping for breath. As our operative numbers shrank, we nonetheless clung to the argument that laparoscopy violated a basic surgical principle: operating with appropriate visibility. What could you see through a tiny scope?

Hans Troidl and Patient-Friendly Surgery

It was at the University of Marburg, Germany, that Hans Troidl first became interested in endoscopy. He developed considerable expertise before moving to Kiel, where he met Kurt Semm. Troidl observed Semm, the forward-thinking gynecologist, perform a laparoscopic appendectomy, and the event was for Troidl "unforgettable."[11] When he joined the Surgical Study Group on Endoscopy and Ultrasound (CAES), Troidl met the movers and shakers in the field and ultimately became one himself. In the mid- to late 1980s, Hans Troidl became involved in two important developments: the idea of creating a separate journal for surgical endoscopy and the creation of the first international conference on surgical endoscopy. The journal became a reality with Troidl as one of the founding editors.[12] It was called *Surgical Endoscopy*. He also became president of the First World Conference on Surgical Endoscopy in Berlin in 1988, the first organized meeting of surgical endoscopists from around the world. His presidential address at what was officially called the International Congress on Surgical Endoscopy noted that surgeons' reasons for failure to adopt endoscopy included concerns about poor light sources, discomfort for patients because of the rigid scopes, and the dangers of perforation and bleeding. He confirmed Gladwell's insistence on the role of context by reaffirming that "another reason for the surgeon's lack of interest in endoscopy was the development of so-called 'major' surgery."[13]

But the eye-catching statement in Troidl's presidential address was this: "Incredibly, laparoscopy has been almost neglected by surgeons, except for pelviscopy, a highly perfected technique used by gynecologists. This procedure has, in fact, revolutionized the science of gynecology. *The degree to which we as surgeons ignore this sophisticated technology and refuse to test its suitability for surgical application, is astonishing* [my italics]."[14] In 1989, Troidl traveled to Bordeaux to observe Jacques Perissat perform his combined lithotripsy-laparoscopic cholecystectomy. From there he went to Paris to watch Francois Dubois do his elegant laparoscopic cholecystectomy. At the April 1989 SAGES meeting in Louisville, Troidl convinced Perissat to show the video of his gallbladder technique to the industry booths.[15] At the Storz booth Perissat played his cassette, and soon the place was crowded with curious surgeons. Interestingly, Perissat's submission of his laparoscopic cholecystectomy technique for a formal podium presentation was rejected by SAGES. Yet his informal video display attracted a larger audience than did the lecturers in the main auditorium.

The notion of not hurting surgical patients is so ingrained in virtually everything we do in the operating room today that Hans Troidl's emphasis on patient-friendly procedures seems archaic. That was hardly the case in the 1980s, a time when the sayings "big surgeons make big incisions," "little incisions are made by little brains," and "the larger the cut, the better the surgeon" ruled the day. These verbal stab wounds were inflicted by surgical giants as well as by regular self-satisfied practitioners in response to the possible benefits of minimally invasive surgery. Ridicule was their defensive posture when confronted with the challenges of adopting the less invasive technology.

Hans Troidl was an innovator. He had done research on patient outcomes looking at patient well-being, acute surgical pain, and quality of life rather than at the usual endpoints for research on new operations, namely, complications, length of hospital stay, and death rates. Troidl performed his first laparoscopic gallbladder removal on October 23, 1989. He became yet another surgeon who would promote the critical mass of practitioners necessary to tip the laparoscopic revolution. In a 1990 report entitled "Surgical Endoscopy and Ultrasonography: Surgery at the Crossroads," Troidl stated: "Incredibly, laparoscopy has been almost neglected by surgeons. . . . Politically motivated arguments against appendectomy via laparoscopy, laparoscopic removal of gallstones with intact gallbladder by means of laparoscopy are neither helpful nor academic. This attitude shows irresponsibility towards patients and the art of surgery."[16] Thus, detractors of less invasive operations had been warned that change in how surgery would be performed in the future was not a fleeting trend.

Thereafter, the general surgery laparoscopic revolution lurched forward and quickly gained momentum. As J. Madeleine Nash reported in *Time* magazine in 1992: "As their skills improve, videoscope surgeons are attempting more daring feats. . . . In the past four years, 28,000 U.S. surgeons have learned how to remove gallbladders laparoscopically. . . . Videoscope surgery may never completely replace open surgery, but it may come closer than anyone a year or two ago might have imagined."[17]

Diffusion of Laparoscopic Surgery—The Ideas of Everett M. Rogers

The story of the spread of laparoscopic gallbladder surgery (as well as the subsequent development of other less invasive procedures) may be framed from the point of view of a classic assessment of the "innovation-decision process." As Everett M. Rogers stated: "This process consists of a series of choices and actions over time through which an individual or a system evaluates a new idea and decides whether or not to incorporate the innovation into ongoing practice. This behavior consists of essentially dealing with the uncertainty that is inherently involved in deciding about a new alternative to an idea previously in existence."[18] Laparoscopy already existed in the practices of many gynecologists and urologists and was performed by some internists. Surgeons were aware of the new minimally invasive technology, but most of them chose not to consider its place in general surgery practice.

In 1962, Rogers defined an innovation as "an idea, practice or object that is perceived as new by an individual or another unit of adoption."[19] In addition, he defined the process of the diffusion of innovation: "The diffusion of innovation is essentially a social process in which subjectively perceived information about a new idea is communicated from person to person. The meaning of innovation is thus gradually worked out through a process of social construction."[20] Thus, as we have seen, the tipping of the laparoscopic surgery revolution reached a point where it became self-sustaining and reached a critical mass of cases as a social phenomenon. Interestingly, despite the lack of Internet connectivity in 1989, the surgeons who were prime movers, the so-called change agents, communicated with each other individually and at meetings. Perhaps the revolution in general surgery sped along its uncontrollable course because the innovators were from several countries and because each served as a change agent, creating a groundswell of enthusiasm. Yet repeatedly the record confirms that most of the early adopters were convinced that they had performed the first laparoscopic cholecystectomy.

In the fifth edition of his book *Diffusion of Innovations*, Rogers outlines five steps in the innovation-decision process. I'll use these steps to interpret the spread of laparoscopic cholecystectomy from Rogers's perspective:

Knowledge: Muhe, Mouret, Dubois, Perissat, McKernan, Saye, Reddick, Olsen, and many others had basic knowledge of urology, gynecology, and the use of the laparoscope. This was knowledge and expertise not possessed by the average general surgeon. They shared, in the words of Rogers, *homophily*, defined by Rogers as "the degree to which two or more individuals who interact are similar in certain attributes."[21] These pioneers shared a real interest in either (or both) gynecology and urology and had cultivated expertise in these specialty areas in their practices. The average general surgeon shared the features of *heterophily*, defined by Rogers as "the degree to which two or more individuals who interact are different in certain attributes."[22] General surgeons in the 1980s made it clear that they were *surgeons*; gynecologists were not. Clearly, the surgeons who began the laparoscopic *general surgery* revolution were homophilious and had cultivated the unique skills of gynecologists and urologists, technical approaches in which they saw potential value for general surgery.

Persuasion: With a positive attitude about the advantages of less invasive surgery, the innovators convinced a small number of other general surgeons (what Gladwell calls "the law of the few") of the value of learning the new gallbladder operation. Around the United States, in France, and in Germany, a minority of general surgeons sought information about the operation. This burgeoning interest was cultivated by the laparoscopic cholecystectomy video shown in Louisville in 1989 by Perissat and by Reddick and Olsen with the display of their laparoscopic cholecystectomy video at the American College of Surgeons meeting in the fall of the same year. Some surgeons were persuaded, some were not.

Decision: A number of general surgeons decided to try to learn the new operation as courses in laparoscopy spread over the surgical world. Many decided to continue performing open gallbladder operations. I decided to learn the operation along with Nick Coe and Chip Alexander, two talented general surgeons (interestingly, one from academia, one from private practice). We traveled to Marietta, Georgia, in June 1990 to work with Eddie Joe Reddick and Bill Saye. After the course we returned to Baystate and worked out how to refine our skills and how to credential other surgeons.

Implementation: This occurred immediately for most of the surgeons who understood that the trend toward less invasive laparoscopic cholecystectomy would catch on with their patients; overall, laparoscopic cholecystectomy was not implemented with patient safety in mind, which is a major point of this book. The scramble was on, and general surgeons everywhere fought to be enrolled in the few courses available. Again, what was not done well was control of the introduction of the operation (e.g., ensuring that surgeons obtained proper training and credentialing and were given specific privileges).

Confirmation: In my own experience the process was safe, and we believed that our results justified further use of the operation for uncomplicated gallbladder disease. All patients were told that they would have an open operation if, at any point in the laparoscopic procedure, we felt that the risk of injury to a vital structure was possible.

Rapid Adoption of Laparoscopic Cholecystectomy with Few Warnings

The two books I've used to describe the incendiary arrival of laparoscopic gallbladder removal around the world join together in their explanation of the word-of-mouth spread of this surgical event. Rogers led the way in defining what Gladwell would later call the "tipping point." Defining *critical mass*, Rogers states, "The *critical mass* occurs at the point at which enough individuals in a system have adopted an innovation so that the innovation's further rate of adoption becomes self-sustaining."[23] Similarly, Gladwell states, "The Tipping Point is the moment of critical mass, the threshold, the boiling point."[24] He further qualifies the crucial moment in an epidemic: "The name given to that one dramatic moment in an epidemic when everything can change all at once is the Tipping Point."[25]

These essentially similar ideas help to frame the swift takeoff of laparoscopic cholecystectomy. What was the magnitude of the critical mass of surgeons performing laparoscopic cholecystectomy in 1990? Exactly how fast did the laparoscopic gallbladder operation tip? Consider a 1992 statement from the Cleveland Clinic Foundation: "Laparoscopic cholecystectomy has taken the United States by storm. Assuming conservatively that 2% to 5% of all cholecystectomies in 1990 were performed with this new technique, then between 10,000 and 25,000 laparoscopic cholecystectomies may have been performed that year."[26] Also, a year earlier, Dr. William Stoney, from Nashville, highlighted the poorly controlled adoption of laparoscopic cholecystectomy when he wrote, "Considering that thousands of patients have now had this procedure, it is curious that so little has been published in the mainstream surgical literature."[27] Thus, a considerable sense of uncertainty surrounded the early adoption of the strange new gallbladder procedure. For example, in a report titled "Retrospective and Prospective Multi-institutional Laparoscopic Cholecystectomy Study Organized by the Society of American Gastrointestinal Endoscopic Surgeons," multiple nationally known authors compared laparoscopic cholecystectomy with open cholecystectomy. They concluded, "LC performed well with sound judgment and awareness of limitations and problems is a safe and feasible surgical procedure compared with the 'gold standard,' of open cholecystectomy."[28] Again, there stands a cautionary note from SAGES insisting that surgeons be well trained and use sound clinical judgment.

Yet warnings about the dangers of laparoscopic cholecystectomy also found their voice.

In a commentary entitled "Laparoscopic Cholecystectomy—Threat or Opportunity," in *Archives of Surgery* in 1990, Ronald K. Tompkins wrote, "It has a steep learning curve and reports of major complications and even fatalities are filtering in. The entrepreneurial exploitation of the procedure in some areas has further complicated objective analysis of the procedure."[29] Now we not only have misgivings about the severity of complications associated with the operation, but we also note a hint of concern regarding surgeons' avarice—practicing surgeons in the community wanted to get the lion's share of the gallbladder cases. Similarly, in an editorial in the *Southern Medical Journal* in 1991, William Stoney warned, "The combination of these forces, i.e., patients seeking the procedure, surgeons pressured to learn, hospitals pushed to buy lasers and laparoscopic instruments, and the manufacturers of this equipment competing for a potentially lucrative large market, has produced for the medical community new problems that need guidelines, but that have evolved rapidly without much input from established resources of medical leadership."[30] Clearly, as the operation reached a critical mass of surgeons performing the procedure, two stumbling blocks were identified: a steep learning curve and profiteering. And the national surgical leadership had little impact on the behavior of these entrepreneurially motivated private clinicians.

Malcolm Gladwell's Tipping Point

Let's examine more closely how laparoscopic cholecystectomy became rapidly adopted by looking at Gladwell's definition of an epidemic. He describes three aspects of an epidemic: (a) they demonstrate "infectious" behavior, (b) small changes have big effects, and (c) both of these changes occur in a hurry. Gladwell observes: "The name given to that one dramatic moment in an epidemic when everything can change all at once is the Tipping Point. . . . Contagiousness, in other words, is an unexpected property of all kinds of things, and we have to remember that, if we are to recognize and diagnose epidemic change."[31] For those of us who experienced the phenomenal spread of laparoscopic cholecystectomy, the word *contagious* perfectly expresses the feelings we experienced. If I were to pick a watershed moment in the history of the laparoscopic revolution to represent the tipping point, it would be when doctors Eddie Joe Reddick and Doug Olsen showed a video of a laparoscopic gallbladder removal at the 1989 annual congress of the American College of Surgeons in Atlanta. They packed the commercial booth where they showed the video with curious surgeons, much as Jacques Perissat had done at SAGES in Louisville, Kentucky, also in 1989.

The videotape they showed of a laparoscopic cholecystectomy was the virus that infected a growing number of general surgeons at the meeting. Not all were impressed. Some walked away in disgust. But enough surgeons caught the laparoscopic cholecystectomy "flu" in response to Reddick and Olsen's enthusiasm. In fact, by the end of the conference they had filled all the slots in their laparoscopic cholecystectomy courses. The years 1988 and 1989 brought about small changes (one-on-one demonstrations of the new operative skill). These small changes would quickly culminate in the tipping of laparoscopy in general surgery in 1990. Consider Gladwell's three rules of epidemics: the law of the few, the stickiness factor, and the power of context.

The Law of the Few

In addition to the videos shown by Reddick, Olsen, and Perissat, a major role was played by George Berci. He had fled Hungary in 1956; traveled to Australia, where he became interested in biliary endoscopy; and ended up at Cedars-Sinai Medical Center in Los Angeles in 1969.

A founding member of the American Association of Gynecologic Laparoscopists as well as of SAGES, Berci became widely published and established contacts throughout the United States and Europe.[32] Speaking several languages, this one individual was what Gladwell calls a connector. There were others, of course, including Alfred Cuschieri, Leon Morgenstern, Frederick Greene, Doug Olsen, Eddie Joe Reddick, Bill Saye, Barry McKernan, Nathaniel Soper, Bob Fitzgibbons, Alexander Nagy, Carol Scott-Conner, Mohan Airan, S. T. Ko, Jonathan Sackier, Edward H. Phillips, Michael S. Kavic, Ralph Ger, and the three Frenchmen Mouret, Dubois, and Perissat. Really, it is a short list of some of the major connectors who worked together (as well as independently) to bring laparoscopic cholecystectomy to fruition.[33]

As Cuschieri and Berci wrote in 1990, "Laparoscopic cholecystectomy has now been performed in several thousand patients worldwide and the early experience indicates that this operation *when performed by the fully trained is safe.*"[34] The operation had tipped by the fall of 1990. Connectors spanned the world of general surgery as well as gynecology, gastroenterology, and urology. Who they knew was important. Cross-fertilization happened only because a few open-minded general surgeons listened to their colleagues in these other specialties. But many of these innovative surgeons were also what Gladwell calls *mavens*—in a word, teachers.[35] And the best of them ran high-quality courses that offered hands-on experience. Mavens possessed the knowledge to make surgery safe. They, and the *salesmen* Gladwell identifies as crucial to a word-of-mouth epidemic, played a major role in the revolutionary expansion of laparoscopic cholecystectomy. In our story the mavens and salesmen were often the same people.[36]

The Stickiness Factor

According to Gladwell, "The Stickiness Factor says that there are specific ways of making a contagious message memorable; there are relatively simple changes in the presentation and structuring of information that can make a big difference in how much of an impact it makes."[37] Inherent in this notion is the withholding of problematic information while actively promoting the positives of the message. For a less invasive gallbladder operation, the major reduction in pain, faster return to daily living activities, and short hospital stays sold the operation. These were the "sticky" advantages that patients quickly recognized and clamored for when asking for the laparoscopic operation. What was concealed from the public and what awaited a more honest assessment of what surgeons could offer was the list of complications. Bile duct injuries tripled. Bowels were perforated, leaking stool into the sterile abdominal cavity. But these facts were not part of the message that spun a new operation into an epidemic.

The Power of Context

Gladwell emphasizes the role of the environment in which an epidemic catches on.[38] Emphasis in the 1980s on heroic operations stands as background for what was to come. When the public discovered less invasive operations, surgeons were literally forced to train themselves in laparoscopy. Patients wanted less traumatic operations. So, the context for change seems to have been a combination of patient and surgeon needs that quickly drove the laparoscopic uprising into its tipping stage.

Further proof that the epidemic of laparoscopic gallbladder removals had indeed tipped came in the form of multiple publications of series of cases. By 1991, Reddick, Olsen, and Spaw reported on a series of 500 laser laparoscopic cholecystectomies with respectful outcomes.[39] The same year a report on the European experience with laparoscopic cholecystectomy appeared. A retrospective study of seven European centers, the report quoted a complication rate of 1.6 percent with a conversion to open gallbladder removal of 3.6 percent, admirable statistics from European experts. The authors confirmed that the tipping point was reached, stating, "Laparoscopic cholecystectomy is well-established, and there have been few instances in the history of surgical practice where the benefits of the procedure became so clearly manifest within such a short period of time."[40]

Then, a 1992 National Institutes of Health (NIH) report appeared to muddy the waters.

Experts Agree—Proceedings of the National Institutes of Health Consensus Development Conference on Gallstones and Laparoscopic Cholecystectomy, 1992

It seems appropriate to revisit the results of a 1992 conference designed to bring together the best minds and the most up-to-date information regarding the treatment of gallstones, including the role of laparoscopic cholecystectomy. A huge amount of information was amassed from 26 experts, various discussants, and audience participants. The material was subsequently evaluated by a panel of 14 physicians, scientists, and laypersons.[41] The planning committee consisted of eight physicians, three nonphysicians, and only three surgeons. Similarly, the actual NIH panel was made up of seven physicians, one PhD, an RN, and only four surgeons. The report stated that the goal of the meeting was to examine the treatment of gallstones (the most expensive gastrointestinal disorder in the

United States) "with a focus on the evaluation of emerging data and contro-
versies surrounding laparoscopic cholecystectomy."[42] The report acknowledged the role of endoscopy, lithotripsy, and gallstone-dissolving technology.
Yet four of the five sections of the conference centered on surgical issues.
These included open versus laparoscopic cholecystectomy, the use of electrocautery versus laser energy in surgery, and methods of creating a pneumoperitoneum (how to get carbon dioxide into the belly cavity without
injuring organs). Also discussed were laparoscopic complications and the
future of laparoscopic cholecystectomy.

As stated in the opening sentence of the conference report, "No other
surgical development has had such a dramatic and pivotal impact on
abdominal surgery as laparoscopic cholecystectomy."[43] Thus, it seems odd
in retrospect that there were so few surgeons on the consensus panel to
address one of the major discussion point of the agenda: "Which patients
with gallstones are candidates for laparoscopic cholecystectomy?" In this
part of the discussion, issues such as the role of laparoscopic cholecystectomy in pregnant patients, in obese patients, in patients with known common bile duct stones, and in patients with chronic obstructive lung disease
were addressed—all basic issues of surgical decision making seldom in
the purvey of nonsurgeons.

I found certain aspects of the report disturbing. For example, given
the newly documented increase in bile duct injuries with laparoscopic
cholecystectomy as compared with the traditional open operation,[44] the
report commented that "the rate of common bile duct injury appears to
be increased."[45] *Appears* to be increased? One report at the time documented
a drop in bile duct injuries from 2.2 percent to 0.1 percent after only 13
cases of experience.[46] That improvement is due either to a major improvement in technique or to better selection of patients. The section of the report
that compares laparoscopic cholecystectomy to open cholecystectomy and
other methods of treating gallstones requires clarification because it is confusing about skills acquisition.

For example, although appropriately identifying weak scientific data
supporting the value of laparoscopic cholecystectomy at the time, the report
then stated, "Moreover, there is a strong consensus that there is a rapid
acquisition of appropriate technical skills associated with laparoscopic cholecystectomy, which is reflected in a widely differing reported rates of
morbidity."[47] This statement appears to be saying that laparoscopic cholecystectomy is easy to learn, but surgeons have widely differing complications. The panel of mostly nonsurgeons decided that it is easy to acquire
laparoscopic skills (rapid learning or acquisition of appropriate laparoscopic
surgical skills) but didn't explain why the results (morbidity) were so

variable. Why aren't all surgeons' outcomes more or less the same if learning the operation is easy? And if acquiring these skills is rapid, why were some results unacceptable (triple the number of bile duct injuries)? Virtually all the surgical studies quoted in this book revealed a steep learning curve as well as significant complications for laparoscopic cholecystectomy in *untrained* hands.

Fortunately, the NIH report appropriately cautioned, "However, the results of laparoscopic cholecystectomy are greatly influenced by the skill and experience of the surgeon performing the procedure and reflect a steep learning curve."[48] What seems to be of more concern in retrospect is the NIH report's statement that "although the rate of common bile duct injuries is increased, this rate appears to be sufficiently low to justify the patient's selecting (with the counsel of a physician) this procedure for the treatment of symptomatic gallstones."[49] Thus, despite knowing the bile duct injury rate following a surgeon's early experience with laparoscopic cholecystectomy could rise to *three times that of open surgery*, the panel was undeterred from stating that the injury rate was "sufficiently low" to recommend the operation for patients.

By the time of the NIH report in 1992, a significant number of patients had already suffered from significant complications because the tipping point had already occurred for laparoscopic cholecystectomy. Thus, a critical mass of general surgeons was performing the operation, which marked a rise in complications not regularly witnessed with open gallbladder surgery.

In summary, laparoscopic cholecystectomy tipped in 1990. The field of general surgery as a specialty tipped as other organ systems were approached with less invasive techniques. The implacable surgical personality that had initially resisted change to less invasive operations developed hairline fractures. As the decade of the 1990s slid forward, the defiant disregard for minimally invasive surgery by entrenched surgeons began to crack under the inexorable pressure exerted by the laparoscope.

PART 4

Crisis in the Operating Room: Surgeons Face Self-Reflection under Bright Lights

CHAPTER TEN

Big Egos, Small Incisions:
The Surgical Personality
Then and Now

Although disruptive physician behavior is widely considered a source of concern in the patient care environment, surgeons have been the specialty most commonly identified as "disruptive physicians."

Amelia Cochran and William B. Elder, *American Journal of Surgery*, 2015

During thirty-three months of research, I observed appalling conduct by venal, careless, and incompetent surgeons. At the same time, I encountered inspiring behavior by exemplary surgeons whose clarity, competence, and caring were acknowledged by patients, colleagues, and subordinates.

Joan Cassell, *Expected Miracles: Surgeons at Work*, 1991

"Scalpel! Swab! Forceps!"
"A little more relaxation, please."
"Too much bleeding!"
This overwrought dialogue barked by a surgeon opens a scene on the first page of Robert G. Richardson's 1968 account of modern surgery, titled *Surgery: Old and New Frontiers.* Explaining the surgeon's persona, Richardson observes: "From time to time he demonstrates an interesting point or a fresh stage to the green-gowned students gathered in awe-inspired reverence round the master. In his hands he holds the balance between life and death; his skill and judgment are on trial."[1] This image of the surgeon as a godlike figure persists in various forms today—especially in the minds of some surgeons. War metaphors are often liberally sprinkled like holy water throughout the action language that surgeons favor. This angst between operating room chaos and mindful exchanges of ideas (back in the day,

mostly one-way exchanges) reflects an irony that defines what it means to be a surgeon. What follows will be a blend of historical dialogue regarding the surgical personality and the reality of surgeon performance today.

A Surgical Personality Paradox

Surgeons are a peculiar lot. We are required to flux emotionally between the cold objectivity demanded in the operating room and the warm empathy of true caring at the bedside. I'll explore this paradox we live with from the perspective of the quality of care you may receive as well as from a patient-safety vantage. Seldom discussed among patients' families and friends beyond a quick "What was she like?" from a friend or relative, the surgical personality has been extensively written about. Your surgeon's caring should be obvious, her lion heart held in reserve until that moment when uncontrollable hemorrhage or other unanticipated catastrophes flip a switch and her single-minded focus on fixing the damage emerges in a heartbeat. Knowing that this paradox is real, you can anticipate, explore, and interpret elements of the particular surgical personality you have to deal with in seeking a safe operation.

We have been analyzed and judged by our peers as well as by anthropologists, internists, anesthesiologists, nurses, other health care workers, and the public. From an array of scientific studies published before as well as over the course of the laparoscopic revolution, from repeatedly expressed formal and informal (undiluted) opinion, and from acidic scorn that regularly bubbles up from nonsurgeons in high-risk areas of the hospital, there emerges the image of a prototypical surgeon as well as of surgeons as a professional group.

One thing is for certain: the attitude of many surgeons in the past—a refusal to accept criticism, a certainty that we were right pretty much all the time—has disappeared to a great extent. For the most part it was a male world, an androcracy of intolerance and aggressive behavior. As a consequence of disasters in the OR resulting from this attitude, among other valuable strategies used today in the operating room there is a two-question rule: if you ask twice about your concern over, say, excessive bleeding, everything stops, and the problem is resolved before the case is allowed to resume.

The tacit sense of admiration for surgeons of all stripes, while often contaminated with recrimination about excessive self-certainty, is nourished by the deep and almost impenetrable roots of the surgical personality. Nonetheless, it must be said that this uncomfortable alliance of bravado mixed with condescension, and its antithesis (a surgeon's empathy), is also the bedrock of the remarkably successful track record built by the daily performances of surgeons around the world.

In the end, surgery is a performing art.

It plays out on a private-public stage referred to as the operating room or operating *theater*. Supporting actors and actresses have historically huddled in silent obedience (one might say hiding in the wings) as the main performance is played out onstage. Of late, these essential members of the operating room cast have finally acquired the recognition they deserve through a more recent emphasis on teamwork. Anesthesiologists, nurse anesthetists, and anesthesia residents, as well as scrub techs, circulating nurses, and surgical trainees, now work with surgeons in a way that approaches but does not quite meet the criteria of true teams.[2]

Despite this progress, one study revealed that nearly 50 percent of physicians and 70 percent of nurses (in a variety of hospital settings) have witnessed disruptive behavior in other physicians and nurses, respectively. The overall sense of these professionals is that disruptive behavior in the operating room and in other high-risk areas of the hospital has a measurable negative impact on patient safety and outcomes.[3] As a consequence, teamwork is a concept we are cultivating today with serious intent. Predictable cooperation across different specialty domains unfortunately remains an unfulfilled goal. Nonetheless, the treatment of the players on the operative stage is more egalitarian today than it was in the past. And shared leadership and teamwork roles are now emerging as fresh possibilities in a more democratic surgical workspace.

When laparoscopic surgery poked its head into the world of radical operations in the late 1980s, there were plenty of practicing surgeons imbued with their own unshakable sense of self-importance. They stood poised to slash viciously at the minimally invasive surgery upstart in diapers bawling at them. To understand why minimally invasive surgery was initially rejected, as well as to gain a deeper understanding of how to obtain reliable information about capable surgeons today, you must appreciate the proclivities of the surgical mind.

Again, consider the surgeon's bipolar enigma: How does a staid surgeon express empathy for a patient lying in bed with a painful incision the surgeon inflicted without emotion? How can the surgeon inspect his or her surgical slash created with indifference and without regret and then become sensitive to the anguish he or she has caused? Can a surgeon flip-flop between objective cutting, wielding an unflinching knife, and sitting at the bedside expressing a caring spirit with a soft touch of the hand? Can surgeons wrestle daily with their emotions without wearing down under the burden of ambiguity?

This challenge—meeting the need for clinical objectivity coupled with the capacity to appreciate suffering—makes the surgeon's work a slurry of contradictions. As a patient you must appreciate the possible added risks you may be exposed to as a consequence of the fallout of a difficult surgical personality. I should state for clarity that competent, caring practitioners constitute the vast majority of practicing surgeons. But not all. And we have the bipolar potential to be a little too harsh and a little too insensitive. Where did the surgical personality come from? Is it real? Is it dangerous? Is it essential? Is it malleable?

The Surgical Personality—Innate or Created?

One does not enter lightly into the sacred temple of the human body. In any other venue in American life, what surgeons do would be considered assault. So how does a focused practitioner pick up a knife and cut into another human being? It's counterintuitive, isn't it? Are surgeons uniquely unshakable emotionally or must we be trained to become indifferent to the painful, debilitating, and often disfiguring consequences of our actions?

This innate ability to act indifferently to chaos in the operating room seems to exist naturally in some individuals. Alternatively, certain people are selected whom surgical educators believe can be taught to develop self-preserving personality traits that allow them to do the cutting while shielding themselves against excessive feelings *in the moment*. Old-time traditional surgeons would bristle at any suggestion that there might be something called doubt in their thoughts before, during, or after an operation. Many older surgeons considered uncertainty (as well as humility) a weakness. For the surgeon grasping the handle of the razor-edged scalpel, there is no room for hesitation. Our surgical literature and folktales are riddled with the notion that medical doctors *think* while surgeons *do*. Surgeons act. These identifiable traits have, in some surgeons, taken on extreme forms.

Richard Selzer has written eloquently about many aspects of the practice of surgery as well as about surgeons in the operating room under sundry conditions.[4,5,6,7,8] He observed over his years at Yale and wrote that the surgical temperament may become pathological in a variety of ways. Regarding a more virulent form of behavior, he wrote: "These martinets infest every hospital to some degree, like rats in a silo. They are recognizable even from the time of their internships, when they can be observed preying upon medical students or barking impolitely at nurses. Invariably these surgeons rise to positions of great authority—Chief Resident,

Professor of Surgery, Dean. Here, a malignant character can flourish unhampered."[9] In 1996, Selzer further observed, "They are all big, good-looking fellows, given to wearing string ties and cowboy boots that can imply virility if need be."[10]

Selzer is not the first surgeon to have observed the self-designation of "cowboy" surgeon. But he is adamant about surgeon hubris when, in *Letters to a Young Doctor*, he added: "Beware contagion from this surgeon. His pox is highly catching. Once so afflicted, you cannot be cured, but must depend ever after upon mere diligence and correctness to keep you out of malpractice courts."[11] Yet despite our somewhat necessary professional arrogance, millions of operations are performed in the United States yearly with remarkable results and with few snafus. There is an unflappable coolness, a detachment that frames the surgeon's psyche. It is a necessary objectivity. And it possesses a dark side.

The Surgical Personality—Back in the Day

The Disruptive Surgeon—When the Surgical Personality Is Out of Control

If the surgical personality were merely annoying, we could dispense with it as a quirk, or possibly as a tolerable curiosity. Once again, this discussion involves the less common but more difficult types of surgeon behaviors. Many patients have endured rude surgeons in order to benefit from their unquestionable technical talents. However, there is a mere molecule-sized gap between quiet confidence and self-centered, manipulative, and disagreeable behavior. Too frequently surgical hubris and disruptive behavior contaminate the operating room atmosphere. As has been well documented, in the past far too many surgeons made the operating room a toxic workplace.

In his presidential address in 2009 to the American Surgical Association, Dr. Anthony D. Whittemore remarked: "In particular, we need to better understand the impact of professional behavior on safe care and the steps we need to consider when that behavior falls short of acceptable norms. . . . Impaired and disruptive behaviors are underemphasized causes for *diminished competency* [my italics] and are often unaddressed, tolerated, and, in some cases, actually rewarded."[12]

Sadly, it is not overreaching to highlight the recent historical record that documents some terrible surgical behavior that ruined operations and killed patients. With displays of arrogant self-importance and uncontrolled rage, surgeons have so upset other members of the operating room team that they have made lethal mistakes. These include upsetting anesthesiologists who administer too little oxygen, rendering patients brain-dead, terrifying circulating nurses who have dropped the organ to be transplanted and thus contaminated and ruined it, and frightening scrub techs who go home to their spouses crying uncontrollably and eventually leaving the health care workforce. For decades, surgeons have been a significant reason for the nursing shortage and for medical students' rejecting surgery as a career.[13]

To dispel cries of foul play—that I am using this format to denigrate surgeons (hardly my intent)—I will examine what experts, anthropologists, and surgeons themselves have to say about the surgical personality. These are classic observational studies.

What Anthropologists Say about Surgeons

Charles Bosk, Anthropologist

In the acknowledgments in his classic and often-quoted 1979 book, *Forgive and Remember: Managing Medical Failure*, detailing his field research on surgeons, Charles Bosk opens by stating: "In what were often very trying circumstances, they were considerate, candid, and courteous beyond the limits of any social and academic obligation. If they taught me nothing else, the surgeons taught me that delivering high-quality humane care is hard work."[14] He summarizes his extensive study of surgeons at a West Coast teaching hospital by making important points about how surgeons are socialized. It's about the way that teaching surgeons handle trainees' mistakes, how surgeons identify errors and then manage them. He stated: "Failure to perform competently as a professional means two different things. First, there is failure to apply correctly the body of theoretic knowledge on which professional action rests. Failures of this sort are errors in techniques. . . . Second, there is the failure to follow the code of conduct on which professional action rests."[15] Bosk makes the unambiguous point that moral failure is punished more harshly than a technical mistake. He further explained: "The professional agrees to apply his expertise to the client's problem in a manner that takes care not to abuse and/or exploit the client's helplessness. . . . Hence the control of technical performance is subordinated to the control of moral performance; without the overarching moral system, the technical system is not amenable to control."[16]

Surgical errors may be of two types. *Technical errors* refer to the application of surgical skills improperly or to not mastering the skills appropriately in the first place. Failure to use one's knowledge correctly may result in a mistake in *judgment* (operating too late in the disease's course, or too early, or when one shouldn't have operated at all).

On the other hand, *moral errors*, according to Bosk, are either "normative" or "quasi-normative." A normative error occurs when a moral mistake is made because the trainee violated a standard that is established for *all* members of the profession (e.g., you will not lie to patients). Bosk clarified the issue: "We are saying that normative, that is, moral, standards are the organizing principle of a professional community."[17] Violations of professionalism represent deficiencies of one of the six ACGME competencies required of all training doctors today. Thus, the seriousness of moral errors has not diminished in the last three decades, and the moral foundation of the surgical personality remains unassailable.

A quasi-normative error occurs when a trainee breaks *someone's personal rule*, a rule that may not apply to any other surgical service. Quasi-normative errors are quirky, individual, and often senseless. For example, rounds start at 5:00 a.m., per the chief of a particular service's rules; other services start at 6:00 a.m. If you don't turn up at five in the morning, you will be held responsible. Quasi-normative errors are someone's closely held idea of what is right.

Bosk observed that the social control of surgical technique is *inconspicuous*.[18] Teaching occurs in various locations, in the OR, on the hospital floor, and in the skills lab today under close supervision. Technique is also ingrained in a number of ways that are not visible, such as one-on-one in an office or locker room with the attending surgeon. Motor skills (technical) training occurs quietly for the most part; it is a matter of private lessons between the surgeon and the resident.

By contrast, the social control of *moral performance*—the way surgeons apply pressure on surgical residents to do the right thing, to behave ethically—is very conspicuous. In such activities as a morbidity and mortality conference, trainees are held responsible for breaches in behavior. For example, if a trainee didn't go to see a sick patient in the middle of the night out of laziness, the trainee will have to answer the charge in that very contentious public forum of the conference room. In fact, the trainee may be fired or placed on probation for such moral violations of patient care.

Joan Cassell, Anthropologist

In 1991, in the free-for-all early phase of the laparoscopic revolution, Joan Cassell published her now classic book *Expected Miracles: Surgeons at*

Work.[19] Her anthropological study of surgeons began in 1983, well before the birth of the laparoscopic revolution in the United States and right after Kurt Semm performed the first laparoscopic appendectomy in the world in Germany. Understanding the surgical personality will allow you to appreciate just how severely Semm, a gynecologist, inflamed the intolerant surgeons of the day with his incursion into the field of general surgery.

Cassell stated: "Surgeons display a specific and recognizable temperament, or ethos, 'a standard system of emotional attitudes' that differ from that of members of other medical specialties. . . . The surgeon must exhibit decisiveness, certitude, control; emergencies must be resolved, unexpected findings anticipated, small advantages exploited."[20] In referring to the temperamental traits of surgeons, Cassell lists the characteristics of surgical operations as a sort of mirror that reflects the surgical personality. These elements of a surgical procedure include: operations are *spectacular*; operations are *definitive* and *irreversible*; operations, like miracles, are *attributable*:[21] attributable to the *visible public performance* of the skills of the surgeon.

Operations are executed with a sense of wonder, unpredictability, and mystery, according to Cassell's observations of surgeons at work. She added: "We might speculate that the kind of person who becomes a doctor is someone who likes to be admired, while the kind of person who becomes a surgeon is someone who *needs* to be admired. . . . The archetypal surgeon is invulnerable, untiring, unafraid of death or disaster."[22]

In the late 1980s, a sea change in the day-to-day practice of surgery was emerging. Laparoscopy was insinuating itself between the clusters of broad-shouldered surgeons bowed over the draped operating room table, holding their dripping knives with bloody gloves. Surgeons, who viewed themselves as members of an elite community that included test pilots and race-car drivers, were facing the end of a way of professional life. But the notion of operating through tiny tubelike sleeves (trocars) pushed through the abdominal wall instead of using huge incisions rattled the self-constructed heroic image surgeons held of themselves.

Laparoscopy? What of the scalpel? Would minimally invasive operations knock the cherished martial menace from the surgeon's psyche? Would surgery no longer be a contact sport? Was that why male surgeons fought to block the entry of women into surgery as vigorously as they battled to refute the value of minimally invasive operations? Was minimally invasive surgery more error prone than open operations? To give surgeons their due, as surgical elder statesman Leon Morgenstern wrote in 2006, "For the great majority of surgeons, ample incisions still afforded the best exposure, the least margin of error, and the best insurance against catastrophic outcomes."[23] Dr. Morgenstern forlornly added a historical note, commenting: "The ideologic bubble around the superiority of big incisions burst in 1986 when Erich Muhe had the temerity to remove a gallbladder through an abdominal 'stab' wound with the aid of a laparoscope and courage akin to foolhardiness. . . . The iconic symbol of the scalpel representing the art and science of surgery was no more."[24]

What are some of those surgical personality characteristics? Arguably the greatest accomplishment of Cassell's 1991 book is her description of the workings of a modern hospital's surgery department as a contemporary version of a medieval morality play. She describes a cast of recognizable characters. You should keep these surgical personalities in mind when seeking surgical care:

- *The Prima Donna Surgeon*— the arrogant, insensitive surgeon who feels he has no peers; everyone else is below him in knowledge and especially in surgical skills
- *The Buffoon Surgeon*—makes technical errors and has poor judgment; often belittled behind his back by other surgeons who gossip about his incompetence
- *The Sleazy Surgeon*—slick, "silver-tongued," cuts corners, does unnecessary operations, money oriented, a psychopath, "a disaster"
- *The Compassionate Young Surgeon*—gentle, kind, thinks about the welfare of his patients, conscientious, competent, loved by trainees
- *The Exemplary Surgeon*—admired by trainees and colleagues, asked to operate on other doctors' families, even deferred to by the prima donnas[25]

Joan Cassell continued her anthropological work by publishing a companion book in 1998 entitled *The Woman in the Surgeon's Body*. In it she noted: "Surgeons can stage spectacular tantrums and many—the men in particular—occupy a lot of psychic space. A temperamental surgeon can complicate the lives and roil the digestion of subordinates; and nurses, residents, medical students, even secretaries tread cautiously when a prima donna is in full voice."[26]

Pearl Katz, Anthropologist

Pearl Katz's anthropological studies were conducted shortly after those of Joan Cassell and, remarkably, reflect many of the same aspects of surgeons' attitudes and personalities identified by Cassell. In Katz's work, surgeons at a Canadian teaching hospital asked her to help them understand why their residents thought the surgeons were not spending enough time teaching. Katz's work culminated in her 1999 book, *The Scalpel's Edge: The Culture of Surgeons.* In one of her observations, Katz identified a major issue of importance to any person seeking surgical care when she wrote, "My initial responses and perceptions became useful to me in subsequently understanding the perspectives of patients who were frightened and bewildered by their illnesses and were recipients of some surgeons' impatience and ill-disguised condescension."[27] Katz identified several characteristics of the surgeons' thinking, including attributing concrete causes to problems with a subsequent need for active solutions. She noted that although the surgeons she studied spent only a quarter of their time in the operating room doing repetitive, mundane tasks, they perceived themselves as somewhat heroic, living in the secretive light of a "surgical mystique." Katz observed, "They reveal their proclivity for action in their use of language which not only prefers using active words and active tense, but also refers to battles and wars, strength and masculinity, while denigrating weakness, passivity, and femininity."[28]

In 1989, women in medical school made up 38.2 percent of the classes, while only 4.6 percent were represented in the surgical specialties. Yet as one report noted, women aspiring to be surgeons were more ambitious and more certain of their specialty choice than women who were not planning a surgical career.[29] Male-oriented thinking about what it meant to be a surgeon reached its zenith in a 1985 editorial in the *American Journal of Surgery*, wherein the statement is made regarding the presumably requisite characteristics of a surgical chairman, "He should be a superman [and] have an attractive understanding wife who will help him achieve his objectives."[30] That was 1985, the year Erich Muhe introduced laparoscopic cholecystectomy into general surgery. There is an obvious question to raise: How could these powerful men who viewed their spouses as chattel (and certainly not up to the rigors of a surgical career) accept the potential of operating through tiny (feminine?) incisions?

They couldn't. And at first, they didn't.

They couldn't imagine it any more than they could imagine their wives standing at the scrub sink beside them as surgeons, equal in knowledge and skills. At that time only a third of medical students were women. By 1993, only 8.6 percent of full professors teaching in medical schools were women. Only 6 percent of the entire surgical workforce was made up of women. The male ego had not undergone the transition it would eventually require to accommodate female surgeons. As of 2016, over 50 percent of our surgical residents at Baystate Medical Center are women.

As Dr. Frances K. Conley wrote in her 1998 book, *Walking Out on the Boys*, about her experiences becoming the first female neurosurgeon in the

United States: "In the early 1990s, surveys of female physicians revealed that 50–80% of them had experienced sexual harassment and/or gender discrimination during their time as students and residents—that is, when they were working in an academic setting. Male surgeons, uniformly, were the most frequent offenders."[31] Conley observed that sexual harassment was virtually never discussed or explicitly defined at Stanford, where she trained. Medical student abuse was emerging as a problem at a time when the laparoscopic revolution was cranking its flywheel. Commenting on the culture of surgery at the time, Conley stated: "It is a culture that breeds arrogance, rigidity, and an inflated sense of self-worth. It is small wonder that many surgeons do not develop an engaging 'bedside manner', and see patients as objects rather than as people with feelings, pain, desires and fear."[32] As her professional life became public spectacle, Conley noted, "But as the media looked inside our peculiar world in the early 1990s, it found that woman, as medical student, physician, nurse, patient, scientist, research subject, clearly was number two in priority and remained vulnerable to abuse by a system which had carefully defined the importance of her role, and, most of all, her limits."[33] Conley also culled stories from other female neurosurgeons across the country, writing about their abuse: "It ranges from inexcusable verbal abuse to rape by a department chair. . . . Another was told she could enhance her chances of becoming a neurosurgeon by having a sex change operation along with a brain transplant."[34]

Katz made an important additional summary point for prospective surgical patients when she wrote about surgeons, "Their penchant for independence, certainty, individualistic action, and optimism also discourages introspection, doubt, and admitting fears and failure."[35] The point is that *certainty squelches insight.* By referring to their cures, some surgeons avoid acknowledging their very human limitations and thus force a more passive role on their patients. In fact, by fostering an attitude of excessive optimism, the surgeon may not only be deluding patients about their chances of cure, but the surgeon may be deluding him- or herself. Katz correctly stated, "Surgeons' optimism and absence of doubt may prevent them from asking critical questions of themselves and others and from learning from their mistakes."[36]

Finally, Pearl Katz analyzed the particular styles used by various surgeons she observed. She noted that a surgeon's style directly affected his or her decision making. And even though referring doctors seldom, if ever, became aware of the surgeon's style of functioning, that style influences most areas of practice. It significantly affects how a surgeon communicates with patients and their families. For example, some surgeons demonstrated a *scientific style* by lacing their discussions with the latest scientific research, as documented in contemporary surgical journals. Their decisions were evidence based. Alternatively, the practicing clinician's approach may be a more *intuitive style*. Neuroscience today supports the notion that many of our decisions as well as biases are unconscious. As Malcolm Gladwell commented on biases in his book *Blink*, "They may bubble up from the unconscious—from behind a locked door inside our brain—but just because something is outside of awareness doesn't mean it's outside of control."[37] Surgeons exhibiting a warm, *patient-oriented style* or approach to informed consent make certain that the patient and his or her family understand the risks and benefits as well as alternatives to a proposed operation. These surgeons have cultivated the habit of thinking about a proposed operation from the patient's point of view as well as from their own operative perspective. However, their unconscious biases regarding particular types of patients may slide into the discussion. An *entrepreneurial style* of surgical practice characterized other surgeons who would adopt a new technology or operation with little evidence that it was better or a significant advance. This style presumes a significant interest in power and possibly in the accumulation of wealth.[38] Katz noted that the entrepreneurial style included spending less time with patients, leaving trainees to operate without supervision, seeking referrals, and often missing rounds on patients. Cassell, referring to these surgeons as venal, observed, "The venal surgeon subordinates what should be the supreme medical good, the welfare of his patients, to a lesser good, money."[39]

The Surgical Personality Today

Imagine a surgeon sitting at a robotic station with her head pressed forward against recessed binoculars built into a huge machine, searching a 3-D screen while her small hands manipulate delicate controls with a wide range of motion. This technical advance gives the surgeon the ability to carefully manipulate delicate tissue, to gently tease out anatomical structures to be saved uninjured (e.g., nerves) as a tumor is removed from its surrounding structures. The view is astonishing, magnified anatomy in clear focus as never seen before. The patient lies hidden under sterile drapes on an operating room table across the room beneath a cluster of sterile instruments. The robotic arms are connected to the surgeon's work station by a thick cable. Beneath sterile blue drapes there is no visible incision, only tiny stab wounds.

The old-school surgeon as fullback has morphed into the surgeon as delicate technical virtuoso. Fewer visible muscles and less or no testosterone are in evidence, and—as in the old adage about one of the best surgical qualities—the operator has the hands of a woman both literally and figuratively. Thus, in the modern era there exists some substantial doubt about the existence of a specific surgical personality. In a 1982 study of the perceived importance of certain personality traits, faculty and surgical residents agreed on the following self-sufficiency traits: admits errors, is well disciplined, considers all facts, is highly motivated, is consistent, and listens. Both groups also agreed on the value of decisiveness, good team participation, fairness, and flexibility.[40]

Alternatively, other doctors agree that although surgeons are talented clinicians, they may be unique only in their own minds. This idea was apparent in a study published in 2010 involving a survey of surgeons who revealed through self-assessment that they see in themselves an excess of achievement orientation and extraversion.[41] Specifically, surgeons' self-assessment showed normal levels of excitability, aggressiveness, and strain, as well as lower values for bodily complaints and health concerns—as was true for the internists studied. However, most interesting in this study was the revelation that there was no difference between internists and surgeons in 12 objectively evaluated (by other health care personnel) personality traits.

Nurses, on the other hand, viewed surgeons as quite different from internists. Specifically, the study showed that nurses felt that surgeons lacked social orientation, were less inhibited, and were more excitable, aggressive, and strained. This study suggested that there continues to exist among health care professionals a strong stereotype about the surgical personality. Regarding the differences in perception between nurses and surgeons, the authors of the 2010 study suggest, "One probable explanation might be the lack of self-awareness among surgeons."[42] It's interesting that in the same study the internists' self-assessments were quite similar to the nurses' evaluations of them.

Other reports highlight such specific personality characteristics as leadership, perseverance, and single-mindedness.[43] But others emphasize the prevalence and seriousness of disruptive behavior in the perioperative period.[44] Also, a 1994 study highlighted a discrepancy between physicians working in "lifestyle" specialties (those less physically challenging than surgery, such as primary care medicine) and surgery.[45] The study revealed that the surgical group rated highest on extroversion ("the stable extrovert") and lowest on the creative factor. More telling was the observation that 62 percent of the surgical group had similar profiles regarding personal and motivational factors, and thus formed a distinct and homogeneous group. The authors concluded: "The most powerful discriminator among the physicians was that of temperament. . . . The surgical group demonstrated the clearest and most consistent personality profile. Surgeons as a group appear to be extroverted, adjusted, practical, social, structured, and competitive."[46]

Think of the battered body of a multiple trauma victim, dying by inches, rushed into the emergency room and into the trauma bay. The broken body parts demand a swift approach that is systematic, organized, certain. Life-saving steps must be executed properly and swiftly. An expeditious workup with minimal testing is followed by rapid transport to the operating room to stanch what appears to be massive hemorrhage. Excessive contemplation of the diagnostic possibilities by the trauma surgeon would spell the death of the patient. Imagine a gunshot wound to the chest, the near-dead victim, as the attending or resident grabs a scalpel, slashes open the chest like a clamshell in the emergency department trauma bay and arrests the hemorrhage.

It is difficult to imagine anyone but a surgeon with the personality attributes I've mentioned doing that kind of work over a long career.

Thus, Dr. J. H. Thomas observed, "It is plausible that the surgical personality is one of the key ingredients in the development of a competent, successful surgeon."[47] It seems that at some level the surgical personality will persist. It appears to have undergone some degree of natural selection for the chores of acute surgical emergencies, as well as for complex elective surgery. And it will understandably continue to evolve as less invasive and more delicate operations replace the more brutal classical open procedures. The rise in the number of women in our surgical ranks will no doubt have an additional positive, moderating influence on the traits surgeons will find useful in the future.

Surgeons have a history punctuated by the behavior of more than a few individuals who meet the criteria of malignant narcissists, self-centered, toxic people who see around themselves only the failure of others. They are immune to criticism. Fault for any of their own failures lies in those around them. Also, a large number of us display elements of the negative side of the surgical personality by periodically losing it. It isn't difficult to understand why other professionals occasionally view surgeons as difficult people.

We need to reflect on our own behavior.[48] This point is supported, for instance, by a report that concluded, "Surgical errors increased significantly with increases in flow disruptions. Teamwork/communication failures were the strongest predictors of surgical errors."[49] Teamwork requires flexible leadership. But we need to be mindful of our nonprofessional lives as well, as a report entitled "Toxic Success and the Mind of a Surgeon" concluded: "Healthy success is related less to time management than attention management. . . . Hard work, time pressure, stress, and a demanding schedule had less of a toxic effect than a lack of mindful engagement with life and those with whom we share it."[50] Finally, when errors or a bad outcome occurs, we must have the humility to apologize. As Lucian L. Leape stated in differentiating between disclosure and apology, "Apology is not an ethical right, but a therapeutic necessity. Apology makes it possible for the patient to recognize our humanity, our fallibility, our remorse for having caused harm."[51]

In the early days of the laparoscopic revolution, the throaty bark "Scalpel!" became a fading echo off the dejected shoulders of older surgeons. Something was in the air besides expletives from irritated surgeons. With less aggressive operations dominating operating room rosters, as well as with the rise in the number of women in surgery, perhaps the character of our profession will continue to moderate and, in a sense, become less invasive.

Almost certainly the traditional surgical personality will continue to lose its voice.

Resident Work-Hour Restrictions and the Destruction of the Culture of Surgery: A Crisis of Commitment, Fatigue, and the Sleep Lobby

After 5 years of experience with resident duty hour restrictions implemented by the ACGME and numerous studies, the available evidence does not support the notion that decreased resident duty hours have improved the safety of surgical patients.

American College of Surgeons Task Force Response to the Institute of Medicine report "Resident Duty Hours: Enhancing Sleep, Supervision and Safety," *Surgery*, 2009

If work hour restrictions remain as they are, and as residents if we aren't pushed to keep going (just looking at the clock to sign out—as I have seen some residents do, even if it means signing out a sick patient) we never get to stretch our fatigue/resilience muscles. . . . Stamina is what needs to be built and used—stamina when it comes to working 48 hours straight, when it comes to operating for 14 hours or more. If we aren't put in those situations repeatedly, we won't build the stamina that we will inevitably need in order to do the right thing for a patient when the time comes.

Saiqa I. Khan, MD, surgical resident, Baystate Medical Center, 2016

A Modern Myth: Tired Surgeons Are Dangerous

A remarkable thing happened to the field of medicine at the beginning of the 21st century. In the process of seeking out reasons to explain why medical mistakes continue to happen at an alarming rate in our hospitals and elsewhere, we've panicked and jumped into the nearest semiscientific warm bed. You could call it *fatigue fear*. In a word, medical educators have become pathologically terrified of being tired. The extensive and incontrovertible research on the negative effects of fatigue by sleep experts supports this anxiety. In fact, being sleepy isn't just a medical dilemma. A major proportion of Americans suffer from chronic sleep deprivation.[1]

The discussion of fatigue among training doctors has incessantly churned with unbridled emotion, hubris, passionate defensiveness, and certitude. Add to this seething brew indignation, intolerance, and ignorance. Studies on fatigue and physician capability are too numerous to document in their entirety in this chapter.

How Did the Fatigue Debate Start?

Volumes have been written about the impact (or lack thereof) of fatigue on physician performance. Much of the public and all training and practicing doctors know of the trial by fire that interns previously endured before entering practice. Add on five to seven or more years of residency training and you have a professional challenge characterized by success, attrition, psychological deterioration, acting out, terrorizing, meanness, exceptional compassion, acts of selflessness, and the birth of some of the world's most magnificent malignant narcissists. No one gets through the medical training meat grinder unscathed, not even with the current 80-hour workweek.

Concern about the demoralizing and dreadful permeation of bone-numbing fatigue on medical trainees was highlighted in 1965 in the book *The Intern* by Dr. X. With candor the author described in detail the abuses training doctors absorbed routinely.[2] Similarly, surgical education giant Dr. Robert E. Condon in 1989 challenged our profession, stating: "A legitimate concern that has as yet to be addressed scientifically is the possibility that long hours have an adverse impact on the ability of residents to retain new information and to fulfill the primary educational objectives of the residency. . . . What is clear is that a patient care deficit or a public health problem does not exist in sufficient magnitude to warrant intrusion by the government into the fundamentally educational endeavors of the residency system."[3] In the meantime, behavioral scientists began to survey trainees who worried about their work hours.[4]

The early New York State experience with duty-hour regulation in the 1980s involved medical residents and was followed by later studies of pediatric residents to identify some of the issues finally being openly discussed.[5] Obstetric and gynecology educators at Columbia Presbyterian Medical Center discovered fundamental themes destined to have mixed reviews as the sleep debate took hold. The authors of a 1991 report following the introduction of the 80-hour workweek commented that the residents' lifestyle had improved by adding midwives and other personnel to help OB/GYN trainees with the workload. But they added: "Although residents commented that they had increased time for reading, this was not reflected in an improvement in the CREOG scores. The quality of patient care was not felt to be improved and the continuity of care was considered adversely affected."[6] The Council on Resident Education in Obstetrics and Gynecology (CREOG) exam would eventually have its surgical equivalent in the ABSITE (American Board of Surgery In-Training Examination); subsequent reports on the ABSITE would demonstrate variable improvements or no change in the overall scores with reduced work hours. More important, to date no objective study has connected these multiple-choice examinations with actual improvement in OB/GYN or surgical outcomes in clinical practice.

What We Knew Then

A 1991 study showed that with duty-hour reductions there was an improvement in patient care and a decrease in the use of health care resources.[7] Perhaps it was this economic measure that medical educators (encouraged by their administrative handlers) found alluring, perhaps a slight softening of our profession's traditional stance against government interference in academic medical affairs. Referring to new directives (established over a decade before they were nationally mandated), the authors state, "These guidelines have been established to regulate the long working hours and consequent sleep deprivation of house officers, the size of the inpatient service, number of admissions per tour of duty, and supervision of house officers."[8] The report, like its innumerable siblings to follow, fails to address concern for the unique challenges of surgical training. This oversight—ignoring the profound differences involved in training capable surgeons as compared to dermatologists or family doctors, for example— echoes as *the* dominant plotline running through the core ideas in this discussion.

In the United Kingdom a 1992 report on the use of a partial-shift system introduced the previously detested concept of doctors working *predetermined shifts* and then going home—regardless of the state of illness of their patients.[9] Today, European trainees are limited to a 48-hour work-week—a result of sweeping reforms that treat training doctors in the same way as plumbers or railroad employees. That same year numerous reports on work-hour violations were cited; some were blamed on inadequate enforcement.[10,11] The specialties most frequently violating work-hour restrictions from the get-go were pediatric surgery, general surgery, colon/rectal surgery, internal medicine, and orthopedic surgery. Clearly, surgeons realized that the idea of shift work was incompatible with their moral obligations to their patients.

Nonetheless, medical mistakes, we were told, resulted from being exhausted. Although the association is real, a complete review is beyond the scope of this book. My primary goal is to make clear that the reality of resident and practitioner fatigue when placed in context in the bigger picture of safe surgical care is little more than a distraction. For example, I laud the dedicated work of the late Thomas J. Krizek, MD, FACS, who in 2002 identified 10 issues he considered to contribute to the profession of surgery as *an impairing profession*. They are:

- The length of training is too long.
- The financial sacrifice is too great.
- *The hours of work are too many.*
- *Sleep deprivation is dangerous.*
- Surgery is emotionally draining.
- There is a "tragic need to suppress emotions."
- Fragmentation of surgeons begins early (into isolated specialties).
- Mistakes are not handled appropriately.
- Impairment may be behavioral, the result of injury, or the product of chemical dependency.
- If the training process is changed, the profession will reap rewards.[12]

Dr. Krizek's concerns have recently been addressed to a large degree by the American College of Surgeons (ACS) and other surgical associations such as the Association of Program Directors in Surgery and the Association for Surgical Education that focus on surgical education and resident well-being. Despite the challenges of training surgeons, surgical educators have been told repeatedly by nonsurgeon "experts" that training a surgeon is the same as training a pediatrician—even though pediatric educators themselves have identified some of the same issues facing surgical educators. For example, a recent report by pediatric educators stated that although working in the outpatient setting wasn't affected by reduced work hours, "inpatient settings were more affected and experienced much more in the way of change."[13]

The vast majority of surgical training occurs in the inpatient (in-hospital) setting. Also, surgical residents are different from other residents with respect to their work ethic, motivation, and commitment to patient-centered care. As a 2004 report noted a year following the introduction of restricted resident duty hours, "Sociologists have previously described surgeons as individuals who, to save human life, are pragmatically oriented, take decisive action, and display value patterns and behaviors that are emblematic of the 'hero' in American society."[14] Many surgical educators worried about the negative impact of work-hour restrictions long before they were instituted. As Dr. Bernie M. Jaffe bemoaned in 2002, a year before mandatory work-hour restrictions were started, "Attendance in clinics or Attendings' offices will almost certainly disappear, so residents will never get to evaluate the long-term effects of their care."[15] He proved to be prescient. Our residents today frequently fail to attend clinic because of other more urgent obligations and with restricted duty hours to complete them. As a result of duty-hour restrictions, too often they do not experience the complex and tortuous preoperative, interoperative, and postoperative course of their patients. Instead, they are told to go home in order to keep the residency program in compliance with national work-hour restrictions and to keep the slathering ACGME watchdogs away from the hospital's front door.

A Revolution Hidden inside the Laparoscopic Revolution

The sleep debate began at about the same time as the early rustlings of the laparoscopic general surgery revolution. In the 1980s several reports documented high in-hospital death rates in the range of 44,000 to 98,000 per year.[16] The trigger in many regards was the 1984 Libby Zion case, mentioned earlier, of a young woman who died after inappropriate treatment by medical residents who were unsupervised. Her tragic case was sold as an extreme example of exhausted trainees. In 1989, a year before the explosion in the use of laparoscopic cholecystectomy, a study of trainees proved that "in the acute sleep-deprived state there were no differences within or between the resident levels on the functional testing in repetitive skills, continuous tasks, clear thinking, judgment, memory or learning."[17]

But a more important issue was identified as duty-hour reductions were introduced. A 1994 study from Brigham and Women's Hospital in Boston examined resident (house staff) coverage schedules and preventable adverse events and concluded: "Potentially preventable adverse events were *strongly associated with coverage by a physician from another team* [my italics], which may reflect management by house staff unfamiliar with the patient. The results emphasize the need for careful attention to the outcome of work-hour reforms for house staff."[18] This newly introduced fly in the fatigue ointment continues to plague on-call schedules today. Damage caused by these information exchanges, referred to as patient handoffs, basically nullified the hoped-for advantages of reduced work hours and better-rested trainees.

Surgeon performance was also looked at in the skills lab. A report in 1998, before the duty-hour restrictions were started, discovered that using simulated surgical tasks, "surgeons awake all night made 20% more errors and took 14% longer to complete the tasks than those who had a full night's sleep and also showed increased stress and decreased arousal."[19] However, the report also highlighted the essential dilemma surrounding the fatigue debate, stating, "Although these changes after sleep deprivation might be seen as dangerous for actual surgical practice, only cognitive and simulated tasks rather than real clinical performance may be affected."[20] Surgeons everywhere understand the profound difference between doing skills in a lab and caring for a dying patient in the middle of the night in the operating room.

It started with the Bell Commission in New York State. That group's activities resulted in the enactment of Code 405 (Public Health Law 405.5) and thereafter the first work-hour restrictions for trainees across the spectrum of medical education were instituted. A 2002 report stated, "The major issue considered by the Bell Commission was the effect of sleep deprivation on the performance of house officers with regard to patient care."[21] Most medical educators assumed that the copious sleep research proving the negative influence of fatigue on human performance would make its application to training doctors self-evident. Yet another 2002 report before the first ACGME work-hour restrictions were implemented sent a mixed message, concluding that "thus far, research findings and published literature reviews of fatigue and sleepiness in medical personnel have not established a consensus on the effects or levels of fatigue or sleepiness, but these studies conflict with findings from other operations settings."[22] And so the idea of sleep deprivation "*from other operations settings*" crept insidiously into the fatigue dialogue.

Harnessed with doubts regarding the prejudice that fatigue kills patients, the authors of the 2002 report regrouped, and their subsequent discussion veers away from medical education toward truck-driving accidents caused by fatigue. They concluded, "Based on the findings from this and other studies, reforms of residents' work and duty hours are justified."[23] The idea of tired truck drivers apparently translates to dangerous surgeons.

Ironically, this conclusion based on speculation arrived from physicians who live and die by the principle of evidence-based medicine.

Thus, the slippery slope plunging to the final work-hour restrictions became greased with the notion that we should heed other operations settings. Multiple reports refer to tired truck drivers, nuclear plant operators, and the sleep lobby's favorite, pilots. These comparisons serve as an insidious onset of a trend toward confusing the reality of sleep deprivation with the reality of dying patients. Both will continue to occur and both are inextricably intertwined. The primary issue for practicing surgeons is the need to operate without delay when faced with dire surgical emergencies. Elective truck driving or piloting a commercial airplane flight are nonurgent activities that can be canceled. Bad weather may ground a flight or delay trucks until the roads are plowed.

Dying patients can't wait for their surgeon to take a nap. Their flights to the operating room can't be canceled, although their lives can certainly be compromised or ended. They have no road to stand beside and hitchhike until a truck rumbles by and takes them to safety. Only an on-call surgeon can help them—whether the surgeon is sleepy or not.

This life-and-death distinction appears nowhere in most reports on resident fatigue. The cultural erosion of surgery as a distinct professional endeavor began when the 2003 ACGME national duty-hour regulations were enforced (Box 11.1).[24]

Box 11.1 The 2003 ACGME Common Program Requirements: National Duty-Hour Restrictions

- Workweek limited to 80 hours total, averaged over four weeks; could add 8 hours for educational needs
- Required one day in seven off from all duties, averaged over four weeks
- Required 10-hour break between work shifts
- In-house night call could occur only every third night
- Limited to 24-hour period of continuous work with an additional 6 hours to complete handoffs and educational needs
- "Internal moonlighting" (extra work by residents, usually to make money in the same hospital where they train) had to be part of the 80 hours, not added to it
- Any hours added when a resident was called in from home were added to the total 80-hour workweek

The ACGME is the organization that accredits and sets standards for about 9,500 U.S. medical residency programs, of which 252 are in general surgery. There are 28 Residency Review Committees with members appointed by the American Medical Association Council on Medical Education. The ACGME identified crucial issues in residency training: "Residency programs are an essential and practical element of physician training in our country. . . . The nation must take a hard look at its residency programs—including hours, schedules, supervision, patient caseloads, and handovers—and ensure that they serve both patient and resident safety today and educational needs for tomorrow."[25] However, as the ACGME work-hour restrictions were instituted, no consideration was given to the special training needs of specialties such as surgery.

One of the studies published in 1993—10 years before the ACGME work-hour restrictions began—found that the New York State duty-hour reductions *increased* in-hospital complications and resulted in delays in getting diagnostic tests performed.[26] The report was ignored. A 2009 study of ICU deaths concluded regarding lower mortality rates, "This decrease was not associated with hospital teaching status, suggesting no net positive or negative association of the resident work hour regulations with a major patient-centered outcome."[27] Work hours, in other words, according to many studies had no effect on death rates, errors, or complications in really sick patients. The ACGME ignored these reports from leading teaching hospitals, which clearly anticipated our current work-hour problems, including the troublesome patient handoffs between shifts of doctors.

Then, in 2010, the second phase of restricted work hours arrived. This occurred despite evolving evidence that the 2003 reduction in duty hours had done little or nothing to improve patient safety and a mixed response from residents regarding their satisfaction with their work. To begin with in September 2010, the ACGME released additional "Common Program Requirements" aimed at improving patient safety. The restrictions were to be instituted on July 1, 2011, despite a lack of clear-cut improvements in patient safety or a reduction in medical errors to date. These changes included the following measures:

- All moonlighting, regardless of where it occurs, must be included in the 80-hour workweek.
- Interns will work no longer than 16-hour shifts (the most contentious issue of the added 2011 restrictions).
- Second-year residents may not exceed 24 consecutive hours and not more than 4 hours for transitions in care.[28]

A recommendation from the Institute of Medicine (IOM) was that shifts longer than 16 hours should include an uninterrupted 5-hour sleep period. The impractical real-world implications for this suggestion for surgical residents are staggering. Again, the IOM seems insulated from the practical issue of life-threatening emergencies. Instead, the ACGME recommended "strategic napping"—presumably what all training and practicing physicians have been doing since the invention of the stethoscope. The added restrictions occurred for all residencies despite a vocal negative response from surgical interns and residents to the original 2003 rules. A 2013 *New England Journal of Medicine* survey of residency program directors concluded: "In a national survey conducted between December 2011 and February 2012, residents reported no improvement in education, total number of hours worked, or the amount of rest they were getting. In fact, many participants described the changes as detrimental, with the majority feeling less prepared to take on more senior roles."[29] And a 2013 survey stated: "The first cohort of surgical interns to train under the new regulations report decreased continuity with patients, coordination of patient care, and time spent in the operating room. Further, suboptimal quality of life, burnout and thoughts of giving up surgery were common, even under the new paradigm of reduced work hours."[30] Clearly, surgical trainees were not benefiting from working fewer hours per week.

Warnings All around Us—A Mixed Bag

The initial New York State and subsequent ACGME work-hour restrictions provoked a flood of research both in the clinical setting and in the sleep laboratory. For example, a 2008 report concluded from its study of surgical residents in both precall and postcall conditions, "Fatigue and sleep deprivation cause a significant deterioration in the surgical residents' cognitive skills as measured by virtual reality simulation."[31] Again, in a *simulated* environment, deterioration of cognitive and motor skills can occur. Another 2008 report on trauma service residents and attendings states: "Both groups (residents and attending surgeons) showed a significant decrement in proficiency measures post call. When tasks were separated based on psychomotor versus cognitive-dominated skills, attending surgeons made 25% fewer cognitive errors than residents postcall."[32] The study demonstrated a near-linear inverse relationship between hours slept and number of errors. Alternatively, a 2010 study concluded: "No performance impairment was found for surgeons with a VSS (virtual surgery simulator) and standardized cognitive tests after a night of relative sleep loss. Although there is no doubt that sleep deprivation ultimately impairs human functioning, typical surgical skills do not necessarily deteriorate with a limited amount of sleep loss under clinical conditions."[33]

Under clinical conditions.

Surgical research on the impact of sleep deprivation focused on the only important issue: real-world outcomes.

Is the Real World Different from the Sleep Lab?

That real work in the real world may *not* be affected by fatigue remains an incompletely assessed problem for all clinicians. In 2000, Dr. Thomas R. Russell, representing the American College of Surgeons, stated emphatically: "Further, in my opinion, constrained work hours do not prepare residents for the real world of surgical practice. Certainly, practicing surgeons cannot deliver care within a set number of hours of work. A surgeon's responsibilities include completing the work at hand regardless of how long they take, and establishing continuity of care at the termination of those obligations."[34] Precisely. Also, the report quoted above regarding the Bell Commission concluded: "Although a few studies have found that performance is affected by fatigue, the majority have not. Most such studies published to date have methodological flaws such as unrealistic definitions of fatigue, and *a failure to recreate realistic medical scenarios* [my italics] with which to evaluate performance. Surgeons may adapt to chronic sleep deprivation, especially for crisis situations and other important tasks."[35]

As early as 1988, the ACS went on record, stating: "The College strongly disagrees that specific hours can be defined for each surgical specialty. Similar hour restraints have never been applied, or even discussed, with either attending or practicing surgeons. Thus, it seems illogical to make specific time-work recommendations without considering the effect on the educational opportunity and experience for those in the residency phase of their career. Lack of familiarity with a patient, not fatigue, is the major cause of errors of judgment."[36] As the most prominent surgical organization in the world, the ACS was, in fact, the association that started the patient safety movement in 1913. It still speaks loudest for the welfare of all patients in the modern era. Yet from the outset, prompted by the sleep lobby, the ACGME ignored the ACS.

The practical necessity of working long hours in everyday practice does not ignore the literature on the negative impact of fatigue. A special article in the *New England Journal of Medicine* in 2002 (one year before the duty-hour restrictions were instituted) entitled "Fatigue among Clinicians and the Safety of Patients" stated: "There is a large body of laboratory data showing beyond a doubt that fatigue impairs human performance. . . . Studies in sleep laboratories show that both at base line and after on-call duty, levels of daytime sleepiness in residents are similar to or higher than those in patients with narcolepsy or sleep apnea."[37] This report establishes the argument that sleep deprivation can be dangerous in certain circumstances, an irrefutable conclusion. The authors do not, however, quote studies supplying the opposite side of the argument and do not connect the dots: surgeons may struggle when tired, but their results are the same as when rested.

Surgeons have always been aware of the tension and anxiety that are the consistent fallout in the conflict between fatigue and the urgency of acute surgical disease. The inconsistency in these next reports is real, and I list them to reflect the ambiguity of the results. For example, a 2004 study concluded that "more than one-third of general surgery residents meet criteria for clinical psychological distress. Surgery residents perceive significantly more stress than social controls."[38] A valuable observation. Is this not like saying that U.S. Navy SEALs perceive more stress than bank tellers? As recently as 2012, a report using specific fatigue-measurement tools on orthopedic residents concluded, "Residents were fatigued during 48% and impaired 27% of their time awake."[39] And yet in 2005, two years following the institution of work hours, a study concluded, "The ACGME regulatory environment is adversely affecting the emergency operative experience of surgical residents."[40] Our trainees weren't around at night and on weekends to participate in trauma cases and acute life-threatening disease care in the operating room. Then, a year later in 2006, a report confirmed this concern by stating, "Fifty-four per cent of respondents believed that trauma education has worsened and 45% believed that patient care has worsened as a result of the work hour restrictions."[41] Also, P. J. Schenarts and colleagues' report showed no difference in patient outcomes with more restricted duty hours.[42] Another 2006 study addressed the ethical issues of limiting patient care: "The Accreditation Council for Graduate Medical Education (ACGME) work-hour restrictions have created an ethical dilemma for residents. Our data show that a significant number of residents feel compelled to exceed work-hour regulations and report those hours falsely."[43]

In a 2009 *New England Journal of Medicine* report entitled "To Nap or Not to Nap? Residents' Work Hours Revisited," the authors responded to the then-new additionally restrictive 2011 duty-hour recommendations by a special panel that released a white paper describing even more draconian work-hour rules. These authors strike a balancing note to what was becoming a one-sided assault on trainee choice. They moved the discussion regarding physician fatigue to its essential core, noting: "The master clinicians who serve as role models for trainees consistently show an overriding commitment to patients' well-being and the determination to follow through on the important details of patient care. The proposed system will signify to our trainees that the overriding consideration is the duration of the shift."[44] Referring to the new IOM work-hour proposals, the authors continued: "The inflexibility of the system proposed by the IOM report is also a cause for concern. In many clinical situations, patients may be better served by a physician who has worked longer than the prescribed limit of 16 hours but who has intimate knowledge of their medical problems than by a physician who has just come on duty and has no direct involvement in their clinical care. . . . Considering the differences in work flow and the responsibilities of the residents between procedural and nonprocedural specialties and between adult and pediatric practices, specialty-specific work-hour rules may be necessary."[45] Thus, for the first time we have a suggestion that more restricted duty hours may be a bad thing. A fatigued doctor who knows the complicated course of a sick patient may be the most capable practitioner. Not all specialties train their charges in the same fashion. Flexibility was needed, according to these authors. It would come in a dramatic study of surgical residents' performance completed in 2016.

Work Hours for Surgeons in Context

In the final analysis, we have a circumstance in which the science documenting the influence of fatigue is solid, but its application to the practice of surgery is seriously flawed. There are therefore two constituencies: on the one hand, there are sleep experts who have informed medical educators about the dangers of fatigue *in the abstract* (using simulation, volunteers, sleep laboratories, etc.); on the other hand are surgeons dealing with fatigue *in the context of rapidly evolving, lethal surgical diseases.* What is remarkable about all this is that these medical educators proclaim their devotion to the notion that everything clinicians do to patients must be evidence based. If this is true, then the impact of sleep deprivation should be measured in terms of educational outcomes (practice-based learning, medical knowledge, patient-care improvements, etc.) as well as of actual clinical improvements reflected in better patient safety. Fatigued practitioners should demonstrate consistently poorer endpoints, such as higher death rates and more complications after surgery.[46]

Just as important is the need to limit studies to the proper subjects working in the appropriate clinical setting. Yet one of the most frequently quoted studies on the negative impact of fatigue involved interns working in the intensive care unit setting. The study revealed that *interns* were responsible for 50 percent of injuries due to medical mistakes while working in medical ICUs. These fresh-out-of-medical-school novices made

36 percent more serious errors working 30-hour shifts as compared with working 16-hour shifts.[47,48] These studies leave a significant intellectual and ethical hole in the authors' arguments to limit work hours. I'm puzzled that educators who promote the need for improved supervision (using the Libby Zion case as an example) allowed rookies in the studies just quoted to manage the sickest hospital patient population, apparently with little oversight. *Why were interns allowed to work without adequate supervision with critically ill ICU patients suffering from complex multiorgan failure?* Thus, we have medical educators demanding better supervision of trainees who should be working fewer hours, while these same instructors make their point by quoting studies of undersupervised interns with no experience caring for sick patients. Was this study not a self-fulfilling prophecy?

Similarly, a 2007 study of malpractice claims and medical errors showed that 27 percent of the cases involved trainees whose role caring for patients was deemed "moderately" important (82 percent were related to inadequate supervision).[49] That leaves over 70 percent of the malpractice cases tied directly to the errors of *practicing doctors*—none of whom have subsequently been subjected to work-hour restrictions. More important, what does any of this have to do with training surgeons?

The acuity and rapid evolution of many surgical diseases, as well as the unique demands of teaching technical surgical skills while being mindful of patient safely, make any discussion of sleep deprivation taken out of context, irrelevant. It's really that simple. All of the cognitive blustering on both sides of the fatigue divide, which leaves everyone scrambling for the moral high ground, will accomplish nothing unless this immovable truth is acknowledged. As the ACS stated in one of its position papers on the specific requirements of surgeon training in the context of resident duty hours, "This intense, immersive model is necessary for residents to acquire the required knowledge and skills to function as independent surgeons. Changes in duty hours that negatively impact this structured surgical education and training model will adversely affect patient safety."[50]

Fatigue erodes and degrades both mental and physical performance. There's certainly enough research on the subject. But to repeat, the crucial issue left out of the dialogue revolving around the implementation of reduced duty hours for training doctors and practicing surgeons is the real world. For example, reports of the brain's ability to adapt to fatigue are absent, save a 2003 report published the year the ACGME restrictions became official. It states, "These results suggest that the brain adapts to chronic sleep restriction. In mild to moderate sleep restriction this adaptation is sufficient to stabilize performance, although at a reduced level."[51] Reports on actual clinical performance, for example, performing cardiac and other types of surgery demonstrate similar results (patient outcomes) for rested and fatigued surgeons.[52,53,54,55,56] These and other reports from the surgical trenches are rarely if ever quoted by the sleep lobby militants.

The media have not helped with their uneven reportage of doctor fatigue. In an article in the November 17, 2011, *New York Times Magazine*, four months after additional duty-hour restrictions were implemented, the author misquoted the work of the surgical genius William Halsted (the originator of the first residency program in surgery at Johns Hopkins in the late 19th century) by stating that Halsted's remarkable work ethic was fueled by cocaine.[57] In fact, Dr. Halsted did accidentally become addicted to cocaine as a consequence of his work on pain management at a time when cocaine's addictive qualities were not well understood. He managed to complete a remarkable career as an academic surgeon—including designing and personally performing hundreds of groin hernia and mastectomy operations, among other procedures—without a drug-related incident.[58] This public assault on a surgical genius reflects poorly on a society that allows it to go unchallenged.

The Cost of Work-Hour Reductions

For the record, I'm not arguing for a return to the horrible work hours we endured in the past, most of which were in the name of scut work—such menial duties as drawing blood samples, finding X-ray folders, transporting patients, starting IVs, and so forth—with virtually no educational value. However, it has been estimated that to meet appropriate safety standards by restricting duty hours further (including an estimate of labor costs to replace training doctors' noneducational duties) would cost an annual $1.6 to $2.5 billion with a needed increase in the resident workforce.[59] Another report suggested that if we attempt to follow the aviation industry's work-hour and retirement standards, it might push additional annual costs up by $10 billion.[60] And, of course, acute surgical emergencies will always challenge our ability to provide timely, cost-effective services. When care is delayed, many really sick surgical patients become even sicker, slipping toward death in the ICU, where their care becomes more complex, futile as a consequence of the delay, and extremely costly—all because of a fear of fatigue.

And Then There Is Lifestyle

Surgery is often (and incorrectly) compared to aviation, and pilots are frequently compared to surgeons. Here's the point I wish to emphasize again: airplanes can be grounded in an emergency (bad weather), but surgeons can't just stop working during an emergency (a massive hemorrhage from a ruptured abdominal aortic aneurysm, overwhelming flesh-eating infections, etc.). To date, there is no conclusive data to support the idea that a rested surgeon has better clinical outcomes than a well-informed and well-trained, if fatigued, surgeon (although they say there are old pilots and bold pilots . . . but no old bold pilots).

The tragedy for modern surgical education is that major decisions regarding resident work (duty) hours were made by nonsurgeons. These medical educators—despite an almost evangelical quest for patient-centered care—are well-meaning, but they have no experience with the challenges presented by sick surgical patients. Nor are they familiar with the extensive recent research on how to teach young surgical trainees complex techniques, instill a special fund of knowledge, or cultivate the elusive and time-consuming juggernaut of surgical judgment.

To the point, in a 2009 report entitled "Should All Duty Hours Be the Same? Results of a National Survey of Surgical Trainees," the authors concluded: "A large subset of surgical residents, particularly senior residents, considered DHR (duty hour regulations) an important barrier to their education and expressed a desire to work longer hours than restrictions allow. These findings suggest that strict and uniform DHR do not allow for optimal training of residents at different levels who have disparate educational goals and needs. Introducing some flexibility into senior residents' limitations should be considered."[61]

National medical education leaders insist on the politically correct position that you can have it all: you can have a controllable lifestyle and at the same time place your patients' interests ahead of your own. (So, do you or don't you leave your kid's soccer game when a text comes in that a patient of yours is having a heart attack?) Medical students are being trained to become physicians who state emphatically that they want an enjoyable lifestyle while insisting that they are providing patient-centered care. A surgeon's life strains the credibility of this tainted philosophy.

A report in the October 2009 *Bulletin of the American College of Surgeons* by Dr. Jacob Moalem addressed the specific issue of restricted duty hours on a surgical chief resident (in the final year of training) by stating: "With increasing stringent hours regulations, chief residents are being stripped of important leadership development opportunities—such as leading the surgical team on afternoon rounds—which are now almost nonexistent. Moreover, we have seen a sharp decline in teaching cases in which the chief residents take their junior colleagues through cases under the watchful eye of an attending surgeon."[62] He also documents several crucial issues for training surgeons and the need for flexibility not addressed with fewer work hours:

- To participate in rare cases and emergencies whenever they arise
- To prepare trainees to operate and respond to emergencies at all hours
- To learn how to cope with sleep deprivation by doing it during training
- To give chief residents more autonomy over their work and to preserve the traditional role of the chief resident[63]

Moalem concludes by defining the core truth of what is wrong with inflexible duty hours: "If a patient takes a turn for the worse, it is the chief, regardless of whether he or she operated on the patient, who is charged with overseeing the restoration of that patient's health. This is not the time to look at the clock; it is a time of commitment to patient care and of invaluable learning opportunities."[64]

The idea that reducing a training doctor's duty hours will make the hospital a safer place simply hasn't occurred. Two representative studies from the surgical literature conclude: "Our data did not provide any evidence to support the contention that resident fatigue leads to increased medical errors. Clinical data supporting a direct relationship between resident fatigue and compromised patient safety must be demonstrated before further work hour restrictions are made."[65] No improvement in patient safety with duty-hour restrictions has been proven. And also consider: "These data show no decrease in junior or senior resident task performance over a twenty-four hour call period, and do not support the 2011 Accreditation Council for Graduate Medical Education maximum duty hour length of 16 hours."[66]

A Summary of the Research on Resident Fatigue and Performance

Since the ACGME's inception of restricted work hours (to 80 hours per week) in 2003, taken together, most studies show one of three patterns: *no improvement* in patient care and doctor education, *some improvement* in care and resident education, or *actual worsening* of patient and educational outcomes. Naps were encouraged in the new 2011 revised work hours. Mandating that trainees take naps seems at best a little silly. The most accomplished nappers in the world are surgeons and surgical residents. Codifying into law that which smart people already do is absurd, yet that was the 2011 ACGME mandate—and once again it was done without specific scientific data.

There are data. They have been deeply mined. Overall, the results are mixed. One of the most reliable studies was a systematic review done in

2011 and published in the *British Medical Journal*.[67] It evaluated 72 studies from 49,084 citations on work hours and trainee fatigue in the literature between 1990 and 2010—the first two decades of the laparoscopic general surgery revolution. Thirty-eight reported training outcomes, 31 reported patient outcomes, and three reported both. I will summarize the 90 references in the report without listing them individually, because a more granular assessment of each report is beyond the scope of our discussion.

Regarding the impact of reducing resident work hours on graduate medical education (training after medical school), two studies showed improvement, 12 studies showed deterioration of education, and 27 showed no change. One of the improvement studies was declared of low methodological quality. Specifically, regarding surgical caseload (operations a resident scrubbed on) only one study (of low methodological quality) showed an increase in caseload, 11 studies showed a decrease in caseloads, and 25 showed no change in caseloads.[68] Patient outcomes, such as complications and length of hospitalization, were also measured. One study revealed fewer complications after laparoscopic cholecystectomy with reduced work hours, while others showed worsening of complications rates and longer hospital stays. Overall, the report concludes, "Most studies showed that duty hour reform did not affect standards of care of patients."[69]

The notion of fatigue fear is perpetrated by sleep experts and nonsurgeon physicians and is based on sleep-deprivation research (a representation of which I have quoted) that is of concern to all of us. That's why dealing with work hours is so difficult—because sleep experts have much to teach us. And we, the surgical experts, must know where to draw the line between fatigue and function. So far we've not been given much of an opportunity to make our case.

In its formal response to the IOM's duty-hour restriction recommendations to the ACGME in 2008, the ACS stated: "The ACS strongly supports optimum education and training of residents to provide patient care of the highest quality, and to inculcate in residents a profound sense of professionalism and responsibility towards patients. . . . In addition, the ACS has specifically focused on technical skills as a seventh core competency in designing and implementing new educational programs because of its relevance to surgery."[70] The ACS further made the following points regarding the uniqueness of training surgeons:

- Optimal training requires a longitudinal, comprehensive curriculum.
- Optimal training produces a progressive transfer of patient responsibility from faculty to resident.

- Optimal training favors retention of skills by requiring periodic reinforcement with structured experiences in a simulated environment.
- Optimal training cultivates a sense of personal responsibility for the care and welfare of patients.
- Optimal training cannot be accomplished with limited experiences (with restricted work hours) between faculty and resident.
- Without optimal training, less qualified surgeons may care for future patients with further training hours restrictions.[71]

The ACS report quotes the European Working Time Directive (EWTD), stating, "With over a decade of experience with the EWTD, it has been considered by the greater medical community as a failure that has resulted in inadequately trained physicians."[72] Also, the report comments on the Association of Surgeons in Training of the Royal College of Surgeons of England regarding the EWTD as being "severely detrimental to surgical training," noting that there was an observed reduction in index operative cases performed in a large study of surgical trainees' logbooks. In other words, surgical trainees in England were not doing as many cases as they were prior to duty-hour restrictions. The study also noted that more medical errors were made with poorer continuity of patient care.[73]

On this side of the pond, a study comparing the educational experiences of medical students before and after the start of work-hour restrictions showed that with less time, students reported:

- A negative impact on their ability to manage patient problems
- Lower levels of clarity about their roles and expectations of them
- Lower quality of feedback to students from residents
- An overall decrease in resident involvement in medical student education
- Diminished opportunities for residents to engage in teaching medical students (most of the teaching of medical students is by residents)[74]

Walking Out On the Dilemma

Unfortunately, the sleep lobby walked away from the patient safety discussion at the very moment we discovered a major new threat to hospitalized patients. It should have been obvious to everyone (and was obvious to those of us who care for sick patients on a daily basis). But nonsurgeons and sleep experts don't understand what practicing surgeons and surgical educators face every day caring for complicated patients. Thus, the nonsurgeon experts created chaos in their wake.

The procedure that now must be carried out more frequently and the primary issue confounding work-hour reductions and patient safety is commonly called a *patient handoff*. They are being improved. But these handoffs or *patient information transfers* are the new and very deadly flaw in the reduced-work-hour paradigm.[75,76,77] Their impact was not fully anticipated by anyone. And as the authors of the large review quoted above (who reported on a major portion of the studies on work-hour restrictions) concluded, "Our study, which summarizes a diverse and sometimes methodologically flawed body of literature, *has been unable to reach firm conclusions* [my emphasis], but we consider that this in itself is an important observation."[78]

A Look at the Real World of Surgical Residents—The FIRST Study

The practice of surgery cannot be standardized. Care of sick surgical patients takes place in an ever-changing and imperfect health care system. To be sure, surgical practice floats precariously on the quicksand of uncertainty. And surgeons deal with more life-threatening emergencies than any other specialty.

The argument for allowing more flexible duty hours for surgical trainees recently received a needed scientific boost. In the February 2016 *New England Journal of Medicine*, a stellar group of surgical educators reported on the FIRST Trial, which assessed expanded duty hours for surgical trainees. Sponsored by the American Board of Surgery, the ACS, and the ACGME, it is referred to as a landmark trial. The study supports additional work hours for surgical trainees.[79] Interns were allowed to work more than 16 hours per shift, second- through fifth-year residents could exceed 28-hour shifts, no residents were required to have 8–10 hours off between shifts, and residents were not required to have 14 hours off after a 24-hour shift. "Flexible-policy" residents were compared to "standard-policy" residents.

The study included 117 U.S. general surgery residency programs and 151 hospitals. It did not demonstrate an increase in death rates or major complications in surgical patients under extended duty hours. Residents working with flexible (additional) hours were significantly less likely to be dissatisfied with or to perceive a negative effect on continuity of care, skills learning, operative volume, conference attendance, time for teaching medical students, and relationships among interns and residents. They were half as likely to leave or miss an operation before it was completed or to hand off a sick patient. The study concluded, "As compared with standard duty-hour policies, flexible, less-restrictive duty-hour policies for surgical

residents were associated with non-inferior patient outcomes and no significant difference in residents' satisfaction with overall well-being and
education quality."[80]

Parenthetically, to repeat for the record, no reasonable surgical educator would argue for the return to the draconian work hours of the past.
Surgical educators have always known intuitively that the burden of unre-
stricted work hours for training surgeons was much more macho bluster
than an intellectually sound educational approach to learning the art and
science of surgery. Because we know that becoming tired is not avoidable,
the real issue is how fatigue can be dealt with safely.

The vital issue for trainees and practicing surgeons alike is the reality
that we never know when an acutely ill patient will arrive in the emergency department, or deteriorate on the floor after an invasive operation
or immediately in the post-anesthesia care unit within minutes or hours
of an operation, or require a second look within 24 hours because of uncertainty regarding tissue viability (Will the dusky-looking colon be dead
tomorrow?). Patients in shock or suffering from overwhelming infection,
whether from advanced appendicitis, perforated (burst) colon, or perforated peptic ulcer, or near death following a traumatic encounter, such as
a car crash or gunshot wound, cannot wait for the on-call surgeon to take
a nap or become fully rested. The surgical disaster must be handled immediately. And for those uninformed voices screaming for shorter call schedules for surgeons or better cross coverage among surgeons: there is an
immediate and *growing surgeon shortage*. There are no backup surgeons! And
because of the advanced age of many surgeons in practice today, this deficiency will grow unless the federal government increases the number of
training slots for surgeons.

Comparing sleep studies involving fatigue in volunteers with the
focused, expert skills of experienced but tired surgeons dealing with deadly
disease lacks credibility. The last thing surgeons in the operating room
need to think about is how tired they are in the moment. *In the moment.*
They aren't engaged in a sleep debate. They are in the zone—a special place
where fatigue can't enter easily. It is how surgeons must perform under
duress because *they have no choice*. It is why I refer to surgical residents as
the special forces of the health care system. As a study on the deadly impact
of overwhelming infections (of all types in general surgery patients, gathered under the umbrella of sepsis) concluded, "These findings emphasize
the need for early recognition through aggressive sepsis screening and rapid
implementation of evidence-based interventions for sepsis and septic shock
in general surgery patients with these risk factors."[81] No waiting to rest.
No nap. As one of our senior surgical residents at Baystate Medical Center

articulated to me regarding operating when exhausted, "You don't even think about peeing. You forget you're sick if you had a cold before you stepped in. Nothing else matters and nothing else exists. It's zen. Almost like meditation. . . . No one thinks about if they're tired or not. It doesn't even cross your mind. I would even argue the opposite—it gives you energy. Something about it enhances your focus, sharpens your mind, and makes you even more laser keen."[82]

I'll conclude with a quotation from Dr. Pauline Chen from her book *Final Exam: A Surgeon's Reflections on Mortality*. She recounts, "I had been up all night because of a difficult transplant; specifically, the recipient patient's hepatic (liver) artery kept shredding. . . . At 4:30, after the operation was essentially done, the attending surgeon left my close friend Susan, also a surgical fellow, and me to finish closing up the patient's skin. Together she and I had been up for over forty-eight hours."[83]

In their conversation at the end of the case regarding the perfection required to do the liver artery connection, Susan said, "Maybe training is doing the thing right so many times over . . . that you cannot accept anything else."[84]

Chen concluded, "No matter how exhausted I was . . . when it came down to that reconstruction, everything disappeared from my mind except for the simple, perfect tension-bearing stitches I had to sew around that pencil-thin artery."[85]

If surgical educators are not allowed to dictate the principles of surgical education and practice, the availability of capable surgeons will get a lot worse. In the face of overwhelming disease, a surgeon's work is nothing less than noble, although at times it may seem flamboyant. The ACGME work-hour restrictions will never work for surgical residents. The 2016 FIRST study shows that they may become tired, but they will not become dysfunctionally fatigued. Not allowing surgical trainees to liberalize their work hours as determined by nonsurgeons is a lethal prescription. In other words, you can't describe the flight characteristics of a Canada goose by studying South American bats.

Unless you have cut into the human body, inflicted necessary damage to cure devastating illnesses such as cancer, or repaired the violations of uncontrolled trauma, you do not understand the *personal commitment* to their patients that surgeons experience. The provision of acute surgical care can be humbling. A surgeon sees, feels, and smells sepsis, cancer, and the ravages of trauma. And despite a variable decay in a surgeon's skills with sleep deprivation, we develop fatigue resistance, as Dr. Chen described. It is born of the exquisite motivation and altruism surgeons live by, a dedication aroused by the need to reverse terribly lethal disease.

CHAPTER TWELVE

A Perfect Surgical Storm Is Brewing for General Surgeons

When we are emotionally exhausted we feel drained, depleted, annoyed, and angry. We question what is happening to us without recognizing that what we are experiencing is a normal response to excessive demands. In trying to cope with this emotional exhaustion, we create a distance between ourselves and others.

Mary L. Brandt, MD, *American Journal of Surgery*, 2009

Administrative hijackers have taken our position of professional responsibility from us and thereby diminished our autonomy, authority, and prestige while often compromising patient care.

John K. MacFarlane, *Archives of Surgery*, 2001

Dark Clouds Gather Overhead

Minimally invasive "Band-Aid" gallbladder surgery grew in sheer volume of cases in the early 1990s at the very moment that the patient-safety movement was gaining momentum. Laparoscopic operations were soon designed and adapted to anatomical areas other than the gallbladder. As I have described, the wormy appendix fell to the laparoscope. Groin hernias were approached less invasively and spawned a debate regarding the best hernia repair that continues to rage in surgical circles today. Spleens, stomachs, colons—even the secretive adrenal glands perched atop the kidneys and buried in fat—were soon displayed on TV screens, teased from their tethering tissues by surgeons using tiny scissors, special bipolar cautery, and other delicate instruments. What surgeons did not anticipate in 1990 was the wholesale transformation of how they would train and practice their art in the 21st century.

We did not anticipate being bought and sold by third parties.

As with its meteorological counterpart, a perfect surgical storm witnessed a joining together of several powerful forces, which have produced a not insignificant amount of disharmony in our ranks. Individually, they would have caused major changes in our profession. But mingled together in a furious gale, these counterproductive constraints ripped through our profession at the very moment we were struggling to adapt to the technical challenges of minimally invasive surgery (MIS).

Across the country, surgeons found themselves in a state of near disbelief as the practice of surgery radiated a brighter and brighter glare of commercialism. At the same time, the government, hospital administrators, and third-party payers began taking over decision making in the clinic—something the U.S. space program had proven can result in a disastrous loss of life. In the words of human factors expert Sidney Dekker, writing about the 1986 space shuttle *Challenger* disaster, "Professional accountability and the dominance of a technical culture and expertise are gradually replaced with bureaucratic accountability by which administrative control is centralized at the top and the focus of decision-makers is trained on business ideology and the meeting of political expectations."[1] In other words, NASA's middle management bean counters made a fatal decision regarding the safety of that fateful flight. It was a classic case of a "drift into failure."[2]

Similarly, today's surgical wisdom is too often replaced by government or other payer decisions to reduce pay or punish doctors for "never" events defined by the bean counters themselves. A "never" event is a complication or adverse event that is not ever supposed to happen, such as postoperative pneumonia, a urinary tract infection, or a patient's falling out of bed. Unrelenting pressure to increase productivity and preserve health care dollars as a consequence of the hospital's business culture has established recognizable features of our own drift to failure. It seemed as though the less certain our grasp on general surgery capability (as minimally invasive operations spread across the country), the more vocal individual hospitals became regarding their institutions' excellence.

The emperor CEO wore no clothes, but no one noticed. He hoisted a shiny new robot overhead and promised excellent care. His subjects eyed each other and the strange technology and nodded their false support. And so, robotic machines became the shiny new technology of the 21st century—just as CT scanners had exploded onto the clinical scene in the 1980s. At first, there were wild claims of technical mastery but only a few real centers of robotic expertise. No concrete description of appropriate credentialing or hospital privileging was available to the public. Average patients knew little or nothing of the levels of robotic surgery expertise at their hospital. Rather, billboards announced the end of painful surgery as we have known it.

Many of today's misleading smoke screens, created by a barrage of advertising about the latest and greatest medical technology, lead the polluted atmosphere surrounding the perfect surgical storm. Of course, none of this is new. False advertising continues to blind us to spotty capability in many health care sectors. And the public's obsession with the new surgery in the 1990s, as laparoscopy caught on, has been reborn today with the advent of sexy, untested robotic and no-incision operations. Having said that, it is important to remember that today's centers of excellence, as well as smaller hospitals with surgeons who have developed expertise with robotic assisted surgery, are far more common than in the Wild West early days of laparoscopic cholecystectomy.

Thus, the collision of events to be described undermined our collective sense of professional well-being. Surgeons and other technologically oriented physicians began using complex instrumentation with minimum training. Unevenly distributed surgical competence insinuated itself into general surgery practice. The public knew little about this aspect of the howling surgical storm outside their doors. However, there were other unsettling aspects of surgical practice in the first decade of the 21st century.

Why a Shift to Surgeons as Employees?

Not the least of the stormy events occurring today is the evolving transition of surgeons from professionals to employees. Burnout among surgeons has skyrocketed. Disgruntled, hard-working surgeons all around the country are struggling to provide safe, effective care to their patients. Our practitioners are getting older, longer in the tooth. There are few replacements in the wings as the government continues to refuse to pay for more training positions. And the profit motive of large insurance entities today may well have irreversibly dampened the otherwise traditionally positive attitude of surgeons. The overwhelming concern of younger surgeons for a good lifestyle seems to many older surgeons a reflection of a recent generational slide toward entitlement. Stated more honestly, the current generation of surgeons—Generation Y, or the millennials—does not accept our past total dedication to our patients. And, of course, they have a very good point. Life balance is needed to avoid the current 30–40 percent burnout rate among surgeons. So, especially in today's highly complex practice environment, the past dedication to selfless patient care contains within it the seeds of harm. Surgeons must limit themselves to their areas of competence and to reasonable work schedules. But a less vigorous work ethic in training (encouraged by reduced work hours and a shift-work mentality) may equate to less technical skill and therefore reduced patient safety.

As it stands, the current impasse on work hours is really a discussion of *shift work*. There is a strong trend today for surgeons to work for a hospital as an employee—presumably fostering the same conduct as other salaried workers. By that I mean surgeons may be practicing without the traditional attitude, characterized by the absolute and unquestioned dedication to the patient—night or day. As surgical educator Dr. Joseph E. Fischer bemoaned in 2005: "Well folks, it's finally happened. The total destruction of medicine, and more specifically general surgery, is upon us as a profession. . . . A professional, in our case a physician or surgeon, takes care of the patient until the job is completed."[3] Not all hospital-employed surgeons take care of the patient until the job is done. We hand off patients like footballs and head for the locker room. Dr. Fischer reminds us that an employee does not have the same level of responsibility as an autonomous professional.

As the feds whittle away at Medicare and Medicaid payments and regulators pile on paperwork, surgeons face the prospect of not being allowed to police themselves. When we lose the ability to regulate our professional activities, such as educational standards and the quality of our clinical activities, we cease to be a profession. We have not yet seen the endgame that will result when surgeons are denied the ability to make treatment decisions for their patients based on their unique wisdom and experience. We will revert back to being a trade—17th-century barber-surgeons without the pole.

Hospital administrators subject full-time surgeons to impossible work schedules. This is occurring at the very time when they and other citizens insist that doctors shouldn't work when fatigued. There is quiet acquiescence by the bean counters to this double standard. While chattering in public from atop the moral high ground of patient safety and about avoiding physician fatigue, the bean counters gleefully whip the faculty like racehorses in private to force them to see more and more patients. The moral decay driving the profit motive that dominates the U.S. health care system is the most forceful of the destructive gusts propelling the perfect surgical storm.

This corporate behavior meets the criteria noted by Sidney Dekker when he describes how complex systems (organizations) drift into failure. Thus, shorter contact time with a patient in the clinic (typically 15–20 minutes) becomes the new normal, potentially leading to errors in history taking or to missing important physical findings that ultimately make a subsequent operation dangerous. Not ordering a test or missing important CT or other imaging findings (to assist in making a diagnosis) may insidiously slip into the surgeon's corporate medical mind-set. This time pressure from the hospital organization nudges practitioners away from attention to detail toward indifference or worse clinical behavior.

Setting standards and enforcing them is what defines surgeons and other professionals as members of a profession. Getting and holding a job and meeting job requirements is what workers (employees) do. But sadly, surgeons are being pressured to downplay the special importance to patients of their knowledge, skills, and behavioral standards. We are insidiously forced to become clock-watchers. I have witnessed the erosion of professional standards by surgeons who are protected by working under the umbrella of large institutions (hospitals) where individual accountability is camouflaged by layers of loose regulations and where staff surgeons dump patients on each other.

Most dedicated surgeons resist this ethically bankrupt trend. I've also witnessed surgeons travel to the hospital from home on their nights off to cover an emergency when the on-call surgeon refused to see a sick patient or the covering surgeon needed their special expertise. It doesn't pay much. But the patient benefits from this traditional brand of professionalism. This commitment to patient care persists in most surgeons and in most of our fine young trainees. Dr. Fischer reminds us: "Only professionals, in the trade-off that is intrinsic in granting a profession its area of expertise and governance, have an obligation to society to do the unpleasant care for all such as trauma and emergency surgery, care for the indigent, practice in rural areas where remuneration and social advantages may not be as pleasant as in the urban setting, and to cover emergency rooms. Employees have no such obligation."[4] In a word, if our middle-management model of health care crushes dedication out of surgeons through heavy-handed regulation, why would surgeons in their right minds attempt to endure in our currently flawed health care system? For that matter, why would those of us in advanced retirement years continue to work (sensitive to the surgeon shortage) when interaction with our patients—the main reason we enjoy our practices—is trivialized?

Employees go home when their shift is over. Surgeons used to go home only after the work was done. Now trainees—and perhaps soon there will follow regulatory restrictions on all practicing surgeons—must leave the hospital before the work is completed. A less savory concern arises at this juncture. Less-motivated surgeons—those without the moral fire in the belly—will be protected in the surgeon-as-employee model. They will become immune to commitment. For them, "My shift's over. Ask someone else" will become the new credo. And, as mentioned earlier, nonsurgeon "experts" with the approval of well-meaning but deluded members of the public have made shift work an integral part of surgical training in the form of the inflexible 80-hour workweek. The deadly cancer that is fatigue fear will consume the host (the health care system) unless all parties return to the negotiating table and reconsider the crucial elements of the dilemma.

In a word, conscientious surgeons don't get paid for doing the right thing. But they do the right thing anyway—rested or fatigued. At least they always have in the past. But regulatory pressures are forcing us into behavior patterns that are hardly characteristic of altruistic practitioners. In other words, it's difficult to get the colossal paperwork tasks done, negotiate the modern regulatory jungle, battle third-party payers, *and* have time to care for sick patients. As a consequence of these outside pressures, surgeons have begun to show signs of wear and tear.[5] Signs of dejection and weariness reflect the battles surgeons have always fought for their patients. Nonetheless, the surgeon shortage now reaching critical proportions will make these practice dilemmas worse.

Elements of the Perfect Surgical Storm

Surgeons practicing in the 21st century must deal with the issues to be described. You should be aware of these pressures when you interact with a surgeon. Most surgeons focus on the patients at hand despite being distracted by the indignity of their perceived loss of professional control. But the following contentious problems surgeons face are the source of much professional dissatisfaction (and may affect patient safety):

- *The surgeon shortage*—projections are scary. If we cannot attract medical students and we lose surgeons to retirement because of the challenges, the shortage may not be fixable; in any event, it will take decades to repair the surgeon shortage even if additional training positions are made available.[6]

- *Public intolerance of medical errors is commendable and an important force for change, but medical errors highlight the uncertain nature of surgical practice as well as the health care system's need to work harder at all aspects of patient safety.* Surgeons know complications will occur; individual patients possess independent risk factors (e.g., obesity, diabetes, high blood pressure) resulting in increased morbidity and mortality. As a corollary, large modern hospitals are highly complex institutions and thus inherently unsafe.[7]

- *Malpractice litigation threatens a surgeon's mental and financial well-being and fails to fix the injured patient's needs, both the victim's compromised health and the victim's financial burden.* American trial lawyers have a strong lobby in Washington that perpetuates inequalities for patients and surgeons alike. Patients who should sue lousy surgeons usually don't; instead, they sue good surgeons with (uncontrollable) bad results. There is no compensation for injured patients who don't sue, but these patients should receive compensation (as in a no-fault system).[8]

- *The introduction of "never" events*—third-party payers and federal regulatory agencies are saving money by insisting that certain postoperative complications (which surgeons can only partly avoid) are solely the surgeon's fault; the added care provided by the surgeon to fix the complication isn't paid for.

- *Pay for performance*—if patients do well, the surgeon gets more money (who decides?); this is a lame attempt to improve quality rather than attack the root causes: inadequate surgical training, questionable certification of practitioners at all levels, and dangerous hospitals fighting to stay afloat financially.

- *Surgeons (as employees) burdened with more work, less pay, less control of their practices, and thus less satisfaction with their lives*—practitioners will inevitably make mistakes, get sued, become more depressed, leave practice, and thus make the surgeon shortage an escalating crisis.

- *The physical and emotional health of many surgeons is at risk* (Box 12.1)—and surgeons, like all doctors, are loath to seek help, which only complicates the precarious status of their ability to care for others.

- *The new generation's work ethic*—the institution of the 80-hour workweek for all medical and surgical residents was necessary, but it has solidly enshrined shift work into the trainee mentality. Millennials' ideas of work and play are not always aligned with patients' coming first, as promoted by the American College of Surgeons' definition of professionalism.

Box 12.1 The Emotional and Physical State of Practicing Surgeons in the 21st Century

- Only 75 percent of practicing surgeons are happy with their work; about the same percentage would *not* recommend a surgical career for their children.
- Over 80 percent of busy laparoscopic surgeons have work-related joint pain.
- 50 percent of surgeons over 50 years of age have a physical disability.
- 30–40 percent of practicing surgeons are burned out (experience depersonalization, loss of empathy, or are not focused on tasks at hand).
- 21 percent of surgeons have been divorced.
- 7 percent of practicing surgeons are alcoholics.
- 6 percent of practicing surgeons have had suicidal thinking.

Shared Decision Making—Is Informed Consent a Victim of the Perfect Surgical Storm?

You have just read about the substantial problems complicating a modern surgical practitioner's daily work. A surgeon's discomfort with unrealistic regulations, coupled with a lack of technical adeptness with some less invasive operations, leaves holes in the way any surgeon may negotiate with his or her patients. In this regard, an issue that is seldom addressed involves how we provide informed consent to patients about to undergo an operation. It has been said that "human inventiveness has created problems because human judgment and humanity's ability to deal with the consequences of its creations lags behind its ability to create."[9] We've created a host of wonderfully less invasive operations. The benefits are huge for patients. But we still haven't dealt adequately with the consequences of the laparoscopic revolution as far as educating our patients about how to negotiate through their many operative choices.

Giving informed consent is not an easy task for surgeons. Our willingness to inform patients about operative choices, to describe the risks involved, and to explain the benefits of a particular procedure are compromised by the complexity of today's laparoscopic operations. Too often the unspoken part of informed consent is the limits of the surgeon's technical skills. Some surgeons are inclined to offer the operation with which they are most familiar. They may not discuss an alternative operation that they are not prepared to perform themselves. And the reason for not discussing an alternative operation is quite possibly that it would require referring the patient to another surgeon.

To begin with, surgeons are appropriately proud of their operative skills. And many feel they can do *any* operation that is needed. This is because they have particular skills, they believe, that can be applied to any operative situation. This is a questionable concept. Therefore, it behooves patients to ask their surgeon about his or her experience, the number of cases the surgeon has done, and the outcomes: "How did your patients do?" True patient safety won't happen while everyone with a laparoscope or robot is yelling "excellence" through their masks while holding their bloodied gloves behind their backs.

What Else Has Changed Since the Laparoscopic Revolution Began?

Many other changes have accompanied the laparoscopic revolution. Just prior to the explosion of less invasive operations in 1990, only 38 percent of medical students were women. Today, over 50 percent of medical students are female. Slowly, women are gaining ground in acquiring academic appointments—although this trend is far too slow.[10] In our surgical residency at Baystate Medical Center, over 50 percent of our trainees are women. There are no gender differences in mental toughness, surgical knowledge, or skills. And our residents display an admirable work ethic—despite the reservations I've expressed. A particular problem for women in surgery is the tendency for female surgeons to work part-time or to share a full-time position. This reduces the workforce and dilutes the output of surgical training programs.

Attitudes have changed. As I stated, Generation Y millennial medical students want better lifestyles. Mentoring third-year medical students in my role as the clerkship director in surgery, I observe students who are considering a surgical career invariably stumble over the huge work demands, the anticipated hours away from family, and the nights and weekends on call. They become worried that they won't be able to handle the stress. And quite possibly, some of them retreat because of their unfavorable experiences with the surgical personality.

Work hours have been significantly reduced, as discussed in Chapter 11. Unfortunately, for surgical residents there has been a significant parallel deterioration in learning opportunities. When asked, surgical trainees will tell you that—despite wanting a better lifestyle—they are extremely unhappy with restricted work hours. They would like to work *more* because they see continuity of patient care compromised. They see their knowledge and skills becoming eroded, for example, when they must leave the hospital just as their patient is about to go to the operating room.

Satisfaction with the work itself has changed for practicing surgeons as well. Box 12.1 tells a sad story, including the fact that only 75 percent of recently surveyed surgeons stated that they enjoyed their work.[11] After studying the tortuous course of the laparoscopic revolution, I think I know what's missing in the way many modern surgeons practice the art and science of surgery today. Sadly, too many surgeons practice without passion.

More critically, studies performed *after* the switch to less invasive operations was well on its way revealed an unexpected truth. A few surgeons just couldn't master the new laparoscopic operations. As nationally renowned surgical educator and 2010 president of the American College of Surgeons, Dr. L. D. Britt wrote in 2005, "While it should be the goal of the training program to finish the chief resident who is able to practice independently, it is highly unlikely that a trainee will reach 'expert' level by the end of the residency or fellowship training."[12] The best minds in American surgical education revealed a surgical competency deficiency that any reasonable person would agree must be shared with the public. A study of trainees demonstrated that 16 percent of *surgical residents* with minimal experience with laparoscopy were not able to reach proficiency in the performance of several laparoscopic operations after training. An additional 8 percent underperformed and never improved with intense training: they couldn't learn the operations.[13]

A similar study showed that 20 percent of *nonsurgical trainees* tested for their ability to learn laparoscopic skills demonstrated that they "had such a low level of innate abilities that they were unable to achieve an acceptable performance in our minimal-access surgery (MAS) simulation."[14] Some of these doctors—who will not become surgeons—will nonetheless work in areas such as interventional radiology and interventional cardiology where innate technical ability is important.

The irony is that despite the problems in surgical education and clinical practice, the care of patients is better today than it has ever been. The MIS mantra says it all: less pain, shorter recoveries, quicker return to daily activities. Patients have experienced huge reductions in postoperative pain and suffering. Hospital stays are shorter. Recovery is swift. Scars are tiny.

The resident surgeon that educators are now cultivating is a trainee who enters the operating room already skilled in many of the basic components of an operation.[15] It is no secret that in the past surgical residents learned on patients exclusively and often without supervision.[16] Today under strict supervision, the trainee, after demonstrating competence in basic skills in the lab, may be allowed to assume increasing responsibility for doing parts of an operation in the OR. This aspect of the perfect surgical storm has abated.

Credentialing the Laparoscopic Surgeon

Historically, hospitals generally let surgeons do whatever operations they (and the program director of their residency program) said they could do. It was a "check the list of operations" mentality. In the day, if a surgeon graduated from a respectable surgical training program, he or she was assumed to know how to operate. Nobody tested the new surgeon (or the older surgeon who took a short course to learn a new operation). And today nobody ever scrubs in to see if the surgeon can actually do the operations he or she checked off on the laundry list of procedures in that specialty.

Hospitals, especially smaller rural hospitals, cannot function without a general surgeon. So these heroic practitioners work in an environment that demands a lot of technical talent. Most of these surgeons are superb. But some may fall prey to the allure of performing less invasive operations with marginal training. Accordingly, Anthony D. Whittemore reminds us,

"Irrespective of certification by the American Board of Surgery, actual credentialing and privileges remains within the domain of the local institution through processes that are neither standardized nor particularly rigorous."[17] This means that the hospital may not require the surgeon to have done anywhere near the 30 to 50 of each of the advanced laparoscopic operations on the hospital's privileges checklist necessary to achieve minimum competency. Nor will the hospital (unable to function without a general surgeon) challenge the surgeon's ongoing operative experience.

Thus, the paradigm shift to less aggressive operations carries with it unresolved issues of how to train surgical residents in order for them to reach a sound level of overall competence. The challenge applies equally to how to credential as fully capable those practicing surgeons in active practice. Our task as surgical educators straddles the imperative to train skilled young surgeons while not subjecting patients to added risks. Twenty years ago, SAGES established guidelines for "privileging qualified surgeons in the performance of general surgical procedures utilizing laparoscopy and/or thoracoscopy."[18]

The surgeon shortage in the United States will place considerable pressure on practicing surgeons to continue to operate into their later years,[19] possibly long beyond the time when their skills begin to deteriorate. And the surgeon shortage may pressure newly minted young surgeons to attempt operations with which they have minimal training. A predictable number of complications will always occur, even in the hands of true surgical masters. But complications should not be confused with medical and surgical errors—mistakes caused by poor judgment or technical errors based on a lack of appropriate skills and training. As far back as 1948, Dr. Robert Zollinger stated, "It should be made clear that the training programs, as they now exist, are at considerable variance with the expressed ideals of the teachers of surgery, and in many instances do not appear to fulfill the needs of the practicing general surgeon."[20]

The challenges facing surgical educators continue to hinge to a real extent on the worries expressed by Dr. Zollinger more than 60 years ago. Our educational dilemmas are different today, but continue to reveal the tension between what we teach our trainees and what a capable practicing surgeon needs to know. What is unchanged is a commitment to the educational principles that anchor our imperative to make all operations safe. Unfortunately, the perfect surgical storm will continue to add layers of complex challenges to daily practice. It will not blow off over the minimally invasive ocean any time soon.

PART 5

The Modern Surgical Toolbox: General Surgery Is Changed Forever

CHAPTER THIRTEEN

Surgical Education Today: Can We Still Train Capable General Surgeons?

Multiple external forces indicate that the magnitude and quality of necessary changes warrant a rebirth of surgical training—a revolution in terms of what training to be a surgeon means and entails.

Edna C. Shenvi, MD, *Bulletin of the American College of Surgeons*, 2014

Many patients still experience the collateral damage that arises from using them to gain experience on them, although it has been known for a very long time that patient harm can be minimized through using simulation.

Harry Owen, MD, *Simulation in Healthcare*, 2012

The operating room falls into deadly silence.

The banter stops. Bob Dylan's howl fades as the circulating nurse turns off the CD, knowing intuitively that something is wrong. With heads bowed, the surgeons plunge their bloody gloved hands into the huge incision. A segment of large intestine, perforated at close range by a 38-caliber slug, spills what at least looks like liquid stool. The surgeons are suddenly distracted from suturing the bowel together. The operative field floods with a gush of blood. The senior resident flaps his hand. Noisy suction sounds fill the room.

"Are you guys OK down there?" the anesthesia resident asks from the head of the table. "His pressure's dropping like a stone!"

"Not sure . . . damn . . ."

The bleeding gets worse. The senior surgical resident probes the wound with a clamp, searching for the bleeder. His gloves and sterile gown sleeve come out of the incision drenched with fresh blood.

"Holy—" The junior resident standing across the draped body from the senior asks, "Where's it coming from?"

"Suction!" The senior resident bends over and focuses his attention in the depths of the wound. "Here . . . you . . . retract like this . . ."

An alarm screams over the suction noise from the anesthesia machine hidden by the drapes. "His pressure's 60 over zip . . ." barks the anesthesiologist behind the wall of sterile drapes at the head of the table. Then she adds in a soft voice, "EKG tracing just shows tachycardia of 130, no other heart problem." "Come on, guys, you gotta get the bleeding under control."

The chief resident stops, twists, and screams, "What the hell you think I'm doing!"

Behind a one-way mirror, I turn to my colleague. She nods. She speaks into her head-mounted microphone. "That's enough, guys. The scenario's over."

For 40 minutes we debrief the two teams sweating in our simulated operating room. Everyone gets his or her say. No pulling rank. No holding back. And we thank each other when it's over.

Today's operating-room simulation exercise reveals several performance problems with our training surgeons attempting to solve the intraoperative bleeding scenario. These issues include individual decision making, poor emotional control, and uneven team performance. For a few minutes we all help clean the simulated operating room (it can also be used to simulate an ER trauma bay or an ICU room). Soon, the mannequin is intact, ready for the next scenario. Our simulation center at Baystate Medical Center is part of one of a growing number of Accreditation of Education Institutes around the country promoted and sponsored by the American College of Surgeons (ACS).

Out-of-the-operating-room technical skills training and patient simulation represent a new core for surgical education and the wave riding us into the future. They're about adapting to the current health care quality-of-care revolution. They're a responsible way of responding to the considerable training demands created by the laparoscopic surgery revolution. They're about honoring today's patients' worries about medical students and training doctors making mistakes on them. Ultimately, improved surgical training is about reducing medical errors across the huge spectrum of medical and surgical care in a system overwhelmed with information.

As a 2009 report concluded: "We need to change! Indeed, we may be on a precipice that without substantial changes to surgical education we may risk, for the first time in the last century, of graduating residents who may be less skilled than the previous generation."[1] This sentiment is echoed in many published reports by leading surgical educators. What we should teach and how to teach it remain big questions in surgical residency programs. However, surgical education has been favorably revolutionized, and every aspect of selecting, pretraining, arduously training (in technical as well as nontechnical skills), and assessing surgical trainees now has a scientific basis. The overwhelming amount of research on surgical education will require me to be selective in choosing topics regarding educational research in order to sketch a broad picture of where we are today.

What Is the Goal of Surgical Education?

The main goal of surgical education is to select, train, and assess the capability of our future surgeons and to assure their competence in the defined areas of clinical activity in which they choose to practice.[2] Remember, we're now dealing with not only laparoscopic and open operations, but also operations performed with an endoscope and through the insides of arteries (endovascular operations). One of our major challenges is to decide what part of general surgery to teach as core principles. Given fewer work hours and the need for more close supervision of residents learning complex skills, we've had to change our teaching methods.

Our challenge as educators rests in the need for a more practical method of defining what is clinically valuable for a trainee to know in an ever-enlarging knowledge pool. To date, our residents spend excessive time, in my opinion, memorizing nonclinical facts. An example is cell biology—the role of DNA polymerase, antiviral protease inhibitors, which cell receptor is most critical in creating new blood vessels in cancers, and so forth—which *has no practical application in the performance of surgery*. Research and scientifically oriented academic surgeons push this menu while residents come to the operating room chock-full of molecular information but can't name the anatomical structure or tissue they are touching with the scalpel or laparoscopic grasper. A review book aimed at preparation for the American Board of Surgery In-Training Exam (ABSITE) runs 535 pages of small-print multiple-choice questions.[3] It also contains abundant information about common diseases that trainees must know about. Thus, the ABSITE exam is a valuable tool for learning about a wide range of diseases and their treatment. My concern is that it also details information unrelated to the practice of surgery and data that residents can retrieve on their cell phones.

The dilemma was summarized recently by a surgical resident in a first-place essay sponsored by the ACS, entitled "Surgical Training: Time for a Revolution." She wrote, "The goal of training should be to get the best care to the patients and not to simply get the most knowledge into the trainee's head; only with a new role for technology and a new professional identity can it be distinguished that these are not synonymous."[4] Training surgeons recognize the wasted energy of memorizing information that has no direct impact on their clinical competence. A major contribution to surgical education has been the Surgical Council on Resident Education (SCORE) program, designed to collect in one online location all the educational material to be covered during a five-year residency in general surgery. Each of the over 800 learning modules contains core didactic material, learning objectives, study questions, text résumés, videos, and self-assessment quizzes. The SCORE program highlights the immense knowledge and skills challenges of modern general surgery. Another essay in the *Bulletin of the American College of Surgeons* stated, "Today, offshoots of general surgery demand mastery of a body of knowledge *as expansive as the parent field* [my italics]."[5] The offshoots are subspecialty areas such as colorectal, pediatric, and breast surgery (over 70 breast-cancer genes have been identified; another 100 or so are associated with inflammatory bowel disease, just two diseases—how many genes will our trainees have to memorize?). The parent field is general surgery. Its ill-defined borders frighten residents who seek not only a controllable lifestyle but a manageable knowledge load as in the surgical subspecialties. And while we are force-feeding our residents this information overload, academic leaders bemoan the dropping pass rate for board certification. It seems to me that this is a self-fulfilling prophecy.

Surgical educators must move beyond the fact-regurgitation mentality and embrace the role of digital storage and *retrieval* as the evolving learning paradigm. Residents can find just about any fact within a minute or less, so mentally retrieving data and its well-documented unreliability is a questionable educational goal. We need to teach our trainees *how* to think, not *what* to think.

The aviation industry uses flight simulators not only for certification but also for ongoing training and retraining of pilots. Surgical educators have been behind the curve using simulation, although the idea isn't new. As Dr. Timothy Eberlein identified in a 2014 report entitled "A New Paradigm in Surgical Training," a "restructuring committee" of American Board of Surgery directors, Residency Review Committee members, fellowship and general surgery program directors, and public members was established to "fix the five" (reconfigure five years of general surgery residency) and consider other, shorter surgical specialty tracks (with fewer training years).[6] A national curriculum employing skills labs and simulation centers now represents the new learning paradigm for surgical residents.

Is Simulation in Medical Education New?

In a fascinating 2012 review by Dr. Harry Owen entitled "Early Use of Simulation in Medical Education," the author sketches out the long history of the use of "phantoms," dolls, mannequins (variously spelled as *manakin*, *maniken*, or *manikin*), carved models, cadavers, dead body parts, and combinations of these simulators in teaching various aspects of patient care.[7] From bronze statues with over 350 holes through which acupuncture was practiced in 1027, through a description of a variety of obstetric simulators made of wood, leather, and rubber, the subject of surgical simulation is covered by Owen as well.

The earliest surgical simulators were described in a classic text from India written by Sushruta between the fourth and sixth centuries BCE. The following quotations highlight the value of simulation then and will be compared to our modern descriptions of simulation in medical education: "To give efficiency in surgical operations (trainees) were asked to try their knives repeatedly on natural and artificial objects resembling diseased parts of the body before undertaking an actual operation";[8] "The art of bandaging or ligaturing should be practically learned by tying bandages around the specific limbs and members of a full-sized doll made of stuffed linen."[9]

According to Owen, little was done to incorporate simulation into a surgeon's training until the 19th century, when a canvas mannequin was used to demonstrate a new hernia operation. Also, between 1870 and 1888, the U.S. government published reports on tens of thousands of Civil War wounds, including suturing intestinal wounds, suggesting that the technique "should not be attempted on the living subject until the operator has acquired some experience by practicing . . . either using the fingers of a glove, or, better still, upon a recent subject, or on intestines placed in a manikin."[10] This portion of Owen's history particularly resonated with me as I worked with the Chamberlain Group in Great Barrington, Massachusetts, in designing an intestinal model (Figure 13.1) for use in learning both laparoscopic and open intestinal anastomosis (sewing the bowel ends together after removing a segment).

Compare Dr. Owen's concluding remarks with those he quoted from hundreds of years ago. He states, "Some comments . . . on using a simulator to learn the new technique are as relevant now as they were in the 19th century; to perform the skill quickly and without causing injury requires a lot of practice, and if you do not practice on a simulator, the first unlucky patient whom you treat will suffer."[11] Finally, Owen concludes: "Simulation was embedded in a surgical training program around 2500 years ago, so

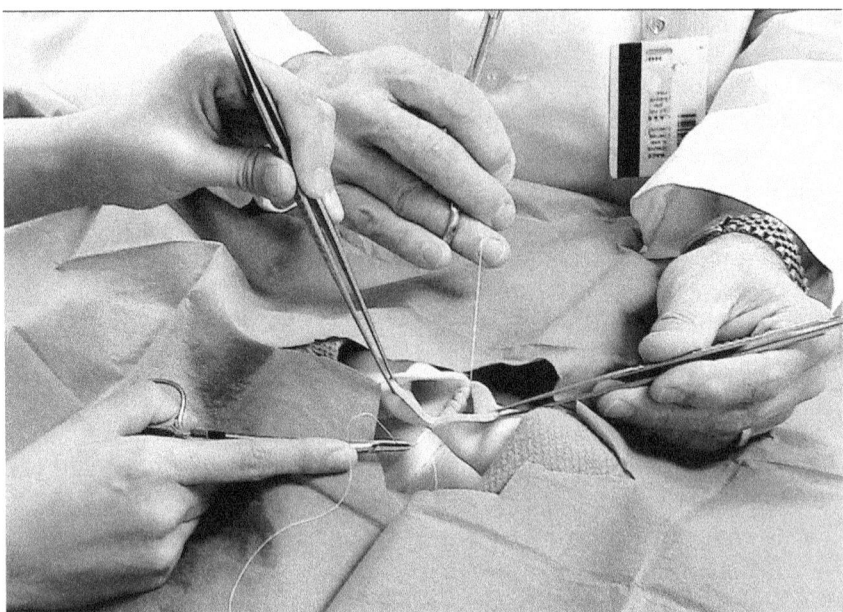

Figure 13.1 Teaching Traditional Open Surgery—Intestinal Anastomosis ("Joining") in the Skills Lab (photo by The Chamberlain Group. Used by permission.)

that students had developed a wide range of skills before commencing clinical practice. . . . The early adopters of simulation described how it facilitated development of procedural skills without risk to patients, that skills could be practiced repeatedly or become expert, that experts could maintain skills, and that uncommon events could be prepared for using simulation."[12]

The surgical education revolution that followed on the heels of the laparoscopic revolution, characterized by simulation and skills lab training, was a true rebirth of ancient simulation training. It has been incorporated into the central nervous system of the teaching of surgery in all its current forms as a necessary rediscovery. It will evolve as robotic surgery and other less invasive approaches to surgical disease are applied to surgical practice from ongoing research and development from both within and outside of the academy. We have eliminated unsupervised trainees where it was service to the hospital that was more important than education and training.[13]

Moving Forward with Surgical Education—A State of Flux

Teaching

Surgical educators haven't completely figured out how to modify and retool the training curriculum for surgical residents. We're struggling with ways to compensate for the impossibility of teaching all the available knowledge and skills now under the umbrella of general surgery. We understand the impact of the explosion of scientific and clinical information birthed by the laparoscopic revolution. The task of training capable graduates using only an apprentice model (one-on-one, on-the-job learning on patients) as done in the past has become especially untenable with the current work hours.

Apprenticeship relationships (one-on-one teaching, as well as a surgeon's modeling proper professionalism and communication skills, among others) are effective if the trainee has prior exposure to skills and adequate basic knowledge. Also, one-on-one teaching *before* working in the operating room is part of deliberate practice. Pretraining in simulation and surgical skills laboratories has become critical because we need to make up for lost operating-room time as well as substitute for less time spent by trainees on the surgical floors and in the clinic directly involved in patient care. The crucial reality seemingly still ignored by some surgical leaders is that, for example, whereas in 2010 medical knowledge doubled in 3.5 years (in 1950 it doubled in 50 years), by 2020 *medical knowledge will double every 73 days!*[14]

What we all agree on is that a well-trained surgeon must be more than a virtuoso technician. Six competencies, as noted earlier (Box 4.1), define for us what our educational goals must be; how to accomplish them is built into the relatively new national surgical education (SCORE) curriculum. Surgical educators everywhere struggle with the continuing gap between our theoretical model of surgical education and the reality on the ground as spelled out by the demands placed on surgical faculty by hospital administrators as well as by today's much sicker patients.

For a moment, let's examine how surgical educators inexorably crept up on the notion that teaching surgery had to change from the pedagogy (teaching methods) of the good old days. In the past we learned on real patients. These patients were often disadvantaged and came to charity and inner city hospitals with no other prospect for receiving medical care than from inadequately supervised trainees. What we have not discussed until recently are the outcomes of those patients cared for by unsupervised surgical trainees. This is the mighty unspoken irony of surgical education today: that the *outcomes-based* (How did the patient actually do?) and *competency-based* (Does the resident actually know how to do this particular case?) modern version of how we teach the six competencies is built on the suppressed truth that the prior pedagogy of "See one, do one, teach one" was lethal for some patients.

Assessing Learning

An important point I've made before is that program directors today sign off on their graduates, assuring the public that the finishing trainee is competent and ready for independent practice just as they did in the past. In truth, some program directors knew that there was inadequate information—and studies have shown that much of our clinical (global) impressions of a trainee's capability were inaccurate—to assure that their graduates were ready for prime time. A 2011 study of general surgery program directors' attitudes regarding testing basic skills in junior residents concluded, "No PD would either prevent residents with demonstrable poor basic skills from going to the operating room or use poor basic surgical skills as a reason to deny promotion."[15] This conclusion implies that the poorly performing resident would be carefully supervised in the operating room and would be offered remediation. Fixing or remediating a trainee is a daunting task. Nonetheless, today we have more objective methods of assessing a resident's progression in the structured program. Still, whether residents are adequately prepared for independent practice remains a challenge even as our methods of assuring trainee capability continue to improve.[16,17,18,19,20]

Recognizing the Need for Change in Surgical Education—A Historical Note

Change has characterized the teaching and practice of surgery since the 17th century. It was Dr. William Stewart Halsted who designed the first American surgery residency at the end of the 19th century after training in Europe. Halsted remarked, "In the German Universities, when chairs of surgery were first created, it was considered beneath the dignity of the physician who taught the doctrines of this art actually to practice it."[21] Could there ever be a bigger change in the field of surgery! Imagine, the masters who taught surgery never wielded a scalpel. When he returned to the United States, Halsted created the idea of a graduated, slow increase in responsibility given to training surgeons under strict supervision as they matured over many years. This method was adopted throughout most of the 20th century. However, surgical residency continued to be a grueling experience but with less emphasis on supervision than Halsted had in mind. Currently, patient-safety failures and an unrelenting cascade of hospital errors have reversed this trend, and we are now oversupervising our trainees.

But let's go back to the mid-20th century and a report from 1958 that serves as background for our discussion of modern surgical education regarding both the educator's beliefs and that of a typical resident back then. The educator states, "Learning the motions, the techniques—a matter of drilling, can be accomplished in a relatively short time, and can be over-emphasized."[22] He states that actual operative skills could be *overtaught*. By comparison, teaching complex motor skills represents one of the most difficult aspects of a surgical educator's job today. However, some things don't change. Describing a surgical resident, the same author explains: "He acquires a feeling that he can do anything better than anyone else and that he can perform the operation better than his chief, although he does make charitable concessions to experience and age. . . . He develops a language of his own. Accepted terms, sentence structure, proper word usage are things which he holds in contempt."[23] The author concludes by making an observation still valuable today: "Maturation takes time and cannot be speeded up by changing the name of the first postgraduate year from internship to assistant residency or by abolishing the last year of college."[24] Residents' overconfidence remains a challenge for us in the modern era but much less so. Nonetheless, a cocky resident who won't accept direction—in essence a trainee who is unteachable—is as dangerous as an ignorant one.

The problem of dealing with the educational challenges of surgical specialization as a consequence of the rapid growth of surgical knowledge after World War II was addressed in the 1960s. Basically, the unsolved problem that has lasted until recently centers on two concerns: (a) How much general surgery training does a resident going into a specialty (orthopedics, plastic surgery, or urology) need before specializing? and (b) How much training (how many years) does a resident in general surgery need before entering practice? As stated in 1961, "Data collected by the American College of Surgeons have indicated that there is considerable support among directors of surgical training programs for the idea of providing more general surgical training for specialty residents, but opinions are divided as to what this training should consist of, how long it should be, and when it should take place in relation to concentrated residency experience of the specialty."[25] These concerns remain today. Another report from 1962 by Owen H. Wangensteen, a giant in surgical circles, anticipated the need for more surgeons based on population projections.[26] Sadly, subsequent attempts to predict the necessary workforce ignored his sage advice. Dr. Wangensteen also noted what now seems like an anachronistic view, stating: "I believe that all surgeons, even those intending to become community surgeons, need to be exposed to the experience of the laboratory. . . . When a young surgeon aspirant has learned to operate successfully and well on a dog, he is ready for operative opportunities on the wards."[27] Animal labs are disappearing as inanimate simulation and skills training have increasingly become commonplace. However, Wangensteen anticipated the value of out-of-the-operating-room training.

This brief historical sketch gives you some background regarding just how stubborn many notions about how best to train surgeons have been over the last five decades.

What Are the New Challenges Facing Surgical Educators?

Who is that doctor introducing herself to you in the pre-anesthesia holding room? Will she review your procedure and provide informed consent as you lie in a gown anxiously awaiting your operation? That is, will she give you enough information in order for you to consent with a comfortable sense that you know what will happen in the operating room and thereafter? Will *she* actually do your surgery? What role will the assistant play? Will she just watch a trainee operate on you? Or will the resident merely hold retractors and learn by observing your surgeon perform every part of your operation? Will there be other trainees, medical students, or other health care observers in the operating room? In other words, what does it mean to be a patient in a teaching hospital?

Innumerable studies have been published on all aspects of surgical education in the last three decades. This vital part of our discussion of surgeon capability must interweave elements of past thinking about teaching surgical skills with the ever-evolving, ever-improving, yet still-incomplete status of surgical education today. I will detail a few topics I believe any potential surgical patient entering a teaching hospital should know about:

- The technology used to teach residents varies in sophistication from basic box trainers to virtual reality machines;[28,29] they have been validated and proven to quickly improve trainees' motor skills learning. First-year residents practice knot tying and basic suturing while more advanced residents do vascular (arterial) anastomosis (sewing together) as well as intestinal anastomosis (Figure 13.1); junior and senior residents practice basic laparoscopic skills (Figure 13.2), as well as remove gallbladders and do other virtual operations on machines. These exercises require *protected learning time*, which places hospitals in a position of needing to hire more expensive midlevel workers (physician assistants, nurse practitioners, etc.) when finances are in a severe belt-tightening mode.

- The requirement to produce a pretrained novice is predicated on the public's awareness of an unacceptable number of medical and surgical errors attributed in the past to a lack of supervision and to trainee fatigue.[30] Surgeons must do the case in less time; this leaves the trainee to do less of the procedure to improve case turnover time—the holy grail of surgical productivity.

- Among other difficulties with work-hour restrictions, some residents struggle to meet the 850 total cases needed to graduate in general surgery, 150 of which must be done in the chief resident's last year; this compares to 1,400 to 1,500 cases we completed back in the day. Thus, some of today's residents do little more than half of the typical intraoperative experience that older surgeons accomplished in their residencies; as a recent report bemoaned: "Junior residents spend the day performing a myriad of apparently aimless tasks with little sense of accomplishment; senior residents often relegate inappropriately or worse, do all the work themselves with even less efficiency. . . . Much of the work done by residents is aimless and noneducational, disparagingly referred to as 'scud.'"[31]

- The ACGME has instituted new "Common Program Requirements" as well as more sophisticated methods to be used in teaching (simulation and skills labs are recommended) and to assess resident knowledge and skills. Added to faculty clinical duties are added hours of committee time; for example, the Clinical Competency Committee must assess every resident on 16 milestones or performance measures related to knowledge, skills, and attitude every six months.[32]

- The federal government has frozen the number of postgraduate medical and surgical residency training slots, thus assuring that the current shortage of surgeons will become much worse. Now and in the future baby boomers will develop more diseases treated by general surgeons. These challenges defeat our teaching efforts, not to mention our efforts to do research.

- Transparency about patient safety and less time to teach in the operating room and elsewhere in the hospital (e.g., in the clinic seeing new and follow-up patients) have resulted in *oversupervision* with graduating surgeons having experienced much *less autonomy*;[33,34] this smothering results in trainees with less clinical judgment than residents in the past.

- The politics of 21st-century surgical care have significantly eroded educational opportunities and include the shift from inpatient to outpatient (daystay) care, in which trainees seldom experience the whole profile of patient management and recovery; fewer work hours producing more handoffs, with the clear implication that it's OK to not follow the patient you just operated on; and fewer work hours reducing the resident's exposure to night and weekend call, when patients in need of resuscitation and dying patients are rushed to the operating room by the residents in-house while the attending surgeon comes in from home.

- In our politically correct world, all trainees, no matter how incompetent, are mandated to have a chance at remediation (in contrast to past decades when the program director dismissed trainees for incompetence, dishonesty, laziness, etc.). Remediation requires endless hours of reteaching by faculty who have little time to begin with; attempting to fix what is often an unfixable trainee takes teaching time away from the solid residents, a waste of everyone's time.[35,36,37,38]

The Need for Changes in Funding for Surgical Education

When Medicare was introduced in 1965, we witnessed the growth of large medical centers populated with huge faculties composed of physicians of all specialties. This beginning of an emphasis on clinical work done began the erosion of surgical education as surgeons spent more time completing cases in less time with trainees doing less and less of the operation. Trainees began to lose their previous autonomy as laws were passed that mandated the surgeon of record be present during the critical parts of the case. All of this was sensible from a patient-safety point of view but represented a major restriction for surgical residents who sought opportunities to operate independently. Also, diagnosis-related groups were introduced; costs were further cut by performing more day-stay operations; surgical residents did not see the patient's pre-op nor experience the patient's post-op progress or the development of complications. This lack of patient contact was aggravated by shorter hospital stays for inpatients. This ongoing trend has dramatically reduced our trainees' exposure to the day-to-day care of surgical patients.

Then, HMOs and for-profit systems placed even more pressure on surgeons to produce more clinical work, further cutting back on their teaching time. Ultimately, a new funding mechanism that includes significantly more contributions from the federal government is needed to support surgical education as the surgeon shortage grows.

Where Do Surgeons Come From?

They all look the same, these third-year medical students. The sheepish grin, the tone of self-deprecation, the uncertain tap on my door. Sure, they're a diverse bunch from different ethnic, cultural, and socioeconomic backgrounds. But they are collectively dedicated to the challenges of becoming proficient doctors. In that regard, in my experience they haven't changed in 40 years.

One of them pushes my door open a crack. "Do you have a moment?"

At times like this I feel like a priest about to confer with a sinner. The medical student sits next to my desk and wears a pained expression. I've seen it before in these incredibly smart and motivated young people. I know they have been advised—often less than subtly very early in medical school—not to consider a surgical career. I'm about to hear a confession. Expecting the verbalization of an epiphany, I ask, "What's on your mind?"

The student exhales, "I can't believe I'm saying this . . . but I think I want to be a surgeon."

And so it begins.

I don't push medical students to choose a career in surgery. The decision is too weighty, too burdened with responsibility and consequences. Only the student can make the call. And yet I savor the energy infused in the student's decision. From this defining moment in my office to board certification there lies a tortuous path strewn with obstacles and triumphs, calamities of unrelenting terror and magical moments of self-satisfaction. For the supercharged students who can't sit still, some who may suffer from some form of attention deficit syndrome (as many if not most surgeons assume they do), they love early morning rounds, the trauma cases, and the allure of that special place—the operating room. They get pleasure from seeing the pathology diagnosed moments earlier, handling the torn spleen, fingering the contours of a colon cancer, feeling the massive, pulsating abdominal aortic aneurysm. It really isn't a choice.

It is a calling.

Students know when they have chosen correctly, just as worried surgical residents experience the pure glee of having decided on a subspecialty for fellowship training or on the desire to practice in the broader field of general surgery. Two questions arise from the wretchedness of medical students' career decision making with the same predictability as snowfall in New England: "Based on your observation of my performance on this rotation," the student sitting beside my desk asks, "do you think I can become a surgeon?"

My answer changes little. "Do you *want* to be a surgeon?"

And then comes the student's more honest and self-reflective inquiry: "Do you really like the lifestyle, you know, being in the hospital so much? . . . I'm not sure if I would like to work this hard all my career."

I talk about my family and my delight in having chosen surgery as a career. I remind them that I'm the oldest faculty member and still at it because I still have work to do—and I point to the student who winces and smiles.

In 2002, a report, "The Modern Medical School Graduate and General Surgery Training," noted that the number of unfilled positions for general surgery training had increased tenfold.[39] Surgeons began introspectively examining their profession: only 10 percent of practicing surgeons were women, as female medical students felt surgery was discriminatory of their gender. Other issues identified were ethnicity (overwhelmingly, white males), Generation X and lifestyle issues, and medical school debt. In a nutshell, the authors reflected that "general surgery training has long been perceived as having a tough, regimented, inflexible and occasionally intimidating atmosphere."[40] Over a dozen years later, we recovered from the 2002 dip in interest in surgery as a career. A study discovered that the role of mentorship (surgeons guiding trainees and medical students in choosing a surgical career) was important.[41] Attrition rates (residents leaving the program for various reasons) were reasonably low at about 6 percent.[42] Today, few general surgery slots go unfilled, largely because we have rehabilitated our attitudes and approaches to millennial medical students.

Applying for Surgical Residency—Matchmaking by Any Other Name Leads to Marriage

Next in line is the application process. Geography may or may not play a role in the student's choice of a residency program. About 250 surgical training programs exist, some with fellowships that may interfere with the overall training experience of the surgical resident. If the specialty surgical fellow doing extra training "steals" the good operations, it leaves the resident short of cases; rules from the Residency Review Committee do apply in this regard. In other words, specialty fellows and chief residents are supposed to navigate separate courses so that they don't become predators and take away each other's cases. Junior residents must be prepared for their initial duties as well. A junior resident's training starts in the last year of medical school with special courses for those entering a surgical residency program.

Interviews are granted to fourth-year medical students based on the students' letters of recommendation, national (Step 1 and Step 2 exams of the United States Medical Licensing Examination [USMLE]) examination scores, and medical school performance. Frankly, test scores don't help much. But the dilemma of how to choose potential trainees dates back to decades ago when neuropsychological predictors of operative skill were pursued, documented, debated, and felt not to be appropriate to use in selecting future residents. For example, a 1984 study demonstrated no correlation between Medical College Admission Test scores and subsequent prediction of surgical resident skill competence as judged by the attending surgeon who rated them. The three factors that correlated most with attending surgeon ratings were complex visual-spatial organization of thinking, stress tolerance, and psychomotor abilities.[43] A commentator on the paper concluded, "One message is that those tests that measure primarily psychometric coordination and ability—so-called manual dexterity, if you will—really do not seem to be so important in the decision of who is and who is not a good operator."[44] In a recent study, although only 55 percent of surveyed programs had laparoscopic skills labs, for example, 88 percent of responders felt that skills lab training would improve operating-room performance.[45] In 2007, a study concluded, "There is strong agreement among respondents that skills laboratories are a necessary and valuable component of residency education."[46] Unfortunately, to date not all programs have truly well-functioning skills labs.

Well, then, what are the "characteristics of highly ranked applicants to general surgery residency programs"? A 2013 report on that subject abstracted data from Electronic Resident Application Service files of the 20 top-ranked applicants to 22 general surgery programs. They found the following characteristics important to the educators selecting applicants: research experience, publications in journals, Alpha Omega Alpha (medical honor society) membership, men who had high USMLE Step 1 scores, and Asian race.[47] A somber comment on the study by Dr. James C. Hebert of the Department of Surgery, University of Vermont, raised the issue of what criteria we should be looking at in this process. As surgical education and the accreditation of surgical programs moves to examining actual patient outcomes, as well as trainees' ability to meet certain performance milestones (of capability), Dr. Hebert agreed that the other competencies should be kept in mind and measured.[48] I would remind you that these include professionalism, communication ability, and an understanding of systems in health care.

A study published in 2004, a year after the work-hour restrictions went into effect, looked at the perceptions of the applicants, the fourth-year medical students. From the applicants' point of view, the study concluded, "The most common factors influencing residency program selection were how much the residency program seemed to care about its trainees (98%), how satisfied the current residents are with their program (98%), how well the applicant thought he or she would fit into the program (97%), the geographic location of the residency (95%), and how well the current residents seem to work with each other."[49] Some programs have tried written examinations to identify applicants who will do well later on the ABSITE.[50] Once again, for most programs, choosing a candidate that is not a "board risk" (poor test taker who may fail the boards) is critical because the ABS judges programs on their board pass rates and will sanction a program if too many graduates fail their boards. Conversely, attrition rates go up with a resident older than 29 at entry, female gender, courses repeated, C grades on the transcript, no team sports participation, and lack of a strong dean's letter.[51]

What happens next is that the various programs submit their top-favorite applicants list. The applicants do the same as part of the National Residency Match Program process. The match occurs after each program has interviewed dozens of candidates (80–100). We try to figure out who they are: Is this person teachable? Psychologically stable? Dedicated to a career in surgery? Or is the candidate just testing the waters and looking at our program as a backup? We meet after each interview day and discuss our impressions of the interviewees, look at test scores, and create a rank list of our favorite candidates. The fourth-year medical students do the same and rank the surgery residency programs in the order of their preference. Then, a computer matches students with programs according to each rank list. We then become married for five to seven years.

The match is administered by the National Resident Matching Program, which is a nonprofit, tax-exempt corporation. It allows both applicants and programs time to consider each other after the interviews and online review of the various programs is completed. Applicants register in August and have until February to submit a list of programs to which they wish to apply (ranked in the order of their interest in the programs). The results come out in March. Although the matching process is done professionally, there are reports that as many as 21 percent of students have felt they had to be dishonest with programs.[52,53]

Preparing for Surgical Residency

Our trainees each bring a different set of knowledge, skills, and attitude to their residency experience. Some residents have really good hands. The issue of innate talent never seems to leave the discussion of surgical resident selection and potential capability. Innate talent or intrinsic capability is quite difficult to prove. Also, most residents who come to residency ready to refine their diagnostic abilities and their problem-solving skills already believe they have a special capacity to do well. The truth is that some trainees just can't seem to figure things out in the clinical setting. They get the wrong impression (diagnostic possibilities) from the available diagnostic clues and come up with the wrong diagnosis. Some can't figure out postoperative complications. A few of these less or differently talented trainees cannot be fixed; they fail remediation and must be let go. Some hopefuls must be redirected into another area of medicine. More often than not, they remain in a medical career and do well.

General surgery isn't the only specialty faced with the need to assess the mastery of special skills for clinical practice. A recent report entitled "How Do You Deliver a Good Obstetrician? Outcome-Based Evaluation of Medical Education" aimed at providing an answer to this question.[54] I'll review this study because I'm convinced it has broad implications for physician education well beyond obstetrics. The authors' results should be important to any patient undergoing a delivery, surgery, or any other skills-based medical intervention. The investigators asked and answered three questions:

- Does it matter where the obstetrician trained? "The *top* quintile of programs produced graduates with an average maternal complication rate of 10.3% but the *bottom* quintile of programs produced graduates whose maternal complication rates were one-third higher, 13.6%. . . . So, some residency programs consistently turn out graduates who take better care of patients."[55]

- Does experience matter? "We found that experience matters. As physicians gained years of experience, their maternal complication rates fell. This was true for complications after vaginal deliveries, and for all of their deliveries combined. We found that these quality improvements continued for three decades after residency."[56]

- Does initial skill matter? "Does initial performance predict future success? Over 15 years, the physicians who start out with relatively poor outcomes never quite catch up to everybody else, meaning that the impact of initial skill persists. In fact, we found that variation in overall quality is determined far more by initial skill than it is by number of deliveries performed."[57]

I find these results compelling and directly applicable to surgical training because both obstetrics and surgery are interventional or "performing" specialties. These authors conclude by examining the ultimate outcome (how well patients do with a particular procedure): "This is an important goal because evaluating educational programs on the basis of the care provided by their graduates provides a more compelling standard against which to judge educational quality than standardized tests of knowledge or rankings based on structural factors like one sees in publications like *U.S. News & World Report*."[58] I am not aware of conclusive evidence-based studies that prove indisputably that test taking and doing well answering multiple-choice questions correlate with actual practitioner outcomes. This, despite the insistence by many surgical educators that multiple-choice questions are the only objective information we have by which to judge our trainees. But if you think surgeons fought mightily to not relinquish their scalpels to the laparoscope, you have seen nothing until you ask an educator to give up multiple-choice questions.

Training to Be Trained—Boot Camp

The complexity of surgical training has redefined how we teach fourth-year medical students basic surgical skills. But before a trainee can begin to learn advanced laparoscopic skills, he or she must be pretrained and master core physician skills. During the fourth year of medical school, students interested in surgery (or any other defined area of practice, such as primary care, pediatrics, etc.) do *subinternships*, usually a four-week rotation in which they gain practical experience. As a position paper published in 2015 stated: "Subinternships are clinical rotations usually completed during the final year of medical school. Subinternships provide medical students with experiential exposure to patient care in the clinical setting with varying degrees of graded autonomy in evaluating patients, creating care plans, and getting involved in various clinical procedures. . . . However, unlike third-year clerkship rotations, subinternships in many institutions lack well-defined structure or explicit curriculum."[59] The Sub-Committee for Surgery Subinternships and the Curriculum Committee of the Association for Surgical Education made concrete suggestions regarding how subinternships should be structured and administered. Among the goals and objectives were emphasizing patient ownership, mastering a core of basic surgical knowledge, focusing on patient-safety issues, understanding quality-control systems, and learning essential communication skills, including patient handoffs and how to conduct difficult conversations.[60] This occurs not only on the floors (wards), but also with protected time in a safe environment with case-based discussions, simulation, and deliberate skills practice. Interestingly, in this regard a 2011 study revealed that senior medical students felt ward-management skills (actually taking care of patients) were more important than operative and technical skills.[61] Presumably, more advanced residents would have already mastered ward skills and would no doubt emphasize the need to practice technical skills.

When the trainee becomes a first-year surgical resident, he or she will in many training programs be required to undergo a basic training experience. This course involves learning suturing, knot tying, central IV access methods, chest tube placement, and other skills that build on early exposure to specific aspects of surgical education offered in medical school. This is done more commonly as a boot camp experience, of which a variety of forms exist. At Baystate Medical Center, we have devised our own version of boot camp.[62] Our program involves learning stations set up around the skills lab where each technical procedure is taught and tested. These techniques are transferable to the operating room, the surgical floors, and elsewhere. I have weekly skills sessions with third-year medical students who often get an opportunity to close a wound in the OR—unheard of before the advent of the pretrained novice. Other programs have instituted Web- and simulation-based curricula for fourth-year medical students to prepare them for their first year as surgical residents.[63]

How Does the Surgery Residency Process Work?

Not all surgical residency programs follow what forward-thinking surgical educators believe is the future of surgical education: simulation and skills lab training *before* operative exposure. As defined and crafted by our national surgical education leadership, accountability regarding objective assessment of knowledge, skills, and attitudes (proving that the resident can do it) is becoming the standard of educational excellence. I believe that in the near future all surgical residents will be required to prove their technical proficiency by doing each essential operation on a virtual-reality machine or other inanimate bench model before being allowed to be trained under supervision in the operating room. We now know that simulation has a positive impact on patient safety.[64] We know simulation works in a broad spectrum of surgical education settings for virtually all subspecialties of surgery. Surgical residents are now required to pass a test called FLS (Fundamentals of Laparoscopic Surgery) before graduation. This entails mechanical skills such as peg transfer using long, skinny laparoscopic instruments and precisely cutting out a circle on premarked gauze inside a box trainer as one would inside a body cavity (a timed exercise; Figure 13.2). FLS also has a cognitive or knowledge component, and before graduation all senior general surgery residents must pass the FLS skills and knowledge test.

Also, practicing surgeons may take the course and the practical test to prove their competency in laparoscopic surgery. In 2011 the Society of American Gastrointestinal Endoscopic Surgeons created a similar educational product called FES: Fundamentals of Endoscopic Surgery through which residents must prove they have mastered endoscopic skills and must pass an FES test. Residents learn the basic techniques of how to maneuver a colonoscope or gastroscope on a mannequin that is interchangeable for each method (Figure 13.3). They also must complete a defined number

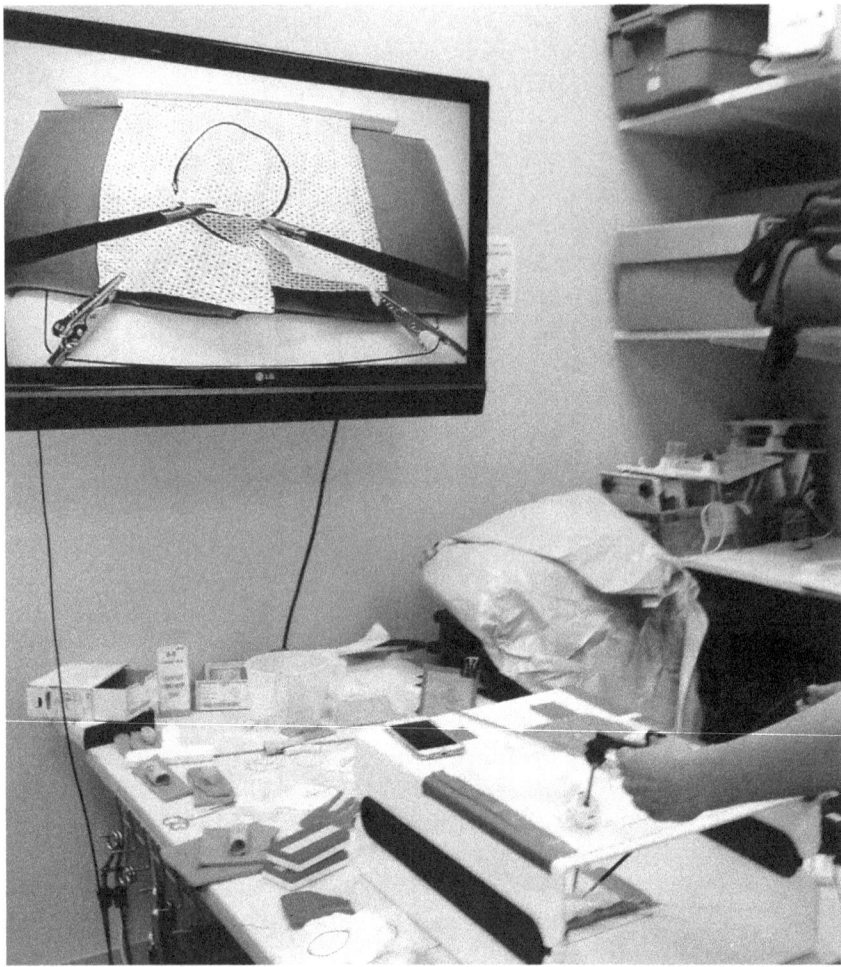

Figure 13.2   Fundamentals of Laparoscopic Surgery—Practicing Cutting Out a Gauze Circle as Part of Basic Minimally Invasive Surgery Training Skill Set (photo by David Page, MD)

of actual endoscopies on patients as part of their graduation requirement. In the future, no doubt, more skills testing will occur throughout the trainees' five to seven years of residency.

However, the often-discussed enigma regarding how many years it takes to train a surgeon has not been definitively settled. As a guide, the following ideas are in the process of being standardized and implemented:

- Five to seven years to train a general surgeon
- Five years of general surgery, then subspecialty training

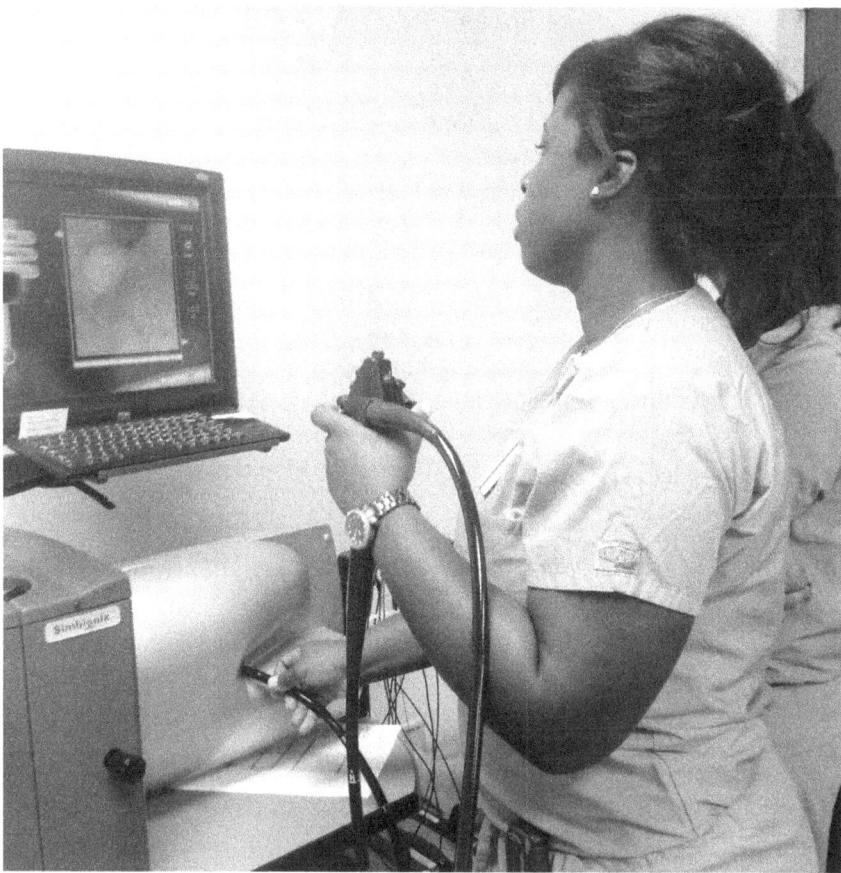

Figure 13.3 Endoscopic Trainer for FES—Learning Basic Endoscope Maneuvers in the Skills Lab (photo by David Page, MD)

- "3 plus 3": three years of general surgery, then three years of vascular or cardiothoracic (heart/chest) training
- Various early specialization pathways or tracks beginning with one or two years of general surgery followed by two to three years of subspecialty training
- Recruiting candidates directly out of medical school into a subspecialty track with no preliminary general surgery training

Obviously, there are numerous factors that determine the capability of any given surgeon. Along the path to competence, surgical trainees scrub with accomplished surgeons such as yours and participate to varying degrees in your operation. Otherwise, we would not have surgeons to care for your grandchildren. A legitimate question is, What might be the impact of having a trainee scrub on my operation?

Does Having a Trainee (Surgical Resident) Assist Your Surgeon Improve or Impair Your Care?

Her gloved hands tapered to long fingers, delicate in touch, decisive in following directions. We dissect out the planes in the man's groin where his hernia hides from sight amid scar tissue and confusing anatomy. My own arthritic fingers with a wealth of sensory memory lead her through the case with the touch and tricks I elected to teach her. She learns quickly. And although I am supervising her closely, she is performing the operation and creating muscle memory upon which she will build additional fine-tuned skills. These are not new maneuvers. She has practiced for hours in the skills lab under supervision.

Can Trainees Judge Their Own Progress?

There are two types of surgical residents: those who know there is much to learn from the program's seasoned teaching faculty, and those who assume that they are innately gifted and who want only to do operative cases without "unnecessary" supervision. The first group usually advances steadily along their learning curves and become master surgeons, especially if they dedicate themselves to deliberate practice in the skills lab before going to the operating room. The second group of trainees stumbles and stalls out on the error-rich steep slope of their learning curves. They struggle to the summit without safety ropes (ignoring surgical faculty advice). They are convinced that they are doing just fine. Over time they improve and remain anchored in mediocre technical performances for a lifetime of practice. Both groups assume that they are equally well trained.

The problem is that we know that more senior and older residents possess more insight into their progress.[65] Another study concluded, "Poorly performing residents appear to lack insight into their abilities."[66] These observations of surgical trainees shouldn't be surprising. In a 1999 study entitled "Unskilled and Unaware of It: How Difficulties in Recognizing One's Own Incompetence Lead to Inflated Self-Assessments," two Cornell psychologists documented that students scoring in the bottom quartile (12th) on certain tests thought they had done much better (in the 62nd percentile).[67] For the most part surgical residents, especially more junior trainees, have difficulty with self-assessment.

Are Teaching Hospitals Safe?

Much has been written about the pros and cons of teaching versus non-teaching hospitals. Only a few years ago in the *New England Journal of*

Medicine a report entitled, "Don't Learn on Me—Are Teaching Hospitals Patient-Centered?" the authored suggested, "It is unknown, for example, how surgeons and procedural specialists in teaching hospitals parry patients' queries about who will wield the scalpel, the scope, or catheter in their care."[68] Questions should be answered with the truth. Often surgeons don't spell out the role of the trainee—although explaining how much or how little a trainee may do in a particular case is often impossible. I have taken the approach—for example, with a hernia case—of explaining that my assistant will help me and do parts of the case depending on how involved it is. I insist, "Whether or not I do every move, you will get *my* operation, even if the resident performs some aspects of it."

It's really about effective communication. As another study concluded: "The ideal teacher has an instructional plan, facilitated surgical independence, and showed support and empathy for the surgical resident. The ideal resident was receptive, prepared, and acknowledged limitations."[69] This means that the teacher sets up the learning goals and objectives and treats the trainees with respect. The residents return the favor, including recognizing when they are in over their head.

So, the real issue for patients in seeking informed consent at a teaching hospital is to ask about what your surgeon expects (in terms of complexity and difficulty) in your particular case and at what level he or she thinks the participating trainee will be involved. *Level of trainee supervision* has been spelled out in a number of reports. One such publication from a VA hospital describes four levels of supervision or lack thereof: *level one* means the attending surgeon is doing the case; *level two* means the resident is performing the operation assisted by the surgeon; *level three* means the resident is doing the case (possibly with a junior resident assisting or doing parts of the case) while the attending surgeon is in the lounge down the hall; *level four* means the resident is operating independently and the attending isn't in the OR but is available if needed.[70] You should remember from my previous remarks that, if anything, we tend to oversupervise surgical residents and give them less autonomy than they would like. Still, it's worth inquiring about your surgeon's expectations regarding resident participation.

Do Residents Cause More Complications?

The majority of studies have shown that having residents involved in your surgical care has no impact on your outcome. At most, some studies show a slight increase in superficial wound infections and slightly longer operating times. But other studies show similar complications but decreased mortality (death rates) with residents involved.[71] One study showed slightly higher complications but again with a lower death rate.[72] A 1999 study is of interest because it bridges training and practice for a complex operative procedure: coronary artery bypass grafting (CABG). In that study a single well-supervised resident had his first 100 CABG patients compared for outcomes with his first 100 CABG patients in independent practice. The complication and mortality rates were the same.[73] This report, although restricted by having only one subject, defines the ultimate goal of surgical education: the opportunity for a trainee to do multiple repetitions of an operation with immediate feedback. I'll review a series of studies that correlate specific operative procedures with the impact of having a trainee participate:

- Residents' and fellows' participation in various types of mastectomy *did not affect early postoperative outcomes*; complications were unrelated to the level of resident or fellow training.[74]

- Resident participation in bilateral breast reduction *did not influence the rate of major postoperative complications.*[75]

- Laparoscopic appendectomy is *safe when performed by residents* as compared with consultant surgeons.[76]

- Laparoscopic inguinal hernia repairs *can be safely performed by supervised surgical trainees.*[77]

- *No difference in complication rate* was seen for laparoscopic inguinal hernia repair between patients operated on by attendings and residents.[78]

- Removal of the adrenal glands *had better outcomes* if surgical residents and fellows participated in the patient's care.[79]

- The large National Surgical Quality Improvement Program was used as a data set, which demonstrated that *for a variety of surgical procedures the participation of surgical trainees was safe.*[80]

How Do We Figure Out Who Is or Isn't Qualified to Progress in the Program?

A 1998 report surveyed practicing surgeons regarding their opinions on how well trainees were being prepared for practice, including how education should best be accomplished and by whom. The authors concluded, "There was agreement by geographic area and academic affiliation that the current system of resident education allows chief residents to graduate with significant gaps in their education, and that the responsibility for correcting these gaps lies with the residency programs."[81] Also, the impact of the Affordable Care Act on surgical education isn't clear.[82] Additional content areas are being recommended such as curricula that address business and practice management topics.[83]

Shortly after the institution of work-hour restrictions in 2003, only about a half of all surgical residency programs had surgical skills labs. By 2008, the FLS program was on its way to universal use as the Residency Review Committee mandated that all programs have skills labs and residents must pass the FLS, FES, and Advanced Trauma and Life Support courses.[84] A national skills curriculum (SCORE) is now in place (created by the ACS and APDS) as a Web-based program and free of charge. Simulation has grown as a teaching method, and assessment of a trainee's progress has become more reliable. Teaching and assessment of skills, knowledge, and the resident's attitude—in essence a quick snapshot of the six ACGME competencies—occur on a daily basis and during protected time (with beepers off). So, Web-based interactive texts, digital media platforms, and video-based instruction and feedback are additional educational tools for surgical educators. Nonetheless, we need better individual surgeon performance measures to educate potential patients.[85]

A Reflection on Case Numbers

In 1971, Joseph A. Kopta, an orthopedic surgeon, became the first surgical educator to articulate the principles that have emerged as the basis for modern surgical education. These include (a) differentiating between ability and learned skills, (b) identifying in the surgical literature for the first time Fitts and Posner's three stages of motor skills learning from 1968, (c) the importance of avoiding "indiscriminate" training (anticipated deliberate practice and the role of immediate expert feedback), and (d) anticipated boot camp. Kopta concluded his historic report with what is a truth all surgical educators live by today when he stated, "Certainly, the operating room cannot be considered the ideal place to learn basic surgical technique when the objective is to accomplish a therapeutic procedure."[86] Thus, learning by performing fewer skills repetitions in a skills lab but with coaching and immediate feedback is much more effective than merely scrubbing on large numbers of operative cases with variable opportunities to participate and receive quality instruction.

Summary: The Two Solutions to the Shortage of Capable General Surgeons

The new distribution of surgical talent may leave you in somewhat of a quandary. If your operation is elective, do you need to take time and explore the Internet and see if there is a subspecialist in your area to do your surgery? Does the surgeon to whom you've been referred have the necessary training and experience with the specific operation you need? Is there other surgical talent in the area that your surgeon can call on if needed? Common operations performed by a capable general surgeon with no subspecialty training beyond residency are safe and effective. Groin hernia repair is a good example. A study revealed that the results of mesh hernia repairs in the hands of a capable general surgeon are comparable to those of specialty surgeons with a more focused interest in hernia repair.[87]

A decade ago, a surgical educator stated: "It is clear that one of our greatest difficulties has been our failure to match our educational products to the needs of our health care system. We must do everything we can to make general surgery attractive and to influence both government and our academic health centers to provide incentives to those who are willing to entertain a career in surgery."[88] The dilemma posed by the overall shortage of general surgeons overlies the more specific problem of a lack of general surgeons in particular geographical areas, including rural and suburban areas, and in the military. The two solutions I have discussed include graduates' choosing one or two extra years of subspecialty training, which narrows and deepens their knowledge; or enrolling in additional residency training called "transition to practice," or similarly joining a group in which they are guided by a more experienced and senior surgeon with a broad understanding of general surgery, for example, in a rural area.

The program Path to Independent Practice: Transition to Practice—From Resident to General Surgeon, sponsored by the ACS, is designed to enhance autonomous experience in broad-based general surgery, often in a rural setting. By comparison, the urban or academic surgeon may have little experience with general surgery beyond his or her subspecialty. The more rural general surgeon may have little experience with complex minimally invasive operations. This reality represents the new normal that all patients must be aware of in the ever-changing world of general surgery.

CHAPTER FOURTEEN

Surgical Competence: A New Definition for the Twenty-First Century

A mammalian biped that has recently been recognized as endangered is *Chirugus generalis,* more commonly known as "the general surgeon."
Leon Morgenstern, MD, FACS, *American Journal of Surgery,* 2010

Deeply rooted in the cultural history of American medicine, this ongoing discourse about the competence of doctors has shaped, as it has been shaped by, the evolution of the profession and the health care system.
Mary-Jo DelVecchio Good, *American Medicine: The Quest for Competence,* 1995

He was my chief resident when I did my internship year at Baystate Medical Center in 1970. Everyone in the department acknowledged his uniqueness—a special surgical talent, almost magical hands. Today, in his eighties, Dr. Sang Rhee has reached legendary status in our department and is still practicing vascular surgery, still addressing residents in his cryptic Korean-tinged English, allowing more autonomy to his learners than most attending surgeons. He is the oldest practicing vascular surgeon in the United States. And so, in a tongue-in-cheek reference to a 1989 novel (Allan Gurganus's *Oldest Living Confederate Widow Tells All*), I suggested to Sang recently that he might become the oldest living Confederate vascular surgeon. What I was acknowledging (gently nudging his subtle sense of humor) was surgical expertise at its zenith, a byproduct of genetics and four and a half decades of vascular surgery practice.

Dr. Rhee is the face of surgical competence. Deep in their anxious hearts, all patients aspire to have a surgeon like him. This is the type of surgeon you are looking for.

Summary Statement—What Do We Know about Surgeon Capability?

As with the chapters in this book on innovation, learning curves, and simulation, I will examine the tortuous history of attempts by clinicians to precisely define the qualities of a capable surgeon. Constant change in the field of surgery is the new normal. Recall the numbers I listed earlier: medical knowledge currently doubles every three years. By 2020 medical facts will double every 73 days.[1] Thus, no one knows what the face of expertise will look like in the very near future. Nor do we know what we will need to know to practice surgery or how we will know it. How will we store knowledge, and how will we retrieve it? Will we use our brains, or will a powerful digital device harvest medical data from the Internet for us in seconds? What new technology will replace laparoscopy?

In Chapter 4, I outlined historical threads our profession has woven into a rich fabric, creating a dialogue regarding how surgical capability emerged over the last decades of the 20th century. Now, we need something more substantial, information that is prescriptive for you, concrete ideas about clinical competence you can use. The ACGME has provided surgical educators with six basic competencies we teach in medical school as well as in all training programs in the United States (Box 14.1). In a real sense, I could end this discussion by reiterating the six competencies as the answer to the question of how best to define surgical capability. However, I believe further teasing out the elements of competence will add to your understanding as a potential patient. Here are the six competencies at the core of surgical capability.[2]

Surgeons are just as capable today in well-defined, specific areas of practice as they were back in the days when I began my practice in the mid-1970s. But they are not competent *in the same way* as we were when we graduated from five years of residency. Then, we knew what we were supposed to know; today, graduates understand that they have not been exposed to a major chunk of general surgery. Thus, any definition of what a capable practitioner is must take into account the shifting training and practice environment of the 21st century.

Also, the *distribution* of surgical expertise is different in today's surgical world. The sheer number and complexity of the operations that may be performed by a general surgeon (listed by the American Board of Surgery) makes mastery of all of them impossible, as I have emphasized as my primary theme.

It seems reasonable for you to inquire about fellowship training if you're seeking a more complicated operation or to ask about transition-to-practice experiences when engaging a younger general surgeon in a smaller

---

Box 14.1 The Six ACGME General Competencies

- *Patient care*—trainees must provide comprehensive, compassionate, and effective care in treating disease and promoting overall health.

- *Medical knowledge*—medical students and residents must be able to demonstrate knowledge about anatomical, biochemical, clinical, epidemiological, and social-behavioral sciences as applied to patient care.

- *Practice-based learning and improvement*—residents must be able to evaluate their own practices (successes and mistakes), appraise and assimilate scientific evidence, and improve their individual practices through self-reflection.

- *Interpersonal and communication skills*—students and training residents must demonstrate interpersonal and communication skills as well as teamwork involving patients and their families and with their professional associates.

- *Professionalism*—students and residents must demonstrate a commitment to ethical behavior that is empathetic, globally aware of the practice environment, and sensitive to diverse patient populations.

- *System-based practice*—trainees must be sensitive to the larger system of health care and be able to employ all resources offered by the system.

---

hospital.[3] It is appropriate to ask about the surgeon's assistant, including the assistant's expertise: Is the assistant a mentor (an experienced surgeon guiding your surgeon)? The American Board of Surgery has also agreed to redesign or "fix the five" years of basic surgical training. At a national level there is recognition of how dramatically the practice of surgery has changed: "The American Board of Surgery directors, representing the breadth of general surgery, agree that now is the time to move forward. The challenges are significant and the issues are complex, but can be overcome with deliberate thought, a collaborative mindset, and a clearly defined process for managing such an undertaking."[4]

You need to do your homework. It will involve finding out who is available in your area and exactly what that surgeon's credentials are and the actual experience the surgeon has with the operation you need. It is no longer appropriate to blindly accept the surgeon's opinion regarding his or her skills. A review of published reports on the ability of doctors to assess their own knowledge and clinical skills concluded, "A number of studies found the worst accuracy in self-assessment was among physicians who were the least skilled and those who were the most confident."[5] Parenthetically, surgeons, in fact, have demonstrated an accurate ability to self-evaluate their own technical skills.[6] Still, when choosing a surgeon, you need some reliable data about his or her outcomes. And this in no way should detract from your developing a trusting relationship with your surgeon.

All surgeons must adapt to their patients' information needs and respect their patients' right to ask about our experience with particular operative procedures. Any "attitude"—especially that of being insulted when asked about one's training and expertise—is not acceptable in today's complex surgical world. The old-time surgical personality has no place in the modern practice of our craft. In fairness to the overwhelming number of compassionate practitioners available to you, this aspect of finding a capable surgeon shouldn't be an issue.

Of critical importance, surgical practitioners must decide what menu of operations they can do safely based on an opportunity to generate a reasonable volume of those particular types of cases. This is a challenge for practicing general surgeons in smaller communities where pressure from both patients and hospitals may nudge them toward performing complex operations, but only in rare circumstances, and thus not providing an adequate volume of cases. Similarly, some (but not all) complex operations should be performed at high-volume medical centers. Unfortunately, this fact will also aggravate the growing surgeon shortage.

You will need to figure out exactly where—that is, in which of the narrowly defined specialties of modern surgery—your surgical problem lies. Finding the appropriate surgeon is critical to your ability to obtain expert surgical care in a field of very complicated operations. To repeat, above all other considerations is the imperative that general surgeons today accept that intelligent patients are going to inquire about their training, experience, and credentials. There is a need for surgeons of all stripes to practice complete informed consent and engage their patients in shared decision making.

For example, suppose you need a valve created at the lower end of your gullet because you have stomach acid refluxing up into your lower esophagus (gullet), causing you severe heartburn. Do you see a general surgeon? A "foregut" or gastrointestinal surgeon? A minimally invasive surgeon? Are they more or less all the same? Are some surgeons all three types of practitioner combined into one superstar? Or are the last two subspecialized examples better trained than the general surgeon who has talent in many other areas unlike the superspecialists, but may have performed only a few fundoplication operations?

How can you tell who is capable of doing your operation flawlessly? Does the anti-reflux valve operation straddle several areas of surgeon training?

Should you see the local surgeon or travel to a larger medical center? The problem is real, because there is plenty of evidence for having your surgery performed safely in a smaller, more rural hospital rather than traveling to a big medical center.

First, We Need Some Definitions

A capable surgeon is a competent surgeon. Definitions parallel each other, like these taken from the online *Merriam-Webster Dictionary*: *Capable* is defined as having the "ability to do something; having the qualities or ability that are needed to do something; skilled at doing something well."[7] *Competence* is similarly defined as "the ability to do something well."[8] Neither of these relatively shallow definitions helps us much in determining the qualities of a surgeon. Under *capability*, *Merriam-Webster* refers to "the ability to do something."[9] The *Random House College Dictionary* defines *capable* as "having intelligence and ability; competent"[10]—all of which makes the terms *capable* and *competent* interchangeable for our purposes. Random House further defines *competence* as "having suitable or sufficient skill, knowledge, experience, etc. for some purpose."[11] Better. Other sources have clarified the definition of a capable person as having intelligence and ability; competent; having the ability, skill, or experience for; or having the personality or character or being in the mood for something. Similarly, competence is considered having suitable or sufficient skill or purpose; being properly qualified; or being adequate but not exceptional. *Roget's Super Thesaurus*, second edition, gives synonyms for *capability* as "ability, knowhow, capacity, proficiency, wherewithal, aptitude, 'the right stuff,' means, power, skill, mind, talent."[12]

We are left with a circular restating of relatively simple word choices. We need more information that refers specifically to the talent excellent surgeons must possess to be considered capable practitioners. A 2015 report addressed this need, stating, "*Competent* and *competence* are terms often used when describing a global, general impression of the adequacy of knowledge, clinical skills, and attitudes of a health care provider to practice independently and autonomously, usually at the end of residency training."[13]

So far we have anemic, circuitous definitions of competence and capability, a broadly defined global definition, and six solid, well-defined ACGME competencies to be mastered by all training doctors in the United States. But are we any closer to understanding what a competent surgeon does in the operating room and elsewhere? Recall from Chapter 4 that Dr. Lawrence Way stated that criticism of a profession centers on the difference between the *actual performance of a practitioner* and the *ideologi-cal claims of the profession* or reasonable expectations of the public.[14] I would submit that this critical difference between what a surgeon can do and what the surgeon says he or she can do will never be completely resolved. In fact, it has been shown that attending surgeons and their trainees dis-agree on many aspects of what is defined as a competency-based training program.[15] And how, for example, do you measure how a surgeon will react in critical situations? A study on the subject of handling an intraop-erative crisis reported that surgeons stated practice and preparation were both important, concluding, "Competence, confidence, composure, prep-aration and experience were most commonly listed as characteristics of behavior that should be encouraged in aspiring surgeons."[16] Managing distractions and remaining vigilant for errors during an operation are also elements of surgeon capability, although not practically measurable.[17,18]

Incompetence—The Unspoken

Psychologists have attempted to define precisely what it is to be capa-ble. In other words, what is incompetence? An important question at the top of the list asks, Is the person who is labeled incompetent really incom-petent? According to authors Langer and Park: "By incompetence we mean the self-perception or that of another of inadequate performance . . . it may refer to specific or global behavior. Further, we believe incompe-tence is socially defined, and thus the difference between actual and per-ceived incompetence is more apparent than real."[19] The issue is a headache for surgical educators. Obviously, competence must be more than a socially defined idea. It hinges on appropriate surgical knowledge, skill, and appro-priate attitude toward proving safe, empathetic care in specific areas of general surgery.

As you have seen, back in the day the evaluation of a resident was global, an overview of performance with little data on how the trainee performed *specific* surgical tasks. The feelings of the surgical teacher toward the pupil played heavily in the final assessment of the resident's competence. That was the social context of trainee evaluation back then. The issue remains today: Is the trainee *truly* incompetent, or is it the *perception* of the teacher that the resident cannot execute skills and demonstrate knowledge prop-erly? The authors quoted above describe the potential damage of helping rather than allowing a learner to figure out the solution to a problem. This is another problematic concept for those dealing with live patients suffer-ing from potentially lethal diseases. For surgical educators the struggle lies in not tarnishing the learner's self-esteem by overteaching (oversupervising) but also in not allowing the resident's autonomy to result in patient harm.

What types of incompetence are we talking about?

Consider the term *precompetence*. This idea is important because it marks a stage in learning in which the student (surgical resident) has not yet mastered certain knowledge or skills. It might apply to an established surgeon learning a new operation. But the teacher must inquire about (observe, objectively test) the learner's experience in order to distinguish precompetence from incompetence. Incompetence exists when learning hasn't occurred despite many opportunities. Precompetence is a milestone on the way toward the state of competence. An intern (first-year resident) is precompetent.

Also, *mindless incompetence* may be defined the way some folks refer to *stupid*: doing something in the same way over and over and expecting a different outcome. One is mindlessly incompetent when one doesn't recognize that there are alternative methods of approaching a problem. *Mindfulness* means being sensitive to all possibilities. Finally, the term *overcompetence* may be applied to learning motor or technical skills to the point of being totally automatic. In this condition, no conscious input is required to execute certain skills. This is true of many surgical skills that are done without thought, such as expert knot tying. It's also referred to as being *unconsciously competent*. It must be balanced with situational awareness.[20] All these concepts illuminate what surgical educators consider to be a 21st-century definition of surgeon capability. We can now measure competence in the skills lab, during simulation, as well as in the operating room using both checklists and global rating scales.

Do Advances in Training and Specialization Improve Patient Outcomes?

Complications and mortality rates after major surgery have dropped significantly in the last 30 or 40 years.[21] Focused training for complex operations improves outcomes through more deliberate practice and increased hospital and surgeon volumes. An example of a measurable improvement in patient safety and better outcomes, based on improved training (and more experienced surgeons), as well as on better postoperative care, is surgery for cancer of the pancreas. The so-called Whipple operation is the bête noire, the biggest technical challenge for general surgeons, who, during their five years of residency, are required to scrub on (mostly to assist, not do the procedure) fewer than half a dozen Whipple operations—a totally inadequate amount of training for that complex operation. Overall, virtually all graduates lack adequate experience to do these operations safely. Yet some relatively inexperienced surgeons perform these complex procedures in practice anyway. Solid data show that since 1990, the era marking the beginning of our story about laparoscopy, death rates after removal of the pancreas for cancer using open methods have decreased by one half, despite patients being older and having more associated diseases (diabetes, hypertension, coronary artery disease, chronic lung disease, kidney disease, etc.).[22] Also, laparoscopic removal of the pancreas has proven to be a reliable cancer operation in selected hands.[23] Both open and minimally invasive pancreatic cancer operations require additional training to assure appropriate capability with this predictably difficult operation.

A large number of reports on surgeon and hospital volume for complex operations prove that more cases and more surgeon experience result in fewer complications and fewer deaths postoperatively for certain vascular, thoracic (chest), and cancer operations. Fellowship-trained surgeons have excellent results when performing an operation for which they were specially trained. However, the other side of the competence argument is that some of these superspecialized surgeons will operate on acute general surgery emergencies out of necessity when on call. And for the same reason of lack of experience, they may not have as good outcomes as general surgeons experienced in a broad number of operations.

How Do We Measure a Trainee's Capability Today?

You must recognize that the transition in the way we train surgeons today will continue to evolve over the next several decades. Therefore, a concise definition of surgical capability is elusive as we continue to experience shifts in our educational priorities and strategies. In a word, we've moved to what was referred to more than 25 years ago as a *competency-based training system*.[24] Years of residency are less important than proof (through rigorous assessments) that the trainee can actually perform the required skills and possesses the appropriate fund of knowledge. Residents moving on to fellowship training can now take the American Board of Surgery exams after four (rather than five) years of training. Although it has taken us a long time to change how we educate surgeons, there still exists in some quarters a stubborn resistance to the new methods of surgical education.

Nonetheless, we now evaluate surgical residents by examining and documenting what they can actually do in the six domains of the listed ACGME competencies. But as for actually defining *competence* (*capability*), a report concluded, "The evaluation of a resident's competency to practice, however, has never been clearly defined, nor has the fixed period of time given for residency training in each specialty been shown to be the right amount of time for every resident to achieve competency."[25]

In 2013, the ACGME ramped up the New Assessment System. It incorporates milestones or levels of competence that trainees must accomplish before they can move on in their pathway to proficiency. For the first time in the history of surgical education, we now have a system that meets the public's needs: to be assured using objective measures that practicing surgeons have completed the training promised by their surgical programs. And yet there are still difficulties with Clinical Competency Committees in terms of how we evaluate residents using milestones and how we promote them in the program. Subcomponents of each of the six competencies are individually considered by the committee, an exhausting task. As one report admitted: "In spite of limited data, we reached consensus on almost everyone in this way, deciding that most of the residents were progressing nicely, identifying a few areas for needed improvement for some. . . . Had we paid enough careful consistent attention to competencies, milestones, and entrustable professional activities, terms we used freely but did not seem to fully understand?"[26]

This diligence on the part of educators today contrasts with how program directors in surgery in the past signed off on surgical residents—they literally signed a graduation certificate as an act of faith that, in some cases, placed them in a moral bind of not really knowing whether the resident was competent after five years of training. A 2001 report stated: "The program director of the program in which the surgeon trained must sign a statement that the applicant for the American Board of Surgery has attained a sufficiently high level of knowledge, has the ability to apply basic science to surgery, has diagnostic and manipulative skills, surgical judgment, technical operative expertise, is considered to have appropriate interpersonal skills, and is fully prepared for independent responsibility as a specialist in surgery."[27] A tall order in the past for a program director with little objective information on a resident's actual residency performance record. Now the question is, do we have the financial support and a talented faculty to make the new assessment system work? The 2001 report concluded, "If financial incentives for clinical productivity prevent the development of critical faculty—student educational relationships, the competency-based assessments will not reach their full potential."[28] In a word, the teaching and assessment of medical students and surgical trainees will suffer if hospital administrators whip the teaching faculty in their single-minded pursuit of ever-increasing billing of patients.

General surgeons are working longer hours and treating more complex patients while their incomes have dropped. This trend was identified in 2004: "In the next twenty years the general surgery workload will increase at a rate that significantly exceeds population growth. Although the population will grow by 18% between 2000 and 2020, the workload of general surgeons will increase by 31%."[29] Competence isn't just about the technical skills you desire in a practitioner. It's also about fatigue and the loss of self-satisfaction. You must listen with your heart when discussing your operation with a surgeon to sense whether he or she is focused on you or disengaged from the process of safe care.

An Example of a Change in (the Perception of) Surgical Competence

My favorite operation is the repair of groin hernias. I've had the privilege of working with talented researchers sorting out particular aspects of inguinal (groin) anatomy,[30,31,32,33,34,35] and I have developed experience over the last 40 years in doing these often challenging operations. But it wasn't always this way with the repair of hernias. The recent microhistory of groin hernia repair accurately reflects the assumptions and glaring deficiencies of the broader old-school surgical education.

The story of the rise of modern hernia surgery as a specialty reflects the ascent of specialization in the overall field of general surgery. When I trained in the early 1970s, a groin hernia was considered a simple operation. It was routinely referred to as an "intern's case." Back in the day, a chief resident in his fifth year of training would scoff at the idea of scrubbing on a groin hernia case. It was below him, below his talent level. He would have rather done complex pancreas and vascular cases.

What happened to hernia surgery? We now have the American Hernia Society. There are many other specialized hernia societies around the globe. Imagine, a national society with its own journal called *Hernia* dedicated to research as well as to addressing the complex clinical decisions and technical issues associated with modern hernia repairs. As you can imagine, there is an unresolved debate about whether an open (traditional) hernia operation is better than a minimally invasive laparoscopic repair.

What happened to the intern's case? With hernia recurrence rates as high as 20 percent, the practice of interns doing hernia repairs went down in flames. Our profession awoke to the realization that we had not only done a poor job of training surgical residents in how to fix a groin hernia, but in the bigger picture we had failed miserably in providing adequate supervision in the teaching of all general surgery operations. The realization arrived, as you now know, when the time came to hand laparoscopic instruments over to a trainee. In a flash, we understood that *that* wasn't going to happen without potentially major consequences. Thus, in the context of hernia surgery there was an immediate disappearance of the intern's hernia case. And in my personal experience, chief residents about to enter private practice now scrub on my cases, in their words, "to see you do another hernia repair before I graduate."

A Framework for Describing a Capable Surgeon

When I scrub on a case with a resident, I know his or her level of training, for example, intern versus chief resident. I observe the vast differences in their knowledge, skills, and decision-making abilities. You will never see your surgeon in action. However, having a grasp of the range of the surgeon's potential abilities may help guide your informed-consent conversation. So, it is useful to understand the categories of competence and the way surgical educators view specific stages in the acquisition of expertise, as well as judge the final (graduate surgeon) product.

In general, these stages of acquiring specific skills apply to all activities, from riding a bicycle to scaling the Matterhorn. For the sake of our discussion, *expertise* includes technical skills, team skills, cognitive or critical thinking skills, and communication skills, among others. For example, a true surgical expert is able to plan an operation, rehearse the steps ahead of time, recognize where danger (of creating errors and complications) lies, and anticipate how to avoid or halt an error in evolution. For a laparoscopic operation, the first steps, for example, would be positioning the patient on the table and prepping and draping the patient. This would be followed by doing a time-out and communicating with all the staff in the operating room. When the operation begins, I would safely insert the trocar and sheaths or tubes through the abdominal wall and inflate the belly cavity with carbon dioxide. That's six individual decisions requiring specific skills—all carried out *before* the challenging part of the operation actually begins. A useful scheme that defines different stages in the process of skills acquisition is the Dreyfus and Dreyfus model:

1. Novice
2. Advanced beginner
3. Competence
4. Proficiency
5. Expertise
6. Master[36]

This sequence of increasing levels of capability describes the learner's progression toward continued improvement and the ultimate goal of mastery. What may also have struck you is the position of two categories we've discussed in this book, namely competence and expertise. They obviously aren't the same thing, nor are they the only levels of learning you may be exposed to as a patient. This is of importance because while I am suggesting there may be a lack of capability in performing certain operations by general surgeons (uneven experience and training), I am also acknowledging the presence of true expertise in surgeons who have mastered the many core operations that make up our specialty.

Now consider each category with examples of what is learned by trainees at each level. The value of understanding these categories is to appreciate that surgeons in practice are *competent* or *proficient* performing many operations; they will also have arrived at the levels of *expertise* and *mastery* for a certain specific number of other operations. This *continuum of skill* defines all trainees and practicing surgeons alike.

Novice. Early learners pick up some facts and rules for applying information. The novice can't put things into a particular situation or context. They don't see the big picture. Thus, ordering intravenous fluid, the novice would prescribe a certain volume of normal saline guided by the patient's weight. If the patient had a history of congestive heart failure, he or she would not tolerate an excessive intravenous fluid load. The novice might miss that point. Also, in the realm of diagnosis, for example, the novice may recognize right lower abdominal pain as being associated with a diagnosis of appendicitis (pattern recognition) without understanding that in a 34-year-old female, the pain could signal an ectopic (tubal) pregnancy.

Advanced Beginner. With a backlog of experiences, the learner now begins to appreciate the bigger world of clinical medicine and pays attention to critical aspects of a particular situation. If the patient receiving IV fluids develops bouncing neck veins and crackly noises in his chest, the advanced beginner will recognize these markers of a failing heart. The advanced beginner will adjust downward the volume of intravenous fluid to be given. The *context* (*who* is the patient, *where* is the encounter, with *what* comorbid conditions) becomes important; a congestive heart failure patient is different from a massively bleeding automobile accident victim in profound shock. The advanced beginner treats a specific patient with a specific problem.

Competence. Additional experience contributes to competence. Experienced surgeons have stored in their memory banks a vast number of specific cases they may draw on to solve clinical problems. These cases, for example, are indexed in various ways so as to be available for pattern recognition ("I've seen that before."). The capable learner knows what facts are important and what information may be ignored for the moment; the trainee is sensitive to the overall situation and *plans ahead* to avoid problems. The 34-year-old woman with right lower abdominal pain may have appendicitis, Crohn's disease, or a gynecological problem such as an ectopic pregnancy, a twisted (possibly dead) tube or ovary, an ovarian cyst, or a tube-ovarian abscess. The choices of diagnosis are *context rich* (a particular 34-year-old female with a specific history and physical findings). The competent surgical practitioner works beyond merely following rules (the sign of a novice). The capable doctor creates a comprehensive treatment plan for which he or she feels personally responsible for the outcome.

Quoting Dreyfus and Dreyfus regarding the two categories of expertise and master, "The two highest levels of skill . . . are characterized by a rapid, fluid, involved kind of behavior that bears no apparent similarity to the slow, detached reasoning of the problem-solving process."[37]

Proficiency. This level of function contrasts with the exacting problem-solving methods of the previous three stages of expertise. As eloquently described by Dreyfus and Dreyfus, "The Hamlet model of decision-making—the detached deliberative and sometimes agonizing selection among alternatives—is the only one recognized in much of the academic literature on the psychology of choice."[38] But there is more to clinical problem solving, according to these authors. It's called *intuition.* Proficient learners can quickly identify certain facts and let go of others. It's fast thinking rather than a measured, slow thinking process.[39]

The proficient clinician is deeply involved with a specific patient and culls certain features of the situation while ignoring others. The 34-year-old woman not only has a negative pelvic (internal) exam, but pushing and releasing the belly wall in the left lower quadrant (away from the appendix) causes severe pain in the right lower quadrant (where the reclusive little worm resides), a strong indicator of acute appendicitis. The clinician may be subliminally absorbing other clues that support the diagnosis. We know that intuitive or fast and frugal thinking is associated with bias and certain errors in thinking. But we also know that proficient and expert physicians make reliable diagnoses with very little information while novices muddle through reams of data only to arrive at less accurate diagnoses despite mountains of evidence.

Expertise. Much of the work of an expert physician is intuitive (fast thinking). From a huge library of indexed and now recalled clinical experiences, the expert matches the present challenge with a pattern he or she recognizes and then comes to a correct conclusion. But the expert also critically reflects on that intuitive call, on the fit of the diagnosis with minimal information, often delving deeper into the facts (slow thinking) only if there is a disparity between his or her initial diagnosis of the situation and a reassessment. But up front, the expert unconsciously matches previous experiences with the new situation, even though his or her intuition may occasionally be wrong.

This applies to how experts function in the operating room, where sorting through various visual and sensory clues regarding anatomy and the patient's pathology is based on prior experience. After teaching detailed skills in the lab, in the operating room we want the case to flow, to transcend mere choppy movements and specific steps. *Flow* in the performance of a surgical operation means the absence of critical self-monitoring of every move. The surgeon focuses on the whole process of operating, feeling tissue and instrument as one, sensing the dissection as a progression through blended movements not individually thought about or felt.

As part of the prescription (questions to ask) regarding the surgeon's level of expertise (e.g., number of cases performed each year, etc.), consider asking about the following issues during your first consultation with a surgeon (you probably won't need to ask all of them):

- What medical school did he or she attend?
- Where did the surgeon train—what residency program?
- Is the surgeon board certified? Has he or she been recertified?
- What are the surgeon's hospital credentials, areas of special expertise, and specialized training?
- Is the surgeon fellowship trained?
- What organizations is the surgeon associated with?
- Has the surgeon won any teaching or patient care awards? Does he or she have any other distinctions?
- Has the surgeon published scientific reports?
- Is the surgeon a member of a local, regional, or national medical or surgical society?
- Has there been any documentation of adverse events—lawsuits, professional reprimands, loss of privileges, and so forth for the surgeon?

What about Health Care Organizations and the Capable Surgeon?

All the training and teaching efforts of surgical educators will fail if the organizations in which they work are tone-deaf to their needs (preoccupied with financial issues). As a 2002 report concluded: "Educational activities for professionals are not sufficient. . . . Those wishing to improve the competence and performance of physicians must be aware of the limitations of educational approaches and know how to integrate these with approaches that focus on teams, organizations, or the political or economic context."[40] Thus, both physicians and the administrators of their hospitals must come together and find common ground in order to accomplish their various goals. A talented surgeon working in a hospital with inadequate equipment or staff will not perform as well as a talented surgeon in a hospital attuned to excellence in all aspects of surgical care. Box 14.2 lists Web sites that may be useful in assessing hospitals.

Summary: Can We Measure Surgical Capability at the Specialist Level?

When all is said, you need to know that your surgeon's level of capability has been evaluated. The message repeated in this book is that today we have the tools to assess trainee and active practitioners' skill and knowledge levels. Board certification is crucial, despite the challenges involved. As a potential surgical patient, you should visit the American College of Surgeons and the American Board of Surgery's Web sites and check out your surgeon.

A 2013 report from Imperial College London appears to have defined the best way to document a surgeon's capability at a high level of accomplishment (specialist). The authors use laparoscopic colorectal surgery in England as their example.[41] The authors created a *competency assessment*

BOX 14.2 USEFUL WEB SITES FOR HOSPITAL EVALUATION

- Medicare's "Hospital Compare" (http://www.medicare.gov/hospitalcompare/search.html)
- Hospital Safety Score (http://www.hospitalsafetyscore.org)
- The Joint Commission's "Quality Check" (https://www.qualitycheck.org)
- Google "health care quality" for several useful sites
- The Leapfrog Group (http://www.leapfroggroup.org)
- Consumers' Checkbook (https://www.checkbook.org)
- Healthgrades (http://www.healthgrades.com)
- WhyNotTheBest.org (http://www.whynotthebest.org)
- MediBid (https://www.medibid.com), where hospitals and doctors bid for your business and discuss prices

tool (CAT) with task-specific elements as well as more general or generic items employed to test a surgeon's clinical performance. The rationale for the National Training Program in England was to eliminate the "unacceptably high conversion and complication rates" documented in the operative experiences of surgeons who were not formally trained to do those procedures.[42] It was the first study on competency assessment of specialists. As the authors concluded: "CAT allows the national training program to identify consultant surgeons who can safely perform laparoscopic colorectal surgery before embarking on independent practice. . . . The concept of a competency-based training curriculum with an exit competency-based assessment has been proven to work on a national level."[43] And I will remind you that the surgeon shortage will seduce older surgeons to keep practicing (or hospitals strapped for surgical talent will encourage them to work on) when their technical skills and cognition may be edging toward incompetence.[44]

Perhaps a new definition of a capable surgeon for the 21st century will eventually have to include results of a CAT-like determination of competence. It appears that this standard ought to be applied throughout the surgical world if and when it becomes available. A new definition of a capable surgeon must include assessment of the practitioner's special knowledge and technical skills with *specific operations* (Box 14.3). You must also be aware of discrepancies in tools on the Internet designed to evaluate surgeon capability. A recent report challenged the ProPublica Surgeon Scorecard for its deficiencies, including statistical errors and other reasons why the tool is unreliable for patients to use to assess a surgeon's competence. The value of the report is that more attention should be focused on surgeon-specific performance reports in the future.[45]

Finally, you should be aware that there is a recent development regarding a surgeon's capability referred to as the "Take the Volume Pledge." Nationally known researchers from Dartmouth-Hitchcock Medical Center, Johns Hopkins Hospital and Health System, and the University of Michigan Health System campaigned to encourage surgeons with low surgical case volumes to not perform certain operations. The reaction was outrage among surgeons. An example is total knee replacement, for which the recommended volume is 50 cases per year per hospital and 25 cases per year per surgeon. For weight-loss surgery, the numbers are 40 cases per year per hospital and 20 per year per bariatric surgeon.[46] But it's not that simple. Who a surgeon selects to operate on (how sick with comorbid conditions?) throws significant bias into the equation. So, hospital and surgeon volume aren't the only criteria for determining safe surgery. The report quoted above entitled "Pledging to Eliminate Low-Volume Surgery" concluded, "Regardless of what happens with efforts to centralize certain

BOX 14.3 SUMMARY OF SAFE SURGICAL CARE ISSUES

- Today, general surgeons must learn more complex operations in less training time; this creates a level of inadequate capability for some operations in general surgeons' practices.

- Five themes of this book: (1) General surgery *knowledge and technical skills have doubled* (undergone mitosis: now laparoscopic operations join traditional open procedures to dilute training and practice opportunities to learn them well); (2) The old school unsupervised 'education' is replaced with *a pretrained novice* approach (surgical education out of the operating room before allowing supervised operative experiences); (3) *Fatigue isn't the problem*; it is the ultimate challenge in the face of deadly surgical disease; (4) *Zero tolerance for belligerent, "malignant narcissist" surgeons* who refuse to be transparent on all issues surrounding surgical care; (5) *True informed consent* must include the surgeon's training, experience (including number of similar cases performed) and outcomes.

- The undisciplined introduction of laparoscopic cholecystectomy into mainstream surgical practice in 1990 was dangerous and caused predictable patient harm; *the potential threat of more new technology* such as robotic surgery in inexperienced hands and causing harm is ever present.

- A brief history of laparoscopic gallbladder removal highlights the ongoing threats to patients because this transitional technology will lead to more new technology that is not easily mastered.

- Realize that although *board certification is vital to surgeon capability* (and serves as a major quality control factor), it alone cannot guarantee that you will receive competent and safe care.

- Be aware that *you may be exposed to surgical innovation* that exceeds the daily modifications all surgeons routinely use to solve an intraoperative problem.

- Recognize that *all surgeons are working on a learning curve*; experienced and expert surgeons (master surgeons) have progressed to the flat part of their curve, where errors rarely occur, just as a younger surgeon may not yet have reached maximum competence (precompetence).

- Do not engage the services of a surgeon who will not listen to your concerns—be they about the operation, the surgeon's experience and track record, your comorbidities, or the best hospital for you; commonly performed minimally invasive operations have a track record, and you should know what it is.

- If a surgeon tells you that you or a loved one needs *an emergency operation*, you should take heed; delay for most acute surgical diseases ultimately spells death. If the decision involves an elderly patient with many comorbidities (you or a loved one), you must *ask about prognosis*— something many doctors with sick patients at the end of life are not good at predicting or providing.

surgeries in large hospitals, some patients will continue to require surgery—and other types of acute care—at small hospitals, and care for these patients will improve only if structures and processes of care in those hospitals can be improved."[47] That is the crux of this entire discussion about surgeon capability: good surgeons exist throughout the country with varying experience with common and complex operations. That is the challenge for general surgery.

An attitude of responsibility on the part of all surgeons to restrict their practice to those areas of expertise proven in training or with competency-based national examinations would seem to be of necessity inherent in any modern definition of surgeon competence. This approach will challenge our traditional notion of what a widely trained general surgeon must know, as well as what that same generally knowledgeable surgeon must not attempt in practice. A truly capable surgeon is technically skilled, knowledgeable, and of necessity humble, insightful, and willing to ask for help from colleagues. Fortunately, this description fits most practitioners working today.

Notes

Preface

1. Ernest Dunn, "The Southwest Surgical Congress: A Seal of Approval," *Am J Surg* 192 (2006): 700.

2. Ibid., 700.

3. Richard H. Bell, "Why Johnny Cannot Operate," *Surgery* 146, no. 4 (2009): 533–541.

4. Hiram C. Polk, foreword to *Complications of Laparoscopic Surgery*, by Robert W. Bailey and John L. Flowers (St. Louis: Quality Medical Publishing, 1995), ix.

5. S. G. Mattar et al., "General Surgery Residency Inadequately Prepares Trainees for Fellowship," *Ann Surg* 258, no. 3 (2013): 440–449.

6. Polk, foreword to *Complications*, x.

7. A. Green et al., "Stress in Surgeons," *Br J Surg* 77 (1990): 1154–1158.

8. T. D. Shanafelt et al., "Burnout and Medical Errors among American Surgeons," *Ann Surg* 251, no. 6 (2010): 995–1000.

9. E. M. Bucholz et al., "Our Trainee's Confidence—Results from a National Survey of 4136 General Surgery Residents," *Arch Surg* 46, no. 8 (2011): 907–914.

10. J. M. Hamdorf and J. C. Hall, "Acquiring Surgical Skills," *Br J Surg* 87 (2000): 28–37.

11. T. E. Williams, E. C. Ellison, and B. Satiani, *The Coming Shortage of Surgeons* (Santa Barbara, CA: Praeger, 2009).

12. J. Airy et al., "Cumulative Operative Experience Is Decreasing During General Surgical Residency: A Worrisome Trend for Surgical Trainees?" *J Am Coll Surg* 206, no. 5 (2008): 804.

13. J. J. Coleman et al., "Early Subspecialization and Perceived Competence in Surgical Training: Are Residents Ready?" *J Am Coll Surg* 216, no. 4 (2013): 764–773.

Chapter One

1. V. Stern, "A Talk with Eddie Joe Reddick: Laparoscopy Pioneer, Recording Artist," *General Surgery News* (September 2013): 13.

2. B. M. Wolfe, B. Gardiner, and C. F. Frey, "Laparoscopic Cholecystectomy—A Remarkable Development," *JAMA* 265, no. 12 (March 1991): 1573.

3. Lawrence Altman, "The Doctor's World: When Patient's Life Is Price of Learning New Kind of Surgery," *New York Times*, June 23, 1992, C3.

4. Judy Licht, "Surgery without Wounds," *Washington Post*, April 28, 1992, Health, Z8.

5. A. Csendes et al., "Late Results of Immediate Primary End-to-End Repair in Accidental Section of the Common Bile Duct," *Surg Gynecol Obstet* 168 (February 1989): 125–130.

6. Philippe Mouret et al., "Laparoscopic Treatment of Perforated Peptic Ulcer," *Br J Surg* 77 (1990): 1006.

7. Alfred Cuschieri et al., "The European Experience with Laparoscopic Cholecystectomy," *Am J Surg* 161 (March 1991): 385–387.

8. J. C. Thompson, comment in *Yearbook of Surgery*, ed. Seymour I. Schwartz et al. (Chicago: Mosby Year Book, 1991), 307.

9. Robert W. Bailey et al., "Laparoscopic Cholecystectomy: Experience with 375 Consecutive Patients," *Ann Surg* 241 (1991): 531–541.

10. H. A. Graves et al., "Appraisal of Laparoscopic Cholecystectomy," *Ann Surg* 213 (1991): 655–664.

11. W. C. Meyes, "A Prospective Analysis of 1,518 Laparoscopic Cholecystectomies," *N Engl J Med* 324 (1991): 1073–1078.

12. E. H. Phillips et al., "The Importance of Intraoperative Cholangiography during Laparoscopic Cholecystectomy," *Am Surg* 56 (1990): 792–795.

13. G. C. Smith and J. P. Pell, "Parachute Use to Prevent Death and Major Trauma Related to Gravitational Challenge: A Systematic Review of Randomized Controlled Trials," *BMJ* 327, no. 7429 (December 2003): 1459–1461.

14. Wolfe, Gardiner, and Frey, "Remarkable Development," 1574.

15. Nathan Soper, "Laparoscopic Cholecystectomy: A Promising New 'Branch' in the Algorithm of Gallstone Management," *Surgery* 109, no. 3 (1991): 342–344.

16. Ibid., 344.

17. Ibid.

18. R. D. Rosin, *Minimal Access: Medicine and Surgery, Principles and Techniques* (Oxford, UK: Radcliffe Medical Press, 1993), xi.

19. Alfred Cuschieri and George Berci, *Laparoscopic Biliary Surgery* (London: Blackwell Scientific Publications, 1990), 1.

20. L. F. Rikkers, preface to *Evidence-Based Approach to Minimally Invasive Surgery*, ed. K. M. Murayama et al. (Woodbury CT: Cine-med, 2012), viii.

21. Jeffrey L. Ponsky, preface to Murayama et al., *Evidence-Based Approach to Minimally Invasive Surgery*, vii.

22. R. S. Chung and N. Ahmed, "The Impact of Minimally Invasive Surgery on Resident's Open Operative Experience," *Ann Surg* 251, no. 2 (2010): 205.

23. J. C. Kairy et al., "Cumulative Operative Experience Is Decreasing during General Surgical Residency: A Worrisome Trend for Surgical Trainees?" *J Am Coll Surg* 206, no. 5 (2008): 804.

24. E. A. Picarella et al., " 'Do One, Teach One' the New Paradigm in General Surgery Residency Training," *J Surg Educ* 68, no. 2 (2011): 126.

25. Leigh Neumayer, "Changing the Surgical Education Paradigm for the 21st Century," *Am J Surg* 203 (2012): 282–286.

26. R. N. Haass, "The Dilemma of Dissent," *Newsweek*, May 11–18, 2009.

Chapter Two

1. Robert Lowes, "Death of Rep. John Murtha Highlights Limitations of Laparoscopic Cholecystectomy," *Medscape Medical News*, February 9, 2010.

2. William D. Haggard, *Surgery—Queen of the Arts* (Philadelphia: W. B. Saunders, 1935), 17.

3. Robert G. Richardson, *Surgery: Old and New Frontiers* (New York: Charles Scribner's Sons, 1968), 37.

4. Joseph B. Lister, *The Collected Papers of Joseph Baron Lister, Volumes I and II* (Oxford, UK: Clarendon Press; repr., Birmingham, AL: Gryphon Editions, 1979).

5. Sherman B. Nuland, *The Origins of Anesthesia* (Birmingham, AL: Classics of Medicine Library, 1983).

6. I. S. Ravdin, "A Surgeon Takes a Second Look at Surgery," *JAMA* 158, no. 7 (1955): 533.

7. Pearl Katz, *The Scalpel's Edge: The Culture of Surgeons* (Boston: Allyn and Bacon, 1999).

8. Joan Cassel, *Expected Miracles: Surgeons at Work* (Philadelphia: Temple University Press, 1991).

9. Charles L. Bosk, *Forgive and Remember: Managing Medical Failure* (Chicago: University of Chicago Press, 1979).

10. David W. Page, "Are Surgeons Capable of Self-Reflection?" *Surg Clin North Am* 91 (2011): 293–304.

11. Claude H. Organ, "Presidential Address: You Can Make a Difference," *Bull Am Coll Surg* 88, no. 12 (2003): 6–12.

12. E. A. Halm, C. Lee, and M. R. Chassin, "Is Volume Related to Outcome in Healthcare? A Systematic Review and Methodologic Critique of the Literature," *Ann Int Med* 137 (2002): 511–520.

13. J. Duffin, *History of Medicine: A Scandalously Short Introduction*, 2nd ed. (Toronto: University of Toronto Press, 2000), 280.

14. Grzegorz S. Litynski, *Highlights in the History of Laparoscopy* (Frankfurt/Main, Ger.: Barbara Bernert Verlag, 1996), 10–21.

15. Lawrence K. Altman, "Complicated Surgery through Tiny Incisions," *New York Times*, August 14, 1990, Science Desk, C1.

16. J. E. A. Wickam, "The New Surgery," *Br Med J* 295, no. 6613 (1987): 1581–1582.

17. Alfred Cuschieri, "Whither Minimal Access Surgery: Tribulations and Expectations," *Am J Surg* 169 (January 1995): 9.

18. Alfred Cuschieri and George Berci, *Laparoscopic Biliary Surgery* (Oxford, UK: Blackwell Scientific Publications, 1990), 4.

19. James M. Hamdorf and J. C. Hall, "Acquiring Surgical Skills," *Br J Surg* 87 (2000): 28–37.

Chapter Three

1. Quoted in Robert E. Berry, *The Association of Program Directors in Surgery: A History of Origin and Maturation, 1966–2001* (Bethesda, MD: Association of Program Directors in Surgery, 2010), 18.

2. Hedley Atkins, *The Surgeon's Craft* (Springfield, IL: Charles C. Thomas, 1965), 34.

3. Caprice C. Greenberg et al., "Surgical Coaching for Individual Performance Improvement," *Ann Surg* 261 (2015): 32–34.

4. Margarett Knott and Dorothy E. Voss, *Proprioceptive Neuromuscular Facilitation: Patterns and Techniques*, 2nd ed. (New York: Harper and Row, 1968).

5. Christopher L. Vaughan, *Biomechanics of Sport* (Boca Raton, FL: CRC Press, 1989).

6. Richard K. Reznick and Helen MacRae, "Teaching Surgical Skills—Changes in the Wind," *N Engl J Med* 355, no. 25 (2006): 2664–2669.

7. Ibid., 2665.

8. Paul M. Fits and Michael I. Posner, *Human Performance* (Belmont, CA: Brooks/Cole, 1967): 115–122.

9. J. A. Kopta, "The Development of Motor Skills in Orthopedic Education," *Clin Orthop* 75 (1971): 70–85.

10. Richard K. Reznick, "Teaching and Testing Technical Skills," *Am J Surg* 165 (1993): 358–363.

11. Eugene J. Gibney, "Performance Skills for Surgeons: Lessons from Sport," *Am J Surg* 204 (2012): 543–544.

12. Mark L. Friedell, "The Carrot and the Stick," *J Surg Ed* 69, no. 6 (November/December 2012): 680–686.

13. Ibid., 683.

14. Alexander Alken et al., "Coaching during a Trauma Surgery Team Training: Perceptions versus Structured Observations," *Am J Surg* 209 (2015): 163–169.

15. Pritam Singh et al., "A Randomized Controlled Study to Evaluate the Role of Video-Based Coaching in Training Laparoscopic Skills," *Ann Surg* 261, no. 5 (May 2015): 862–869.

16. Stacey C. Carter et al., "Video-Based Peer Feedback through Social Networking for Robotic Surgery Simulation," *Ann Surg* 261, no. 5 (2015): 870–875.

17. Thomas Dent, "Training, Credentialing and Granting of Clinical Privileging for Laparoscopic General Surgery," *Amer J Surg* 161 (1991): 399–403.

18. M. Borten, *Laparoscopic Complications: Prevention and Management* (Toronto: B. C. Decker, 1986).

19. Dent, "Training, Credentialing," 339.

20. Grzegorz S. Litynski, "Erich Muhe and the Rejection of Laparoscopic Cholecystectomy (1985): A Surgeon before His Time," *JSLS* 2 (1998): 341–346.

21. Dent, "Training, Credentialing," 339.

22. Society of American Gastrointestinal Endoscopic Surgeons, "Granting Privileges for Laparoscopic General Surgery," *Amer J Surg* 161 (1991): 324–325.

23. Grzegorz S. Litynski, *Highlights in the History of Laparoscopy* (Frankfurt/Main, Ger.: Barbara Bernert Verlag, 1996), 261.

24. Ibid.

25. E. W. Archibald, "Higher Degrees in the Profession of Surgery," *Trans Meet Am Surg Assoc* 53 (1935): 1–15.

26. Dent, "Training, Credentialing," 399–403.

27. Alfred Cuschieri, "The Laparoscopic Revolution—Walk Carefully before We Run," *J Royal Coll Surg Edinb* 34 (December 1989): 295.

28. Ibid.

29. Dent, "Training, Credentialing," 339.

30. "Health Letters: Patients Should Ask Questions," *Washington Post*, June 30, 1992.

31. Charles Zacks and John Hoepner, "Ethical Considerations in Learning and Teaching Surgery," *Ophthalmology Clinics of North America* 13, no. 1 (March 2000): 63.

32. A. Johnson, "Laparoscopic Surgery," *Lancet* 349 (1997): 634.

33. John L. Gollan, "Proceedings of the NIH Consensus Development Conference on Gallstones and Laparoscopic Cholecystectomy," *Am J Surg* 165 (April 1993): 387–398.

34. Kurt Semm, *Operative Manual for Endoscopic Abdominal Surgery: Operative Pelviscopy, Operative Laparoscopy* (Chicago: Year Book Medical Publishers, 1987).

35. Lucien L. Leape, "The Preventability of Medical Injury," in *Human Error in Medicine*, ed. Marilyn S. Bogner (Hillsdale, NJ: Lawrence Erlbaum, 1994), 13.

36. T. A. Brennan et al., "Incidence of Adverse Events and Negligence in Hospitalized Patients: Results from the Harvard Medical Practice Study I," *New Engl J Med* 324 (1991): 370–376.

37. Lucien L. Leape et al., "The Preventability of Medical Injury," *Quality Review Bulletin* (May 1993): 144–149.

38. Linda T. Kohn and Janet M. Corrigan, eds., *To Err Is Human: Building a Safer Health System* (Washington, D.C.: National Academy Press, 2000), 26.

39. John T. James, "A New Evidence-Based Estimate of Patient Harms Associated with Hospital Care," *J Patient Saf*, no. 3 (September 2013): 122–128.

40. Christopher P. Landrigan et al., "Temporal Trends in Rates of Patient Harm Resulting from Medical Care," *N Engl J Med* 363, no. 22 (2010): 2124–2133.

41. Ibid., 2130.

42. Bogner, "Human Error in Medicine: A Frontier for Change," in *Human Error in Medicine*, 94.

43. J. Perper, "Life-Threatening and Fatal Therapeutic Misadventures," in Bogner, *Human Error in Medicine*, 46.

44. Lawrence Altman, "The Doctor's World: When Patient's Life Is Price of Learning New Kinds of Surgery," *New York Times*, June 23, 1992.

Chapter Four

1. Richard Bell, "Why Johnny Cannot Operate," *Surgery* 146, no. 4 (2009): 533–542.

2. John D. Birkmeyer et al., "Surgical Skill and Complication Rates after Bariatric Surgery," *New Engl J Med* 369 (2013): 1434–1442.

3. K. A. Ericsson, "Deliberate Practice and the Acquisition of Expert Performance: A General Overview," *Acad Emerg Med* 151 (2008): 988–994.

4. R. S. Chung, "How Much Time Do Surgical Residents Need to Learn to Operate?" *Am J Surg* 190 (2005): 351–353.

5. Sonal Arora et al., "What Makes a Competent Surgeon? Experts and Trainees' Perceptions of the Roles of a Surgeon," *Am J Surg* 198 (2009): 726–732.

6. D. Klass, "A Performance-Based Conception of Competence Is Changing the Regulation of Physicians' Professional Behavior," *Acad Med* 82, no. 6 (June 2007): 529–534.

7. Pearl Katz, *The Scalpel's Edge: The Culture of Surgeons* (Needham Heights, MA: Allyn and Bacon, 1999), 28–35.

8. J. B. Prystowsky, "Are Young Surgeons Competent to Perform Alimentary Tract Surgery?" *Arch Surg* 140 (2005): 495–502.

9. J. F. Waljee et al., "Surgeon Age and Operative Mortality in the United States," *Ann Surg* 244, no. 3 (2006): 353–362.

10. G. L. Freed, K. M. Dunham, and D. Singer, "Health Plan Use of Board-Certification and Recertification of Surgeons and Nonsurgical Subspecialists in Contracting Policies," *Arch Surg* 144, no. 8 (2009): 753–758.

11. G. L. Freed, K. M. Dunham, and D. Singer, "Use of Board-Certification and Recertification in Hospital Privileging," *Arch Surg* 144, no. 8 (2009): 746.

12. S. A. Shikora et al., "Laparoscopic Roux-en-Y Gastric Bypass: Results and Learning Curve of a High Volume Academic Program," *Arch Surg* 140 (2005): 362–367.

13. C. C. Passerotti et al., "Comparing the Quality of the Suture Anastomosis and the Learning Curves Associated with Performing Open, Freehand, and Robotic-Assisted Laparoscopic Pyeloplasty in a Swine Animal Model," *J Am Coll Surg* 208 (2009): 576–586.

14. Theodore P. Grantcharov and P. Funch-Jensen, "Can Everyone Achieve Proficiency with the Laparoscopic Technique? Learning Curve Patterns in Technical Skills Acquisition," *Am J Surg* 197 (2009): 447–449.

15. Loyal Davis, *Fellowship of Surgeons: A History of the American College of Surgeons* (Chicago, IL: Charles C. Thomas, 1960), 248.

16. Ibid.

17. H. S. Pritchett, introduction to "Medical Education in the United States and Canada: A Report to the Carnegie Foundation for the Advancement of Teaching," by A. Flexner, *Bulletin* (Boston), no. 4 (1910).

18. E. Passaro and Claude H. Organ, "Ernest A. Codman: The Improper Bostonian," *Bull Am Coll Surg* 84, no. 1 (1999): 19.

19. Ibid., 20.

20. Lawrence W. Way, "General Surgery in Evolution: Technology and Competence," *Amer J Surg* 171 (January 1996): 3.

21. Ibid.

22. Ibid.

23. Ibid., 4–6.

24. D. Casarett and C. Helms, "Systems Errors versus Physicians' Errors: Finding the Balance in Medical Education," *Acad Med* 74, no. 1 (January 1999): 19–22.

25. Ibid., 21.

26. Anthony Whittemore, "The Competent Surgeon: Individual Accountability in the Era of 'Systems' Failure," *Ann Surg* 250, no. 3 (2009): 357.

27. Ibid., 359.

28. C. J. Parsa, Claude H. Organ, and H. Barkan, "Changing Patterns of Resident Operative Experience from 1990 to 1997," *Arch Surg* 135 (May 2000): 570–575.

29. Ibid., 572.

30. David L. Narwold, "The Competency Movement: A Report on the Activities of the American Board of Medical Specialties," *Bull Am Coll Surg* 85, no. 11 (2000): 17.

31. Ibid., 16.

32. Wallace P. Ritchie, "The Measurement of Competence: Current Plans and Future Initiatives of the American Board of Surgery," *Bull Am Coll Surg* 86, no. 4 (April 2001): 11.

33. Ibid.

34. Ibid., 14.

35. Ibid., 15.

36. A. Darzi and S. Mackay, "Assessment of Surgical Competence," *Qual Health Care* 10, suppl. 2 (2001): ii64–ii69.

37. Ibid., ii64.

38. Ibid., ii68.

39. Richard M. Satava, Anthony G. Gallagher, and Carlos A. Pelligrini, "Surgical Competence and Surgical Proficiency: Definitions, Taxonomy, and Metrics," *J Amer Coll Surg* 196, no. 6 (June 2003): 933.

40. Ibid., 933.

41. R. W. Beart, "We Are Not All the Same—What Are We Going to Do about It?" *Contemp Surgery* 60, no. 11 (November 2004): 502.

42. R. M. Epstein and E. M. Hundert, "Defining and Assessing Professional Competence," *JAMA* 287, no. 2 (2002): 226.

43. Ibid., 227.

44. Arora et al., "Competent Surgeon," 726–732.

45. Ibid., 727.

46. Ibid., 731.

Chapter Five

1. J. S. Barkun et al., "Randomized Controlled Trial of Laparoscopic versus Mini Cholecystectomy," *Lancet* 340 (November 7, 1992): 116–119.

2. P. J. O'Dwyer, J. J. Murphy, N. J. O'Higgins, "Cholecystectomy through a 5 cm Subcostal Incision," *Br J Surg* 77 (October 1990): 1189–1190.

3. L. M. Stinton and E. A. Shaffer, "Epidemiology of Gallbladder Disease: Cholelithiasis and Cancer," *Liver* 6, no. 2 (2012): 172–187.

4. R. P. Nenner et al., "Increased Cholecystectomy Rates among Medicare Patients after the Introduction of Laparoscopic Cholecystectomy," *J Commun Health* 19 (1994): 409–415.

5. M. J. Kellett, J. E. A. Wickham, and R. C. G. Russell, "Percutaneous Cholecystolithotomy," *Br Med J* 296 (1988): 453.

6. American Medical Association, "Council Report—The Future of General Surgery," *JAMA* 262, no. 22 (December 8, 1989): 3178–3183.

7. Ibid., 3181.

8. Joseph E. Fischer, "The Impending Disappearance of the General Surgeon," *JAMA* 298, no. 18 (November 14, 2007): 2191–2193.

9. Steven B. Golden, "The Dying Field of General Surgery: When Do We Intervene? Why Residents Choose to Specialize in Fields outside Surgery," *J Surg Research* 159 (2010): 487–488.

10. Jacques Perissat, "Laparoscopic Cholecystectomy, a Treatment for Gallstones: From Idea to Reality," *World J Surg* 23 (1999): 328–331.

11. U. Leuschner, "Endoscopic Therapy of Biliary Calculi," *Clin Gastroenterol* 15, no. 2 (April 1986): 333.

12. J. Terblance et al., "Gallstones in the Gallbladder, In or Out and How? A Panel Presentation," *Surg Endosc* 4 (1990): 127–140.

13. R. F. Danzinger et al., "Dissolution of Cholesterol Gallstones by Chenodeoxycholic Acid," *N Engl J Med* 286 (1972): 1–8.

14. M. J. Allen et al., "Rapid Dissolution of Gallstones by Methyl Tert-Butyl Ether, Preliminary Observations," *N Engl J Med* 312 (1985): 217–220.

15. Alfred Cuschieri, Abd El Ghany, and M. P. Holley, "Successful Chemical Cholecystectomy: A Laparoscopic Guided Technique," *Gut* 30 (1989): 1786–1794.

16. Terblance et al., "Gallstones in the Gallbladder," 127–132.

17. I. A. D. Boucher, "Dissolution of Gallstones," *Curr Surg Pract* 1 (1990): 213–117.

18. M. Podda et al., "Efficacy and Safety of a Combination of Chenodeoxycholic Acid and Ursodeoxycholic Acid for Gallstone Dissolution: A Comparison with Ursodeoxycholic Acid Alone," *Gastroenterology* 96 (1989): 222–229.

19. Leslie J. Schoenfield et al., "Chenodiol (Chenodeoxycholic Acid) for Dissolution of Gallstones: The National Cooperative Gallstone Study," *Ann Int Med* 95 (1981): 257–282.

20. Kellett, Wickham, and Russell, "Percutaneous Cholecystolithotomy," 453.

21. American College of Surgeons, "Statement on Laparoscopic Cholecystectomy," *Bull Am Coll Surg* 75, no. 6 (1990): 6.

22. David W. Page, "Immediate Enteral Feeding and Early Discharge following Cholecystectomy" (abstract), *J Am Coll Nutr* 2, no. 3 (1983).

23. Grzegorz Litynski, *Highlights in the History of Laparoscopy* (Frankfurt/Main, Ger.: Barbara Bernert Verlag, 1996), 1185.

24. Grzegorz Litynski, "Erich Muhe and the Rejection of Laparoscopic Cholecystectomy (1985): A Surgeon ahead of His Time," *JSLS* 2 (1998): 342.

Chapter Six

1. Grzegorz Litynski, *Highlights in the History of Laparoscopic Surgery* (Frankfurt/Main, Ger.: Barbara Bernert Verlag, 1996), 243.

2. Timothy Johnson, "Shattuck Lecture—Medicine and the Media," *New Engl J Med* 339, no. 2 (July 1998): 88.

3. Ibid., 89.

4. H. Troidl, "Endoscopic Surgery a Fascinating Idea Requires Responsibility in Evaluation and Handling," in *Surgical Technology International III*, ed. Zoltan Szabo, Morris D. Kerstein, and James E. Lewis (San Francisco: Universal Medical Press, 1994), 113.

5. Robert G. Richardson, *Surgery: Old and New Frontiers* (New York: Charles Scribner's Sons, 1958), 65–66.

6. Ibid., 65.

7. Ibid., 66.

8. Leon Morgenstern, "Carl Langenbuch and the First Cholecystectomy," *Surg Endosc* 6 (1992): 113–114.

9. H. E. Stephenson, "Justus Ohage—America's Premier Cholecystectomy Surgeon," *Missouri Medicine* 69, no. 2 (1972): 86–91.

10. Ibid., 89.

11. Ibid., 90.

12. Walker Reynolds, "The First Laparoscopic Cholecystectomy," *JSLS* 5 (2001): 89–94.

13. Litynski, *Highlights*, 186.

14. Ibid., 184.

15. Ibid., 166.

16. Ibid., 167.

17. Ibid., 166.

18. Ibid., 184.

19. Ibid., 172–173.

20. Ibid., 173.

21. Ibid., 189.

22. Malcolm Gladwell, *Outliers: The Story of Success* (New York: Little, Brown, 2008), 37.

23. Grzegorz S. Litynski, "Kurt Semm and the Fight against Skepticism: Endoscopic Hemostatsis, Laparoscopic Appendectomy, and Semm's Impact on the 'Laparoscopic Revolution,'" *JSLS* 2 (1998): 311.

24. Litynski, *Highlights*, 136–137.

25. Ibid., 151.

26. Ibid., 218.

27. Ibid., 219.

28. Francois Dubois et al., "Coelioscopic Cholecystectomy," *Ann Surg* 211 (1990): 60–62.

29. Litynski, *Highlights*, 221.

30. Jacques Perissat, "Laparoscopic Cholecystectomy: A Treatment for Gallstones—from Idea to Reality," *World J Surg* 23 (1999): 328–331.

31. Litynski, *Highlights*, 225.

32. J. Barry McKernan, "Origin of Laparoscopic Cholecystectomy in the USA: Personal Experience," *World J Surg* 23 (1999): 332–333.

33. Ibid., 332.

34. Ibid.

35. Litynski, *Highlights*, 228.

36. Ibid., 229.

37. Ibid., 230.

38. Ibid.

39. Barry McKernan, "Origin of Laparoscopic Cholecystectomy," 332.

40. Litynski, *Highlights*, 231.

41. Ibid.

42. Eddie J. Reddick and Douglas O. Olsen, "Laparoscopic Cholecystectomy," *Surg Endosc* 3 (1989): 131–133.

43. Litynski, *Highlights*, 233.

44. Ibid., 234–235.

45. Ibid., 236.

46. Ibid., 239.

47. Ibid., 243.

48. Ibid., 246.

49. Ibid.

50. Ibid., 253.

51. Ibid., 247.

52. Barry McKernan, "Origin of Laparoscopic Cholecystectomy," 333.

Chapter Seven

1. Linsey Lyon, "Gallbladder Out, No Incision Required," *U.S. News and World Report*, October 2008, 68.

2. Martin F. McKneally, "Ethical Problems in Surgery: Innovation Leading to Unforeseen Complications," *World J Surg* 23 (1999): 786–788.

3. Christina Frangou, "Patient Enthusiasm for NOTES Is Tempered by Caution," *General Surgery News* (September 2007): 8.

4. R. Tevlin et al., "Impact of Surgical Innovation on Tissue Repair in the Surgical Patient," *BJS* 102 (2015): e41.

5. McKneally, "Ethical Problems," 787.

6. Ibid.

7. R. J. Siewert et al., "Reoperation following Failed Fundoplication," *World J Surg* 13 (1989): 791.

8. Monica J. Smith, "You Want to Take Out My Gallbladder, *How?*" *General Surgical News* (September 2007): 8.

9. Mary Beth Nierengarten, "Tuning into NOTES," *General Surgery News* (October 2006): 27.

10. Ryan Childers, Pamela A. Lipsett, and Timothy M. Pawlik, "Informed Consent and the Surgeon," *J Am Coll Surg* 208, no. 4 (April 2009): 627.

11. Faiz Gani et al., "Potential Barriers to the Diffusion of Surgical Innovation," *JAMA Surg* 151, no. 5 (March 16, 2016): 403–404, doi:10.1001/jamasurg.2016.0030.

12. Anees B. Chagpar, "Innovation in Surgery: From Imagination to Implementation," *Am J Surg* 202 (2011): 641.

13. Ibid., 644.

14. H. David Banta and Stephen B. Thacker, "The Case for Reassessment of Health Care Technology," *JAMA* 264, no. 2 (July 11, 1990): 236.

15. Ibid., 237.

16. Ibid., 239.

17. Victor R. Fuchs and Alan M. Garber, "The New Technology Assessment," *N Engl J Med* 323, no. 10 (September 6, 1990): 677.

18. B. Wolfe, B. Gardiner, and C. Frey, "Laparoscopic Cholecystectomy—A Remarkable Development," *JAMA* 265, no. 12 (March 27, 1991): 1573–1574.

19. Ibid., 1574.

20. Gordon M. Stirrat et al., "The Challenge of Evaluating Surgical Procedures," *Ann Royal Coll Surg Engl* 74 (1992): 80–84.

21. David A. Grimes, "Technology Follies—The Uncritical Acceptance of Medical Innovation," *JAMA* 269, no. 23 (June 16, 1993): 3030–3032.

22. Ibid., 3030.

23. Ibid., 3031.

24. Ibid., 3031–3032.

25. Ibid., 3032.

26. Ibid.

27. Richard I. Cook and David D. Woods, "Adapting to New Technology in the Operating Room," *Human Factors* 38, no. 4 (1996): 593–613.

28. Martin F. McKneally, "Ethical Problems," 786–788.

29. Ibid., 787.

30. Ibid., 786.

31. Ibid., 787.

32. F. William Heer, "The Place of Trust in Our Changing Surgical Environment," *Arch Surg* 132 (August 1997): 809.

33. Kenton C. Bodily, "Surgeons and Technology," *Am J Surg* 177 (1999): 352.

34. Angelique M. Reitsma and Jonathan D. Moreno, "Ethical Regulations for Innovative Surgery: The Last Frontier," *J Am Coll Surg* 194 (2002): 792.

35. Ibid., 792.

36. Ibid., 795.

37. Angelique M. Reitsma and Jonathan D. Moreno, "Ethics in Innovative Surgery: US Surgeons' Definitions, Knowledge and Attitudes," *J Am Coll Surg* 200 (2005): 103–110.

38. Ibid., 108.

39. Ibid., 103.

40. Walter A. Biffl et al., "Responsible Development and Application of Innovations: A Position Statement of the Society of University Surgeons," *J Am Coll Surg* 206, no. 6 (June 2008): 1204.

41. Ibid.

42. Deborah Korenstein, Salomeh Keyhani, and J. S. Ross, "Physician Attitudes toward Industry—A View across the Specialties," *Arch Surg* 145, no. 6 (2010): 575.

43. Jo Buyske, "Invited Critique," in Korenstein, Keyhani, and Ross, "Physician Attitudes," 577.

44. Stephen P. Sagar et al., "Hey, I Just Did a New Operation! Introducing Innovative Procedures and Devices within an Academic Health Center," *Ann Surg* 261, no. 1 (January 2015): 30–34.

45. Lindsey A. McNair and Walter L. Biffl, "Assessing Awareness and Implementation of a Recommendation for Surgical Innovation Committees," *Ann Surg* 262, no. 6 (December 2015): 941–948.

46. Katrina Hutchison et al., "Getting Clearer about Surgical Innovation—A New Definition and a Tool to Support Responsible Practice," *Ann Surg* 262, no. 6 (December 2015): 949–954.

Chapter Eight

1. John Carreyrou, "Surgical Robot Examined in Injuries," *Wall Street Journal*, May 4, 2010, 1–8.

2. Robert H. Wozniak, *Classics in Psychology, 1885–1914: Historical Essays* (Bristol, UK: Thoemmes Press, 1999).

3. Charles J. Teplitz, *The Learning Curve Deskbook: A Reference Guide to Theory, Calculations, and Applications* (Westport, CT: Quorum Books, 1991), 7.

4. Ibid., 3.

5. M. P. Schijven and J. Jakimowicz, "The Learning Curve on the Xitact LS 500 Laparoscopy Simulator: Profiles in Performance," *Surg Endosc* 18 (2004): 126.

6. Theodore P. Grantcharov and P. Funch-Jensen, "Can Everyone Achieve Proficiency with the Laparoscopic Technique? Learning Curve Patterns in Technical Skills Acquisition," *Am J Surg* 197 (2009): 447–449.

7. Schijven and Jakimowicz, "Learning Curve," 121.

8. Anthony G. Gallagher et al., "Psychomotor Skills Assessment in Practicing Surgeons Experienced in Performing Advanced Laparoscopic Procedures," *J Am Coll Surg* 1971 (2003): 479–488.

9. Elena A. Gates, "New Surgical Procedures: Can Our Patients Benefit while We Learn?" *Am J Obstret Gynecol* 176, no. 6 (June 1997): 1293.

10. Ibid.

11. J. F. Hulka et al., "Open Hysterotomy: American Association of Gynecologic Laparoscopists 1991 Membership Survey," *J Reproductive Med* 38 (1993): 572–573.

12. Phillip R. Schauer, "Who Will Help Surgeons Climb the Learning Curve?" *Contemp Surg* 59, no. 11 (November 2003): 502.

13. "Spotlight on Robotic Surgery," *General Surgery News* 42, no. 11 (October 2015): 8–12.

14. Justin Kruger and David Dunning, "Unskilled and Unaware: How Difficulties in Recognizing One's Own Incompetence Lead to Inflated Self-Assessments," *J Personality and Social Psychology* 77, no. 6 (1999): 1121.

15. Ibid., 1121.

16. Schijven and Jakimowicz, "Learning Curve," 121–127.

17. Edward D. Gifford et al., "Variation in the Learning Curve of General Surgery Residents Performing Arteriovenous Fistulas," *J Surg Ed* 72, no. 4 (July/August 2015): 761–766.

18. Alfred Cuschieri, "Whither Minimal Access Surgery: Tribulations and Expectations," *Am J Surg* 169 (January 1995): 11.

19. Eddie Joe Reddick and Douglas O. Olsen, "Laparoscopic Laser Cholecystectomy—A Comparison with Mini-Lap Cholecystectomy," *Surg Endosc* 3 (1989): 131–133.

20. Erich Muhe, "Long-Term Follow-Up after Laparoscopic Cholecystectomy," *Endoscopy* 24 (1992): 754–758.

21. Eddie Joe Reddick et al., "Safe Performance of Difficult Laparoscopic Cholecystectomies," *Am J Surg* 161 (March 1991): 377–381.

22. Jeffrey H. Peters et al., "Safety and Efficacy of Laparoscopic Cholecystectomy," *Ann Surg* 213, no. 1 (January 1991): 3–12.

23. Joaquin Sariego, Larry Spitzer, and Teruo Matsumoto, "The 'Learning Curve' in the Performance of Laparoscopic Cholecystectomy," *Int Surg* 78 (1993): 1–3.

24. Burt Cagar et al., "The Learning Curve for Laparoscopic Cholecystectomy," *J Laparoendoscopic Surg* 4, no. 6 (1994): 419.

25. David C. Wherry et al., "An External Audit of Laparoscopic Cholecystectomy Performed in Medical Treatment Facilities of the Department of Defense," *Ann Surg* 220, no. 5 (1994): 633.

26. Andrus J. Voitk, G. S. Smiley, and S. I. Tsao, "The Tail of the Learning Curve for Laparoscopic Cholecystectomy," *Am J Surg* 182 (2001): 250–253.

27. The Southern Surgeons Club, Michael J. Moore, and Charles L. Bennett, "The Learning Curve for Laparoscopic Cholecystectomy," *Am J Surg* 170 (July 1995): 55–59.

28. Larry Dashow et al., "Initial Experience with Laparoscopic Cholecystectomy at the Beth Israel Medical Center," *Surg Gynecol Obstet* 175 (1992): 25–30.

29. Charles L. Bennett et al., "The Learning Curve for Laparoscopic Colorectal Surgery," *Arch Surg* 132 (1997): 41.

30. Twomo K. Rantanen et al., "Complications in Anti-reflux Surgery," *Arch Surg* 143 (April 2008): 359–365.

31. Gunnar Ahlberg et al., "Is the Learning Curve for Fundoplication Determined by the Teacher or Pupil?" *Am J Surg* 189 (2005): 184–189.

32. Anders Ericsson and Robert Pool, *PEAK: Secrets from the New Science of Expertise* (New York: Houghton Mifflin Harcourt, 2016), 84–114.

Chapter Nine

1. Malcolm Gladwell, *The Tipping Point: How Little Things Can Make a Big Difference* (New York: Little, Brown, 2000).

2. Everett M. Rogers, *Diffusion of Innovations*, 5th ed. (New York: Free Press, 2003).

3. Roy Porter, *The Greatest Benefit to Mankind: A Medical History of Humanity* (New York: W. W. Norton, 1997), 369.

4. Gladwell, *Tipping Point*, 7.

5. David Rosin, *Minimal Access Medicine and Surgery* (Oxford, UK: Radcliffe Medical Press, 1993), xi.

6. K. Michael Hughes et al., "A Crew Resource Management Program Tailored to Trauma Resuscitation Improves Team Behavior and Communication," *J Am Coll Surg* 219 (2014): 545–551.

7. Steven K. Howard and David M. Gaba, "Anesthesia Crisis Resource Management Training: Teaching Anesthesiologists to Handle Critical Incidents," *Aviat Space Environ Med* 63, no. 9, sec. 1 (September 1992): 763–770.

8. Grzegorz S. Litynski, *Highlights in the History of Laparoscopy—The Development of Laparoscopic Techniques: A Cumulative Effort of Internists, Gynecologists and Surgeons* (Frankfurt/Main, Ger.: Barbara Bernert Verlag, 1996), 177.

9. Ibid.

10. Gladwell, *Tipping Point*, 160.

11. Litynski, *Highlights*, 209.

12. Ibid.

13. H. Troidl, "Surgical Endoscopy and Sonography: Surgery at the Crossroads," *Surg Endosc* 4 (1990): 41.

14. Ibid., 43.

15. Litynski, *Highlights*, 238.

16. Troidl, "Surgical Endoscopy and Sonography," 43.

17. J. Madeleine Nash, "The Kindest Cuts of All," *Time*, March 23, 1992.

18. Rogers, *Diffusion*, 168.

19. Ibid., 12.

20. Ibid., xxi.

21. Ibid., 19.

22. Ibid.

23. Ibid., 343.

24. Gladwell, *Tipping Point*, 12.

25. Ibid., 9.

26. R. S. Chung and T. A. Broughan, "The Phenomenal Growth of Laparoscopic Cholecystectomy: A Review," *Clev Clin J Med* 59, no. 2 (1992): 186.

27. William Stoney, "Laparoscopic Cholecystectomy: Problems of Rapid Growth," *Southern Med J* 84, no. 6 (1992): 681.

28. Mohan Airan et al., "Retrospective and Prospective Multi-institutional Laparoscopic Cholecystectomy Study Organized by the Society of American Gastrointestinal Endoscopic Surgeons," *Surg Endosc* 6 (1992): 169.

29. R. K. Tompkins, "Laparoscopic Cholecystectomy—Threat or Opportunity," *Arch Surg* 125 (1990): 1245.

30. Stoney, "Laparoscopic Cholecystectomy: Problems," 681.

31. Gladwell, *Tipping Point*, 10.

32. Litynski, *Highlights*, 148–152.

33. Ibid., 227–258.

34. Alfred Cuschieri and George Berci, *Laparoscopic Biliary Surgery* (Oxford, UK: Blackwell Scientific Publications, 1990), viii.

35. Gladwell, *Tipping Point*, 69.

36. Ibid., 84–87.

37. Ibid., 91.

38. Ibid., 160.

39. Albert T. Spaw, Eddie J. Reddick, and Douglas O. Olsen, "Laparoscopic Laser Cholecystectomy: Analysis of 500 Procedures," *Surg Endosc and Endosc* 1, no. 1 (1991): 2–7.

40. Alfred Cuschieri et al., "The European Experience with Laparoscopic Cholecystectomy," *Am J Surg* 161 (March 1991): 387.

41. John L. Gollan et al., eds., "Proceedings of the NIH Consensus Development Conference on Gallstones and Laparoscopic Cholecystectomy," *Am J Surg* 165 (April 1993): 387–397.

42. Ibid., 388.

43. Ibid.

44. Andrew M. Davidoff et al., "Mechanisms of Major Biliary Injury during Laparoscopic Cholecystectomy," *Ann Surg* 215, no. 3 (March 1992): 196–202.

45. Gollan et al., "Proceedings of the NIH Consensus Development Conference," 388.

46. The Southern Surgeons Club, "A Prospective Analysis of 1,518 Laparoscopic Cholecystectomies Performed by Southern US Surgeons," *N Engl J Med* 324 (1991): 1073–1078.

47. Gollan et al., "Proceedings of the NIH Consensus Development Conference," 390.

48. Ibid., 393–394.

49. Ibid., 393.

Chapter Ten

1. Robert G. Richardson, *Surgery: Old and New Frontiers* (New York: Charles Scribner's Sons, 1968), 3.

2. David W. Page, "Teams and Professionalism," in *Professionalism in Mental Health: Experts, Expertise, and Expectations*, ed. D. Bhugra and A. Malik (Cambridge, UK: Cambridge University Press, 2011), 101–114.

3. A. H. Rosenstein and M. O'Daniel, "Disruptive and Clinical Perceptions of Behavior Outcomes," *Am J Nursing* 105, no. 1 (2005): 54.

4. Richard Selzer, *Letters to a Young Doctor* (San Diego: Harcourt Brace, 1982).

5. Richard Selzer, *Confessions of a Knife* (New York: Touchstone / Simon and Schuster, 1979).

6. Richard Selzer, *Mortal Lessons—Notes on the Art of Surgery* (New York: Touchstone / Simon and Schuster, 1974).

7. Richard Selzer, *Taking the World in for Repairs* (New York: Penguin, 1986).

8. Richard Selzer, *The Exact Location of the Soul* (New York: Picador / St. Martin's Press, 2001).

9. Selzer, *Letters*, 42.

10. Ibid., 43.

11. Ibid.

12. Anthony D. Whittemore, "The Competent Surgeon—Individual Accountability in the Era of 'Systems' Failure," *Ann Surg* 250, no. 3 (2009): 359.

13. Amelia Cochran and William B. Elder, "Effects of Disruptive Surgeon Behavior in the Operating Room," *Am J Surg* 209 (2015): 65–70.

14. Charles Bosk, *Forgive and Remember: Managing Medical Failure* (Chicago: University of Chicago, 1979), ix.

15. Ibid., 168.

16. Ibid., 169–171.

17. Ibid., 172.

18. Ibid., 173–177.

19. Joan Cassell, *Expected Miracles: Surgeons at Work* (Philadelphia: Temple University Press, 1991).

20. Ibid., 20.

21. Ibid., 38–39.

22. Ibid., 39.

23. Leon Morgenstern, "Final Reflections—The Decline and Fall of the Surgical Incision," *Surg Innovation* 13, no. 3 (September 2006): 207.

24. Ibid., 208.

25. Cassell, *Expected Miracles*, 72–80.

26. Joan Cassell, *The Woman in the Surgeon's Body* (Cambridge, MA: Harvard University Press, 1998), 11.

27. Pearl Katz, *The Scalpel's Edge: The Culture of Surgeons* (Boston: Allyn and Bacon, 1999), 4.

28. Ibid., 21.

29. Raylene Gordon, Steven J. Jacobsen, and Alfred A. Rimm, "Similarities in the Personalities of Women and Men Who Were First-Year Medical Students Planning Careers in Surgery," *Acad Med* 66, no. 9 (1991): 560.

30. H. Schumacker, "What Do We Want in a Surgical Chairman?" *Am J Surg* 150 (1985): 292.

31. Frances Conley, *Walking Out on the Boys* (New York: Farrar, Straus and Giroux, 1998), 6.

32. Ibid., 50.

33. Ibid., 135.

34. Ibid., 209.

35. Katz, *Scalpel's Edge*, 31.

36. Ibid., 40.

37. Malcolm Gladwell, *Blink: The Power of Thinking without Thinking* (New York: Little, Brown, 2005), 96.

38. Katz, *Scalpel's Edge*, 77–82.

39. Cassel, *Expected Miracles*, 163.

40. A. G. Greenburg, D. K. McClure, and N. E. Penn, "Personality Traits of Surgical House Officers: Faculty and Resident Views," *Surgery* 92, no. 2 (1982): 368–372.

41. M. Warschkow et al., "A Comparative Cross-Sectional Study of Personality Traits in Internists and Surgeons," *Surgery* 148, no. 5 (November 2010): 901–907.

42. Ibid., 906.

43. James McGreevy and D. Wiebe, "A Preliminary Measurement of the Surgical Personality," *Am J Surg* 184 (2002): 121–125.

44. Alan H. Rosenstein and Michelle O'Daniel, "Impact and Implications of Disruptive Behavior in the Perioperative Arena," *J Am Coll Surg* 203 (2006): 96–105.

45. Richard W. Schwartz et al., "Defining the Surgical Personality: A Preliminary Study," *Surgery* 115, no. 1 (1994): 62–68.

46. Ibid., 66.

47. J. H. Thomas, "The Surgical Personality: Fact or Fiction," *Am J Surg* 174 (1997): 576.

48. David W. Page, "Are Surgeons Capable of Introspection?" *Surg Clin N Am* 91 (2011): 293–304.

49. Douglas A. Wiegmann et al., "Disruptions in Surgical Flow and Their Relationship to Surgical Errors: An Exploratory Investigation," *Surgery* 142 (2007): 658.

50. Paul Pearsall, "Toxic Success and the Mind of a Surgeon," *Arch Surg* 139 (August 2004): 879.

51. Lucian L. Leape, "Full Disclosure and Apology—An Idea Whose Time Has Come," *Physician Executive* (March-April 2006): 16.

Chapter Eleven

1. D. L. Bliwise et al., "Prevalence of Self-Reported Poor Sleep in a Healthy Population Aged 50–65," *Soc Sci Med* 34 (1992): 49–55.

2. Dr. X, *The Intern* (New York: Harper and Row, 1965).

3. Robert E. Condon, "Resident Hours: Only Work?" *Arch Surg* 124 (October 1989): 1121–1122.

4. Leora R. Lewittes and Victor W. Marshall, "Fatigue and Concerns about Quality of Care among Ontario Interns and Residents," *CMAJ* 140 (January 1, 1989): 21–24.

5. Gerald E. Daigler, Robert C. Welliver, and Bruder Stapleton, "New York Regulation of Residents' Working Conditions," *AJDC* 144 (July 1990): 799–802.

6. Amalia Kelly et al., "The Effect of the New York State Restrictions on Resident Work Hours," *Obstet Gynecol* 78, no. 3, pt. 1 (September 1991): 469–473.

7. Daniel J. Gottlieb et al., "Effect of a Change in House Staff Work Schedule on Resource Utilization and Patient Care," *Arch Int Med* 151 (October 1991): 2065–2070.

8. Ibid., 2065.

9. D. J. Vassallo et al., "Introduction of a Partial Shift System for House Officers in a Teaching Hospital," *BMJ* 305 (1992): 1005–1008.

10. Ruth A. Potee, "Letter to the Editor," *JAMA* 288, no. 23 (December 18, 2002): 2973–2974.

11. Jay Greene, "More Residencies Cited for Work Violations," *American Medical News*, March 6, 2000.

12. Thomas J. Krizek, "Surgery: Is It an Impairing Profession? A Summary of the Ethics and Philosophy Lecture," *Bull Amer Coll Surg* (February 2002): 29.

13. Ronald C. Samuels et al., "Lessons from Pediatric Residency Program Director's Experience with Work Hour Limitations in New York State," *Acad Med* 80, no. 5 (May 2005): 467.

14. Willie Underwood et al., "Viewpoints from Generation X: A Survey of Candidates and Associate Viewpoints on Resident Duty-Hour Regulations," *J Am Coll Surg* 198 (2004): 991.

15. Bernard M. Jaffe, "Collision Course," *Surgical Rounds* (August 2002): 379.

16. L. Kohn et al., *To Err Is Human: Building a Safer Health Care System* (Washington, D.C.: National Academy Press, 2000).

17. Andrew I. Light et al., "The Effects of Acute Sleep Deprivation on Level of Resident Training," *Curr Surg* (January-February 1989): 29.

18. Laura A. Petersen et al., "Does Housestaff Discontinuity of Care Increase the Risk for Preventable Adverse Events?" *Ann Int Med* 121, no. 11 (December 1, 1994): 866.

19. N. J. Taffinder et al., "Effect of Sleep Deprivation on Surgeon's Dexterity on Laparoscopy Simulator," *Lancet* 352 (October 1998): 1191.

20. Ibid.

21. Catharine B. Barden et al., "Effect of Limited Work Hours on Surgical Training," *J Am Coll Surg* 195 (2002): 531.

22. Steven K. Howard et al., "The Risks and Implications of Excessive Daytime Sleepiness in Resident Physicians," *Acad Med* 77, no. 10 (October 2002): 1019.

23. Ibid.

24. *Resident Duty Hours: Enhancing Sleep, Supervision, and Safety* (Washington, D.C.: Institute of Medicine of the National Academies, 2008).

25. Ibid., 3.

26. C. Laine et al., "The Impact of a Regulation Restricting Medical House Staff Working Hours on the Quality of Patient Care," *JAMA* 269 (1993): 374–378.

27. Meeta Prasad et al., "The Effect of Work-Hours Restrictions on ICU Mortality in United States Teaching Hospitals," *Crit Care Med* 37, no. 9 (2009): 2565.

28. Accreditation Council for Graduate Medical Education, "Common Program Requirements," ACGME approved focused revision, September 29, 2013; effective July 1, 2016.

29. Brian C. Drolet, Mamoona T. Khokhar, and Staci A. Fischer, "The 2011 Duty Hour Requirements—A Survey of Residency Program Directors," *N Engl J Med* 3368, no. 8 (2013): 694.

30. Ryan M. Antiel et al., "Effect of Duty Hour Restrictions on Core Competencies, Education, Quality of Life, and Burnout among General Surgery Interns," *JAMA Surg* 148, no. 5 (May 2013): 448.

31. Kanav Kahol et al., "Effect of Fatigue on Psychomotor and Cognitive Skills," *Am J Surg* 195 (2008): 195.

32. Jodi Gerdes et al., "Jack Barney Award: The Effect of Fatigue on Cognitive and Psychomotor Skills of Trauma Residents and Attendings," *Am J Surg* 196 (2008): 813.

33. Kai S. Lehmann et al., "Impact of Sleep Deprivation on Medium Term Psychomotor and Cognitive Performance of Surgeons: Prospective Cross-over Study with a Virtual Surgery Simulator and Psychometric Tests," *Surgery* 147 (2010): 246.

34. Thomas R. Russell, "From My Perspective," *Bull Am Coll Surg* 85, no. 12 (December 2000): 5.

35. Barden, Specht, and McCarter, "Effect of Limited Work Hours," 535–536.

36. "Statement on Fundamental Characteristics of Surgical Residency Programs (ST-4): The American College of Surgeons," *Bull Am Coll Surg* 73 (1988): 22–23.

37. David M. Gaba and Steven K. Howard, "Fatigue among Clinicians and the Safety of Patients," *N Engl J Med* 347, no. 16 (October 17, 2002): 1249.

38. S. Mahmood Zare et al., "Psychological Well-Being of Surgical Residents before the 80-Hour Work Week: A Multiinstitutional Study," *J Am Coll Surg* 198 (2004): 633.

39. Frank McCormick et al., "Surgeon Fatigue—A Prospective Analysis of the Incidence, Risk, and Intervals of Predicted Fatigue-Related Impairment in Residents," *Arch Surg* 147, no. 5 (May 2012): 430.

40. Mark A. Feanny et al., "Impact of the 80-Hour Work Week on Resident Emergency Operative Experience," *Am J Surg* 190 (2005): 947.

41. Mathew C. Byrnes et al., "Impact of Resident Work Hours on Trauma Care," *Am J Surg* 191 (2006): 338.

42. Paul J. Schenarts et al., "The Effect of a Night-Float Coverage Scheme on Preventable and Potentially Preventable Morbidity at a Level 1 Trauma Center," *Am J Surg* 190 (2005): 147–152.

43. Robert O. Carpenter et al., "Work Hour Restrictions as an Ethical Dilemma for Residents," *Am J Surg* 191 (2006): 527.

44. Melvin S. Blanchard, David Melzer, and Kenneth S. Polonsky, "To Nap or Not to Nap? Residents' Work Hours Revisited," *N Engl J Med* 360, no. 21 (May 21, 2009): 2242.

45. Ibid., 2242.

46. Ibid., 2242–2244.

47. C. P. Landrigan et al., "Effect of Reducing Intern Work Hours on Serious Medical Errors in Intensive Care Units," *N Engl J Med* 351, no. 18 (October 2004): 1838–1848.

48. Steven W. Lockley et al., "Effect of Reducing Intern's Weekly Work Hours on Sleep and Attentional Failures," *N Engl J Med* 351, no. 18 (October 2004): 1829–1837.

49. H. Singh et al., "Medical Errors Involving Trainees: A Study of Closed Malpractice Claims from 5 Insurers," *Arch Int Med* 167 (2007): 2030–2036.

50. L. D. Britt et al., "Resident Duty Hours in Surgery for Ensuring Patient Safety, Providing Optimum Resident Education and Training, and Promoting Resident Well-Being: A Response from the American College of Surgeons to the Report of the Institute of Medicine, 'Resident Duty Hours: Enhancing Sleep, Supervision, and Safety,'" *Surgery* 146, no. 3 (September 2009): 403.

51. Gregory Belenky et al., "Patterns of Performance Degradation and Restoration during Sleep Restriction and Subsequent Recovery: A Sleep Dose-Response Study," *J Sleep Res* 12 (2003): 1.

52. Peter I. Ellman et al., "Sleep Deprivation Does Not Affect Operative Results in Cardiac Surgery," *Ann Thorac Surg* 78 (2004): 906–911.

53. Michael W. H. Chu et al., "Prospective Evaluation of Consultant Surgeon Sleep Deprivation and Outcomes in More Than 4000 Consecutive Cardiac Surgical Procedures," *Arch Surg* 146, no. 9 (September 2011): 1080–1085.

54. Meeta Prasad Kerlin et al., "A Randomized Trial of Nighttime Physician Staffing in an Intensive Care Unit," *N Engl J Med* 368, no. 23 (June 2013): 2201–2210.

55. Jeffrey M. Rothchild et al., "Risks of Complications by Attending Physicians after Performing Nighttime Procedures," *JAMA* 302, no. 14 (2009): 1565–1572.

56. Colin Schieman et al., "Does Surgeon Fatigue Influence Outcomes after Anterior Resection for Rectal Cancer?" *Am J Surg* 195 (2008): 684–688.

57. Darshak Sanghavi, "Young Doctors Are No Longer Working Long, Stupor-Inducing Hours. So Why Aren't Hospitals Any Safer?" *New York Times Magazine*, November 17, 2011, 28–29.

58. Gerald Imber, *Genius on the Edge* (New York: Kaplan, 2010), 90–94.

59. Teryl K. Nuckols et al., "Cost Implications of Reduced Work Hours and Workloads for Resident Physicians," *N Engl J Med* 360 (2009): 2202–2215.

60. Michael Payette, Abhishek Chatterjee, and William B. Weeks, "Cost and Workforce Implications of Subjecting All Physicians to Aviation Industry Work-Hour Restrictions," *Am J Surg* 197 (22009): 820–825.

61. Jacob Moalem et al., "Should All Duty Hours Be the Same? Results of a National Survey of Surgical Trainees," *J Am Coll Surg* 209 (2009): 48.

62. Jacob Moalem, "Why Resident Work Hours Must Be Flexible: One Young Surgeon's View," *Bull Am Coll Surg* 94, no. 10 (October 2009): 15.

63. Ibid.

64. Ibid.

65. Christopher D. Mitchell et al., "Resident Fatigue: Is There a Patient Safety Issue?" *Am J Surg* 198 (2009): 811.

66. Maria Veronica Hegar et al., "Resident Fatigue in 2010: Where Is the Beef?" *Am J Surg* 202 (2011): 727.

67. S. R. Moonesinghe et al., "Impact of Reduction in Work Hours for Doctors in Training on Postgraduate Medical Education and Patient Outcomes: Systematic Review," *BMJ* 342 (2011): 1–13, doi:10.1136/bmj.d1580.

68. Ibid., 4–5.

69. Ibid., 6.

70. Britt et al., "Resident Duty Hours in Surgery," 399.

71. Ibid., 400.

72. Ibid., 401.

73. Ibid.

74. George Miller et al., "Impact of Mandatory Resident Work Hour Limitations on Medical Students' Interest in Surgery," *J Am Coll Surg* 199 (2004): 615–619.

75. J. Sharit et al., "Examining Links between Sign-Out Reporting during Shift Changeovers and Patient Management Risks," *Risk Anal* 28, no. 4 (2008): 969–981.

76. C. C. Greenberg et al., "Patterns of Communication Breakdowns Resulting in Injury to Surgical Patients," *J Am Coll Surg* 204, no. 4 (2007): 533–540.

77. Jeanne M. Farnan et al., "Hand-Off Education and Evaluation: Piloting the Observed Simulation Hand-Off Experience," *J Gen Intern Med* 25, no. 2 (2009): 129–134.

78. Moonesinghe et al., "Impact of Reduction in Work Hours," 10.

79. Karl Y. Bilimoria et al., "National Cluster-Randomized Trial of Duty-Hour Flexibility in Surgical Training," *N Engl J Med* 374 (2016): 713–727, doi:10.1056/NEJMoa1515724.

80. Ibid., 713.

81. Laura J. Moore et al., "Sepsis in General Surgery: A Deadly Complication," *Am J Surg* 198 (2009): 868.

82. Saiqa I. Khan, personal communication, 2016.

83. Pauline W. Chen, *Final Exam: A Surgeon's Reflections on Mortality* (New York: Knopf, 2007), 86.

84. Ibid., 87.

85. Ibid.

Chapter Twelve

1. Sidney Dekker, *Patient Safety: A Human Factors Approach* (Boca Raton, FL: CRC Press / Taylor and Francis, 2011), 16.

2. Sidney Dekker, *Drift into Failure: From Hunting Broken Components to Understanding Complex Systems* (Burlington, VT: Ashgate, 2011).

3. Joseph E. Fischer, "Surgeons: Employees or Professionals?" *Am J Surg* 190 (2005): 1.

4. Ibid., 3.

5. Charles M. Balch, Julie A. Freischlag, and T. A. Shanafelt, "Stress and Burnout among Surgeons—Understanding and Managing the Syndrome and Avoiding the Adverse Consequences," *Arch Surg* 144, no. 4 (2009): 371–376.

6. T. E. Williams, B. Satiani, and E. C. Ellison, *The Coming Shortage of Surgeons: Why They Are Disappearing and What That Means for Our Health* (Santa Barbara, CA: ABC-CLIO, 2009).

7. T. A. Brennan et al., "Incidence of Adverse Events and Negligence in Hospitalized Patients—Results of the Harvard Medical Practice Study I," *N Engl J Med* 324 (1991): 370–376.

8. N. P. Couch et al., "The High Cost of Low Frequency Events—The Anatomy and Economics of Surgical Mishaps," *N Engl J Med* 304 (1981): 634–637.

9. R. Ornstein and P. Ehrlich, *New World, New Mind: Moving toward Conscious Evolution* (New York: Doubleday, 1989), 9.

10. Kevin Wayne Sexton et al., "Women in Academic Surgery: The Pipeline Is Busted," *J Surg Ed* 69, no. 1 (January/February 2012): 84–90.

11. Balch, Freischlag, and Shanafelt, "Stress and Burnout," 374.

12. L. D. Britt, "A Major Challenge for Graduate Medical Education," *Arch Surg* 140 (2005): 250–253.

13. Teodor P. Grantcharov and P. Funch-Jensen, "Can Everyone Achieve Proficiency with the Laparoscopic Technique? Learning Curve Patterns in Technical Skills Acquisition," *Am J Surg* 197 (2009): 447–449.

14. M. P. Schijven and J. Jakimowicz, "The Learning Curve on the Xitact LS 500 Laparoscopy Simulator: Profiles in Performance," *Surg Endosc* 18 (2004): 121.

15. K. R. Van Sickle, M. Ritter, and C. Daniel-Smith, "The Pre-trained Novice: Using Simulation-Based Training to Improve Learning in the Operating Room," *Surg Innovation* 13, no. 3 (2006): 198–204.

16. C. S. McArdle and D. Hole, "Impact of Variability among Surgeons on Postoperative Morbidity and Mortality and Ultimate Survival," *BMJ* 302 (1991): 1501.

17. Anthony D. Whittemore, "The Competent Surgeon: Individual Accountability in an Era of 'Systems' Failure," *Ann Surg* 250, no. 3 (2009): 359.

18. "Guidelines for Granting Privileges for Laparoscopic and/or Thoracoscopic General Surgery, Recommendations from Society of American Gastrointestinal Endoscopic Surgeons (SAGES)," *Surg Clin N Am* 80, no. 4 (August 2000): 1145.

19. T. E. Williams, B. Satiani, and E. C. Ellison, *The Coming Shortage of Surgeons* (Santa Barbara, CA: Praeger, 2009).

20. Robert M. Zollinger, "The Postwar Trends in the Training of the General Surgeon," *Surgery* 24, no. 2 (1948): 164.

Chapter Thirteen

1. Teodor P. Grantcharov and Richaed K. Resnick, "Training Tomorrow's Surgeons: What Are We Looking For and How Can We Achieve It?" *ANZ J Surg* 79 (2009): 104.

2. Ibid., 106.

3. Steven M. Fisher, *The ABSITE Review: Practical Questions* (Richmond, VA: Handcock Surgical Consultants, 2004), 4–5.

4. Corey Wright, "Surgical Training: Time for a Revolution," *Bull Am Coll Surg* 99, no. 11 (November 2014): 18.

5. Jahan Mohebali, "Reformation of Current Surgical Residency and Fellowship Training Is the Best Solution," *Bull Am Coll Surg* 99, no. 11 (November 2014): 24.

6. Timothy Eberlein, "A New Paradigm in Surgical Training," *J Am Coll Surg* 218, no. 4 (2014): 511–518.

7. Harry Owen, "Early Use of Simulation in Medical Education," *Soc for Sim in Healthcare* 7, no. 2 (April 2012): 102–116.

8. Ibid., 110.

9. Ibid.

10. Ibid., 111.

11. Ibid.

12. Ibid., 112.

13. R. A. Cobb et al., "What Constitutes General Surgery Training? Evidence from the Log Books of Trainees in One District General Hospital," supplement, *Ann R Coll Surg Engl* 76 (1994): 117–120.

14. Peter Densen, "Challenges and Opportunities Facing Medical Education," *Trans Am Clin Climatol Assoc* 122 (2011): 48–58.

15. Hilary Sanfey and Gary Dunnington, "Basic Surgical Skills Testing for Junior Residents: Current Views of General Surgery Program Directors," *J Am Coll Surg* 212 (2011): 406.

16. Joseph R. Schneider et al., "Patient Assessment and Management Examination: Lack of Correlation between Faculty Assessment and Resident Self-Assessment," *Am J Surg* 195 (2008): 16–19.

17. Vivek Datta et al., "The Use of Electromagnetic Motion Tracking Analysis to Objectively Measure Open Surgical Skill in the Laboratory-Based Model," *J Am Coll Surg* 1193 (2001): 479–485.

18. Jeffery H. Peters et al., "Development and Validation of a Comprehensive Program of Education and Assessment of the Basic Fundamentals of Laparoscopic Surgery," *Surgery* 135, no. 1 (January 2004): 21–27.

19. Matthew B. Blood et al., "Virtual Reality Applied to Testing: The Next Era," *Ann Surg* 237, no. 3 (2002): 442–448.

20. Reed G. Williams et al., "A Template for Reliable Assessment of Resident Operative Performance: Assessment Intervals, Number of Cases, and Raters," *Surgery* 152 (2012): 517–527.

21. Lindsay E. Beaton, "Psychiatric Necessities in Surgical Education," *Am J Surg* 110 (July 1965): 28–34.

22. John H. Mulholland, "Learning to Be a Surgeon," *Ann Surg* 148 (September 1958): 297.

23. Ibid., 300.

24. Ibid., 301.

25. H. William Scott, "Basic Surgical Education," *Surgery* 50, no. 1 (July 1961): 4.

26. Owen H. Wangensteen, "Some Present-Day Problems in Surgical Education," *J Med Ed* 37 (June 1962): 620–631.

27. Ibid., 630.

28. David T. Cooke et al., "The Virtual Surgeon: Using Medical Simulation to Train the Modern Surgical Resident," *Bull Am Coll Surg* 93, no. 7 (July 2008): 26–31.

29. Thomas M. Krummel, "Surgical Simulation and Virtual Reality: The Coming Revolution," editorial, *Ann Surg* 228, no. 5 (1998): 635–637.

30. K. R. Van Sickle, M. Ritter, and C. Daniel-Smith, "The Pre-trained Novice: Using Simulation-Based Training to Improve Learning in the Operating Room," *Surg Innovation* 13, no. 3 (2006): 198–204.

31. Raphael S. Chung and Naveed Ahmed, "How Surgical Residents Spend Their Time—The Effect of a Goal-Oriented Work Style on Efficiency and Work Satisfaction," *Arch Surg* 142 (2007): 251.

32. Colleen Y. Colbert, Elaine F. Dannefer, and Judith C. French, "Clinical Competency Committees and Assessment: Changing the Conversation in Graduate Medical Education," *J Grad Med Ed* (June 2015): 162–165.

33. Chryssa McAlister, "Breaking the Silence of the Switch—Increasing Transparency about Trainee Participation in Surgery," *N Engl J Med* 372, no. 26 (2015): 2477–2479.

34. Gutjit Sandhu, Nicholas R. Teman, and Rebecca M. Minter, "Training Autonomous Surgeons: More Time or Faculty Development?" *Ann Surg* 261, no. 5 (May 2015): 843–844.

35. Yvonne Steinert and Cheryl Levitt, "Working with the 'Problem' Resident: Guidelines for Definition and Intervention," *Fam Med* 25 (1993): 627–632.

36. Andrew S. Resnick et al., "Patterns and Predictions of Resident Misbehavior—A 10 Year Retrospective Look," *Curr Surg* 63 (2006): 418–425.

37. Brian V. Reamy and Jefferson H. Harman, "Residents in Trouble: An In-Depth Assessment of the 25-Year Experience of a Single Family Medicine Residency," *Fam Med* 38 (2006): 252–257.

38. Laura Torbeck and David F. Canal, "Remediation Practices for Surgery Residents," *Am J Surg* 197 (2009): 397–402.

39. Steven Evans and Babak Sarani, "The Modern Medical School Graduate and General Surgery Training," *Arch Surg* 137 (March 2002): 274–277.

40. Ibid., 275.

41. Mary E. Klingensmith et al., "Factors Influencing the Decision of Surgery Residency Graduates to Pursue General Surgery Practice Versus Fellowship," *Ann Surg* 262, no. 3 (September 2015): 449–455.

42. Walter E. Longo et al., "Attrition of Categoric General Surgery Residents: Results of a 20-Year Audit," *Am J Surg* 197 (2009): 774–778.

43. Arthur L Schueneman et al., "Neurophysiologic Predictors of Operative Skill among General Surgery Residents," *Surgery* 96, no. 2 (August 1984): 288–295.

44. Ibid., 294.

45. J. R. Korndorffer, D. Stefanidis, and Dan J. Scott, "Laparoscopic Skills Laboratories: Current Assessment and a Call for Resident Training Standards," *Am J Surg* 191 (2006): 17–22.

46. Muneera R. Kapadia et al., "Current Assessment and Future Directions of Surgical Skills Laboratories," *J Surg Ed* 64, no. 5 (September/October 2007): 260.

47. Steven C. Stain et al., "Characteristics of Highly Ranked Applicants to General Surgery Residency Programs," *JAMA Surg* 148, no. 5 (2013): 413–417.

48. James C. Hebert, "Characteristics of Highly Ranked Applicants to General Surgery Residency Programs," comment, *JAMA Surg* 148, no. 5 (2013): 413–417.

49. Francis S. Nuthalapaty, James R. Jackson, and John Owen, "The Influence of Quality-of-Life, Academic, and Workplace Factors on Residency Program Selection," *Acad Med* 79, no. 5 (May 2004): 417.

50. Daniel T. Farkas et al., "The Use of a Surgery-Specific Written Examination in the Selection Process of Surgical Residents," *J Surg Ed* 69, no. 6 (November/December 2012): 807–812.

51. Rebekah A. Naylor, Joan S. Reisch, and James Valentine, "Factors Related to Attrition in Surgery Residency Based on Application Data," *Arch Surg* 143, no. 7 (July 2008): 647–652.

52. Karen R. Borman, "Professionalism in the Match Process: The Rules and Ethics of Recruitment," *Surg Clin N Am* 84 (2004): 1511–1523.

53. K. D. Anderson, D. M. Jacobs, and A. V. Blue, "Is Match Ethics an Oxymoron?" *Am J Surg* 177, no. 3 (1999): 237–239.

54. David A. Asch et al., "How Do You Deliver a Good Obstetrician? Outcome-Based Evaluation of Medical Education," *Acad Med* 89 (2014): 24–26.

55. Ibid., 24.

56. Ibid., 25.

57. Ibid., 25–26.

58. Ibid., 26.

59. Nabil Issa et al., "Surgical Subinternships: Bridging the Chiasm between Medical School and Residency: A Position Paper Prepared by the Subcommittee for Surgery Subinternship and the Curriculum Committee of the Association for Surgical Education," *Am J Surg* 209 (2015): 8–9.

60. Ibid., 11.

61. Mara B. Antonoff and Jonathan D'Cunha, "PGY-1 Surgery Preparation Course Design: Identification of Key Curricular Components," *J Surg Ed* 68, no. 6 (November/December 2011): 478–484.

62. Gladys L. Fernandez et al., "BOOT CAMP: Implementation of an Intensive Simulation-Based Educational Curriculum for New Surgical Interns" (abstract, podium presentation, Baystate Medical Center, New England Surgical Society, September 2008).

63. Andreas H. Meier et al., "Implementation of a Web- and Simulation-Based Curriculum to Ease the Transition from Medical School to Surgical Internship," *Am J Surg* 190 (2005): 137–140.

64. Neal E. Seymour et al., "Virtual Reality Training Improves Operating Room Performance: Results of a Randomized Double-Blinded Study," *Ann Surg* 236 (2002): 458–463.

65. Catharine de Blacam et al., "Are Residents Accurate in Their Assessments of Their Own Surgical Skills?" *Am J Surg* 204 (2012): 724–731.

66. Kenneth W. Gow, "Self-Evaluation: How Well Do Surgery Residents Judge Performance on a Rotation?" *Am J Surg* 205 (2013): 557.

67. Justin Kruger and David Dunning, "Unskilled and Unaware of It: How Difficulties in Recognizing One's Own Incompetence Lead to Inflated Self-Assessments," *J Personal and Social Psych* 77, no. 6 (1999): 1121–1134.

68. Brendan M. Reilly, "Don't Learn on Me—Are Teaching Hospitals Patient-Centered?" *N Engl J Med* 371, no. 4 (July 2014): 294.

69. Elena A. Vikis et al., "Teaching and Learning in the Operating Room Is a Two-Way Street: Resident Perceptions," *Am J Surg* 195 (2008): 594.

70. Kamal M. F. Itani et al., "Surgical Resident Supervision in the Operating Room and Outcomes of Care in Veterans Affairs Hospitals," *Am J Surg* 190 (2005): 725–731.

71. Antoine N. Saliba et al., "Impact of Resident Involvement in Surgery: (IRIS-NSQIP): Looking at the Bigger Picture Based on the American College of Surgeons-NSQIP Database," *J Am Coll Surg* 222 (2016): 30–40.

72. Mehul V. Raval et al., "The Influence of Resident Involvement on Surgical Outcomes," *J Am Coll Surg* 212 (2011): 889–898.

73. Charles S. Roberts and Ruben Bocanegra, "Comparison of the First 100 Coronary Bypass Patients of a Supervised Resident with His First 100 as an Attending Surgeon at the Same Institution," *Am J Surg* 178 (1999): 348–350.

74. Abhishek Chatterjee et al., "Resident and Fellow Participation in Breast Surgery: An American College of Surgeons NSQIP Clinical Outcomes Analysis," *J Am Coll Surg* 221 (2015): 988–994.

75. Shaun P. Patel et al., "Resident Participation Does Not Affect Surgical Outcomes, Despite Introduction of New Techniques," *J Am Coll Surg* 211 (2010): 540–545.

76. K. Wong, T. Duncan, and A. Pearson, "Unsupervised Laparoscopic Appendectomy by Surgical Trainees Is Safe and Time-Effective," *Asian J Surg* 30 (2007): 161–166.

77. Bengamin Zendejas et al., "Long-Term Outcomes of Laparoscopically Totally Extraperitoneal Inguinal Hernia Repairs Performed by Supervised Surgical Trainees," *Am J Surg* 201 (2011): 379–384.

78. Roberto Hernandez-Irizarry et al., "Impact of Resident Participation on Laparoscopic Inguinal Hernia Repairs: Are Residents Slowing Us Down?" *J Surg Ed* 69, no. 6 (November/December 2012): 746–752.

79. Carolyn D. Seib et al., "Adrenalectomy Outcomes Are Superior with the Participation of Residents and Fellows," *J Am Coll Surg* 219 (2014): 53–61.

80. Ravi Pokala Kiran et al., "Impact of Resident Participation in Surgical Operations on Postoperative Outcomes," *Ann Surg* 256, no. 3 (September 2012): 469–475.

81. John Weigelt et al., "Opinions of General Surgeons on Surgical Education," *Am J Surg* 176 (1998): 481.

82. Paris D. Butler, Benjamin Chang, and L. D. Britt, "The Affordable Care Act and Academic Surgery: Expectations and Possibilities," *J Am Coll Surg* 218, no. 5 (2014): 1049–1062.

83. Vincent C. Lusco, Serge A. Martinez, and Hiram C. Polk, "Program Directors in Surgery Agree That Residents Should Be Formally Trained in Business and Practice Management," *Am J Surg* 1189 (2005): 11–13.

84. Charles T. Klodell et al., "Advanced Surgical Technology Experience—Valuable to the Basic Education of General Surgery Residents," *Bull Am Coll Surg* 86, no. 6 (June 2001): 1115.

85. Todd A. Jaffe, Steven J. Hasday, and Justin B. Dimmick, "Power Outage—Inadequate Surgeon Performance Measures Leave Patients in the Dark," *JAMA Surg* 151, no. 7 (2016): 597–600, doi:10.1001/jamasurg.2015.5459.

86. Joseph A. Kopta, "The Development of Motor Skills in Orthopaedic Education," *Clin Orthop Relat Res* 75 (March-April 1971): 80.

87. A. G. Shulman, P. K. Amid, and I. L. Lichtenstein, "A Survey of Non-expert Surgeons Using the Open Tension-free Mesh Patch Repair for Primary Inguinal Hernias," *Int Surg* 80, no. 1 (January-March 1995): 35–36.

88. James A. O'Neal, "Surgical Education: Foundations and Values," *J Am Coll Surg* 208, no. 5 (May 2009): 659.

Chapter Fourteen

1. Peter Densen, "Challenges and Opportunities Facing Medical Education," *Trans Am Clin Climatol Assoc* 122 (2011): 48–58.

2. Carlos M. Mery et al., "Teaching and Assessing the ACGME Competencies in Surgical Residency," *Bull Am Coll Surg* 93, no. 7 (July 2008): 39–48.

3. J. David Richardson, "ACS Transition to Practice Program Offers Residents Additional Opportunities to Hone Skills," *Bull Am Coll Surg* (September 1, 2013), http://bulletin.facs.org/2013/09/acs-transition-to-practice-program-offers-residents-additional-opportunities-to-hone-skills/.

4. "ABS Statement Regarding Residency Redesign," American Board of Surgery, April 25, 2016, http://absurgery.org/default.jsp?news_resredesign0416.

5. D. A. David et al., "Accuracy of Physician Self-Assessment Compared with Observed Measures of Competence," *JAMA* 296, no. 9 (2006): 1094.

6. S. K. Sarker et al. "Self-Appraisal Hierarchical Task Analysis of Laparoscopic Surgery Performed by Expert Surgeons," *Surg Endos* 20 (2006): 636–640.

7. *Merriam-Webster.com*, s.v. "capable."

8. *Merriam-Webster.com*, s.v. "competence."

9. *Merriam-Webster.com*, s.v. "capability."

10. *Random House College Dictionary*, rev. ed., s.v. "capable."

11. *Random House College Dictionary*, rev. ed., s.v. "competence."

12. *Roget's Super Thesaurus*, 2nd ed., s.v. "capability."

13. David P. Sklar, "Competencies, Milestones, and Entrustable Professional Activities: What They Are, What They Could Be," *Acad Med* 90, no. 4 (April 2015): 396.

14. Lawrence W. Way, "General Surgery in Evolution: Technology and Competence," *Am J Surg* 171 (January 1996): 4.

15. Cornelis J. Hopmans et al., "Surgeons' Attitude Toward a Competency-Based Training and Assessment Program: Results of a Multicenter Survey," *J Surg Ed* 70 (2013): 647–654.

16. Katie Wiggins-Dohlvik et al., "Surgeons' Performance during Critical Situations: Competence, Confidence, and Composure," *Am J Surg* 198 (2009): 817.

17. Craig Szafranski et al., "Distractions and Surgical Proficiency: An Educational Perspective," *Am J Surg* 198 (2009): 804–810.

18. Bin Zheng et al., "Surgeons' Vigilance in the Operating Room," *Am J Surg* 201 (2011): 667–671.

19. Ellen J. Langer and Kwangyang Park, "Incompetence: A Conceptual Reconsideration," in *Competence Considered*, ed. Robert J. Sternberg and John Kolligian Jr. (New Haven, CT: Yale University Press, 1990), 149.

20. Ibid., 149–166.

21. Bulletin, American College of Surgeons, Division of Education (May 2013).

22. S. C. Mayo et al., "Management of Patients with Pancreatic Adenocarcinoma: National Trends in Patient Selection, Operative Management, and Use of Adjuvant Therapy," *J Am Coll Surg* 214 (2012): 33–45.

23. Chinnasamy Palanivelu et al., "Laparoscopic Pancreaticoduodenectomy: Technique and Outcomes," *J Am Coll Surg* 205 (2007): 222–230.

24. Donlin M. Long, "Competency-Based Residency Training: The Next Advance in Graduate Medical Education," *Acad Med* 74, no. 12 (December 2000): 1178–1183.

25. R. Spence et al., "Training for Professional Competence in General Surgery," *Curr Surg* 44, no. 4 (July-August 1987): 273–278.

26. Sklar, "Competencies," 395.

27. Donald D. Trunkey and Richard Botney, "Assessing Competency: A Tale of Two Professions," *J Am Coll Surg* 92, no. 3 (March 2001): 391.

28. Sklar, "Competencies," 397.

29. Jerome H. Lui et al., "The Increasing Workload of General Surgeons," *Arch Surg* 139 (April 2004): 426.

30. David W. Page, "The Real Anatomy Lesson: Differential Diagnosis in the First Year Anatomy Course," *Clin Anat* 4, no. 1 (1991): 51–55.

31. Anne M. Gilroy et al., "Anatomical Characteristics of the Iliopubic Tract: Implications for Repair of Inguinal Hernias," *Clin Anat* 5 (1992): 255–263.

32. Lynn M. DiBenedetto et al., "Variations in the Inferior Pelvic Pathway of the Lateral Femoral Cutaneous Nerve: Implications for Laparoscopic Hernia Repair," *Clin Anat* 9 (1996): 232–236.

33. Sandy C. Marks Jr., Anne M. Gilroy, and David W. Page, "The Clinical Anatomy of Laparoscopic Inguinal Hernia Repair," *Singapore Med J* 37, no. 5 (1996): 519–521.

34. David W. Page, Anne Gilroy, and Sandy Marks, "The Iliopubic Tract: An Essential Guide in Teaching and Performing Groin Hernia Repairs," *Contemp Surg* (October 1996).

35. Anne M. Gilroy et al., "The Variability of the Obturator Vessels," *Clin Anat* 10 (1997): 328–332.

36. Hubert L. Dreyfus and Stuart E. Dreyfus, *Mind over Machine: The Power of Human Intuition and Expertise in the Era of the Computer* (New York: Free Press, 1986), 19–40.

37. Ibid., 27.

38. Ibid., 28.

39. Daniel Kahneman, *Thinking Fast and Slow* (New York: Farrar, Straus and Giroux, 2011).

40. Richard Grol, "Changing Physicians' Competence and Performance: Finding the Balance between the Individual and the Organization," *J Contin Educ Health Prof* 22 (2002): 244.

41. Danilo Miskovic et al., "Is Competency Assessment at the Specialist Level Achievable? A Study for the National Training Programme in Laparoscopic Colorectal Surgery in England," *Ann Surg* 257, no. 3 (March 2013): 476–482.

42. Ibid., 481.

43. Ibid., 476.

44. Linas A. Bieliauskas et al., "Cognitive Changes and Retirement among Senior Surgeons (CCRASS): Results from the CCRASS Study," *J Am Coll Surg* 207 (2008): 69–79.

45. Christina Frangou, "Surgeon Scorecard Garners More Criticism after Studies Uncover Flaws," *Gen Surg News* 43, no. 7 (July 2016): 1, 30.

46. David R. Urbach, "Pledging to Eliminate Low-Volume Surgery," *N Engl J Med* 373, no. 15 (October 2015): 1388–1390.

47. Ibid., 1390.

Glossary

Attending surgeon
Medical school faculty or private surgeon working in a supervisory role with surgical residents.

"Band-Aid" surgery
Another name for laparoscopic or minimally invasive operations in which the incisions are small enough to be covered with a Band-Aid.

Boot camp
A series of learning experiences for interns (first-year residents) that focus on technical skills (chest tube placement, suturing and knot tying, central intravenous access lines, etc.) as well as on basic applied knowledge, such as how to respond to a floor call from a nurse about a particular problem.

Capability
Used interchangeably with competence; the ability to do something (e.g., technical surgery) well; midway in ability between novice and master performance; assumes skill and knowledge in specific areas of surgical practice.

Comorbid conditions
Such medical conditions as diabetes, high blood pressure, obesity, COPD and smoking, cancer, malnutrition, and so forth that will make the possibility of complications higher.

Failure to rescue
Death after postoperative complications due to a delay in diagnosis, often of acute heart, lung, kidney, and other complications (e.g., heart attack, stroke, pneumonia) that progress to a lethal level and are not reversed by the actions of a rapid response team.

Frailty
A condition of the elderly characterized by diminished resiliency and loss of adaptive capacity in dealing with the stress of an operation; often characterized by

weight loss, diminished muscle strength and walking speed, depression, impaired thinking, poor nutrition, and social vulnerability.

General surgeon
A surgical specialist trained to perform the wide range of operations that include but are not limited to removal of the appendix, gallbladder, colon, stomach, breast, thyroid, and parathyroid glands; cancer surgery for the above organs; emergency operations for such complications of diseases as hemorrhage, perforation (burst appendix, intestines, etc.), bowel blockage, proctology (hemorrhoids, rectal abscesses, fistulas, etc.); and in smaller rural communities, C-sections and sub-specialty procedures in orthopedics, urology, and other areas.

Imaging
Refers to any type of X-ray or scanning (CT, MRI, etc.), ultrasound, angiography (dye study of blood vessels), nuclear scans, and so forth.

Insufflate
To put carbon dioxide into the belly cavity through a special needle called a Veress needle, which is spring loaded to avoid bowel injury; also, a Hasson technique involving a small belly-button incision and direct visualization of the belly cavity, placing a Hasson trocar/sleeve and introducing carbon dioxide; the flow of gas is controlled and pressures are measured and kept within a certain range; the process creates a pneumoperitoneum or belly cavity distended with carbon dioxide.

Laparoscopic cholecystectomy
The first general surgery operation devised in the 1980s to avoid a large incision; learned on the run by general surgeons with little or no laparoscopic experience; the unreported increase in bile duct injuries then has been a cautionary story for surgeons working with innovations now.

Minimally invasive surgery
Interchangeable term for laparoscopic surgery and other forms of operations using small incisions, miniaturized cameras, and TV screens to visualize the operative field.

Morbidity
Such complications as wound infections, pneumonia, urinary tract infections, leg blood clots (deep vein thrombosis [DVT] or venous thrombo-embolism [VTE]), and so forth.

Mortality
Death rate.

Pretrained novice
A trainee who has practiced and mastered basic surgical skills in the skills lab setting before scrubbing on live patients.

Resident

A trainee of one to seven or more years in any specialty including pediatrics, medicine, OB/GYN, surgery; originally derived from the long hours a training doctor spent as a "resident" of the hospital.

Risk factors

Conditions that make an operation more complication prone; poor nutrition, smoking, psychological issues, as well as comorbid conditions such as diabetes, COPD, cancer, poor conditioning (lack of exercise), obesity, and so forth.

Rounding

Doctors', nurses', and trainees' individual or collective evaluation of patients in the morning and at night to assess their progress and to seek out potential complications before they progress; reviewing and documenting patient status; sometimes called *chart rounds*.

Supervision

As related to surgical education, the presence and involvement of an attending surgeon in a case being done partly or completely by a trainee; in the past there was too little supervision, today perhaps too much (less resident autonomy).

Trocar

A sharp, pointed, removable internal obturator inside a cannula, hollow tube, or sheath used to enter the abdominal or chest wall; placed through the wall and acts as a sleeve through which laparoscopic instruments are slid through one-inch or smaller incisions.

Index

About the Author

David W. Page, MD, MFA, FACS, is the surgical patient's advocate. He has made it his mission to inform and educate people about the perils of surgery so they can make choices that will increase their chances of having a successful surgical outcome. A board-certified surgeon and professor of surgery at Tufts University School of Medicine in Boston, he is also director of undergraduate programs in surgery at Baystate Medical Center, Tufts' western campus, in Springfield, Massachusetts. He's a member of the American College of Surgeons, the Association of Surgical Education, the New England Surgical Society, and the American Hernia Society, and he's a founding member of the American Association of Clinical Anatomists.

Dr. Page has 40 years of experience in teaching, performing surgery, and doing research in surgical anatomy and surgical simulation. He has conducted surgical education and research projects and presented the results at national meetings. Calling on his master of fine arts background, he's also published more than 35 scientific papers on surgical topics, numerous lay articles, and two reference books: *Body Trauma: A Writer's Guide to Wounds and Injuries*, which was awarded a Silver Medal by the Independent Book Publishers for the second edition (Behler Publications, 2006) in 2007; and *Code Blue: A Writer's Guide to the Modern Hospital*, written with Keith Wilson, MD (1999). He has also written three surgical-textbook chapters and self-published a novel.

Dr. Page's honors have been many since the Baystate Medical Center surgical residents awarded him his first Golden Apple, recognizing him as teacher of the year in 1979; he received another in 2009. At the Tufts University School of Medicine, medical students have honored Dr. Page with more than 20 Excellence in Teaching Awards over the course of his career. He received the Lifetime Teaching Award from Baystate in 2001 and the Outstanding Clinical Teacher Award from Tufts in 2004. Tufts medical school's graduating classes of 2006 and 2011 honored him with the Special Faculty Recognition Award, which was established to recognize a faculty member who has "made medical school a more enjoyable experience through his exemplary teaching and genuine concern for students' interests both inside and outside of the classroom." In 2010, Dr. Page was one of three surgical educators in the United States to receive that year's Philip J. Wolfson Outstanding Teacher Award from the Association for Surgical Education. In 2013, he received the Dean's Outstanding Mentor Award from the Tufts medical school's class of 2013. For the years 2013 and 2016,

he won a prestigious Professional Research Consultants, Inc., patient satisfaction award for his clinical work, and he sat on an expert panel at the
American College of Surgeons' annual meeting in Washington, D.C. In
2015, Dr. Page won the Tufts University School of Medicine's Milton O.
and Natalie V. Zucker Clinical Teaching Prize for Accomplishments in
Medical Education.

CPSIA information can be obtained
at www.ICGtesting.com
Printed in the USA
JSHW050934300422
25138JS00002B/48